Encyclopedia of Phytochemicals: Nutraceuticals and Impact on Health

Volume IV

Encyclopedia of Phytochemicals: Nutraceuticals and Impact on Health

Volume IV

Edited by **Vivian Belt**

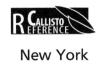

New York

Published by Callisto Reference,
106 Park Avenue, Suite 200,
New York, NY 10016, USA
www.callistoreference.com

Encyclopedia of Phytochemicals: Nutraceuticals and Impact on Health
Volume IV
Edited by Vivian Belt

International Standard Book Number: 978-1-63239-285-5 (Hardback)

This book contains information obtained from authentic and highly regarded sources. Copyright for all individual chapters remain with the respective authors as indicated. A wide variety of references are listed. Permission and sources are indicated; for detailed attributions, please refer to the permissions page. Reasonable efforts have been made to publish reliable data and information, but the authors, editors and publisher cannot assume any responsibility for the validity of all materials or the consequences of their use.

The publisher's policy is to use permanent paper from mills that operate a sustainable forestry policy. Furthermore, the publisher ensures that the text paper and cover boards used have met acceptable environmental accreditation standards.

Trademark Notice: Registered trademark of products or corporate names are used only for explanation and identification without intent to infringe.

Printed in the United States of America.

Contents

Preface

Every book is a source of knowledge and this one is no exception. The idea that led to the conceptualization of this book was the fact that the world is advancing rapidly; which makes it crucial to document the progress in every field. I am aware that a lot of data is already available, yet, there is a lot more to learn. Hence, I accepted the responsibility of editing this book and contributing my knowledge to the community.

This book extensively examines phytochemicals and the impact on human health. Phytochemicals can be referred to as any of the various biologically active compounds found in plants. None of the thousands of naturally occurring constituents so far found in plants are considered to be dangerous towards human health at the present low levels of intake when used as flavoring substances. Genetic as well as environmental factors often influence the chemical composition of the plant essential oils because of their natural origin. Factors like geographical location, species and subspecies, harvest time, plant part used and technique of isolation all influence the chemical composition of the crude material detached from the plant. The screening of natural products and plant extracts for antimicrobial and antioxidative activity has unveiled the potential of higher plants as a source of novel agents, to serve the processing of natural products.

While editing this book, I had multiple visions for it. Then I finally narrowed down to make every chapter a sole standing text explaining a particular topic, so that they can be used independently. However, the umbrella subject sinews them into a common theme. This makes the book a unique platform of knowledge.

I would like to give the major credit of this book to the experts from every corner of the world, who took the time to share their expertise with us. Also, I owe the completion of this book to the never-ending support of my family, who supported me throughout the project.

Editor

Biological Oxidations and Antioxidant Activity of Natural Products

Xirley Pereira Nunes et al.*
Universidade Federal do Vale do São Francisco,
Brazil

1. Introduction

Oxygen is the most prevalent element in the earth's crust. It exists in air as a diatomic molecule, O_2. Except for a small number of anaerobic bacteria, all living organisms use O_2 for energy production and it is essential for life as we know it. Energy production by organisms from food material requires "oxidation", which implies the loss of electrons. However the potential of O_2 to oxidize also makes it toxic. Oxidation can inactivate important enzymes, and anaerobes that do not have antioxidant mechanisms do not survive in an O_2 environment (Magder, 2006).

Life under aerobic conditions is characterized by continuous production of free radicals, which is counterbalanced by the activity of antioxidant enzymes and non-enzyme defences. Under physiological conditions oxidising agents and antioxidant defences are in balance. Living cells can either produce or take in anti-oxidative defense molecules which include enzymes such as catalase, superoxide dismutase, glutathione peroxidase, and non-enzymatic antioxidants such as glutathione, and vitamins C and E. However, if the production of free radicals exceeds the antioxidant capacity of a living system, these reactive oxygen and nitrogen species can react with lipids, proteins, and DNA causing structural and/or functional damage to the cell's enzymes and genetic material (Barreiros et al., 2006). The predominance of oxidants, and their consequent damage is called oxidative stress. Oxidants are generated in normal metabolism, in mitochondria, in peroxisomes, as cytosolic enzymes such as xanthine oxidase which is present in the cytosol of many tissues, and also can be found in the blood circulation bound to glycosaminoglycan sites in the arterial wall (Magder, 2006).

According to Sanchez et al. (2003), the body's mechanisms against the excess of reactive oxygen species (ROS), and oxidative stress may be classified as follows: (I) preventive mechanism; proteins which have a coordinated nucleus of iron or copper with the capacity to

* Fabrício Souza Silva[1], Jackson Roberto Guedes da S. Almeida[1], Julianeli Tolentino de Lima[1],
Luciano Augusto de Araújo Ribeiro[1], Lucindo José Quintans Júnior[2] and José Maria Barbosa Filho[3]
[1]Universidade Federal do Vale do São Francisco, Brazil
[2]Universidade Federal de Sergipe, Brazil
[3]Universidade Federal da Paraíba, Brazil

bind (albumin, myoglobin, metallothionein, ceruloplasmin, ferritin, transferrin,), which prevents the overproduction of HO•, (II) repairing mechanism; enzymes which repair or eliminate damaged biomolecules by ROS, like glutathione peroxidase, glutathione reductase, and methionine-sulphoxide reductase, and (III) scavenger mechanism; enzymes with capacity to scavenge excess ROS like superoxide dismutase, glutathione peroxidase, catalase, other metalloenzymes, and chemical entities with scavenging capacity like polyunsaturated fatty acids, vitamins C and E, uric acid, bilirubin, carotenoids, and flavonoids.

The term reactive oxygen species (ROS) includes radicals or chemical species that take part in radical type reactions (i.e. gain or loss of electrons) but are not true radicals in that they do not have unpaired electrons. Examples of non-radical ROS include hydrogen peroxide (H_2O_2), hypochlorous acid (HOCl), ozone (O_3) and singlet oxygen ($^1O_2$). Examples of radical ROS include super oxide anion radicals ($O_2^{•-}$) and hydroxyl radical species (•OH). Besides oxygen-based radicals, there are also reactive nitrogen species such as nitric oxide (NO) and nitrogen dioxide (NO_2). An important product of the two radicals $O_2^{•-}$ and NO is peroxynitrite (ONOO-), this reaction occurs at a diffusion limited rate (Halliwell & Gutteridge, 2007; Magder, 2006). ROS may be generated through endogenous processes like mitochondrial respiration, the activation of polymorphonuclear leukocytes, arachidonic acid metabolism, enzymatic functions, and iron or copper mediated catalysis, among others. The human organism produces these ROS as a functional part of the harmonic balance between several physiological processes (Gupta & Verma, 2010).

Oxidative stress, caused by an imbalance between ROS and the anti-oxidative defense systems is considered to be a major etiological or pathogenic agent of cardiovascular and neurodegenerative diseases, cancers, Alzheimer's, diabetes and aging. Because they inhibit or delay the oxidative process by blocking both the initiation and propagation of oxidizing chain reactions, antioxidants for the treatment of cellular degenerations are beginning to be considered (Jang et al., 2010). Oxidative stress and its effects on human health have become a serious issue. Under stress, our bodies end up having more reactive oxygen species than antioxidant species, an imbalance that leads to cell damage (Krishnaiah et al., 2011). Cell degradation eventually leads to partial or total functional loss of physiological systems in the body. Currently, the incidence of free radical imbalance at the onset and during the evolution of more than 100 diseases (cardiovascular, neurological, endocrine, respiratory, immune and self-immune, ischaemia, gastric disorders, tumor progression and carcinogenesis, among others) has been demonstrated (Gupta & Verma, 2010).

Oxidation is essential to most living organisms for the production of energy and biological processes such as metabolic regulation, metabolic energy control, and activation/inactivation of biomolecules, signal transduction, cell exchange, endothelium-related vascular functions and gene expression. Reactive oxygen species are produced *in vivo* during oxidation. Free radical-scavenging is one of the known mechanisms by which antioxidants inhibit lipid peroxidation (Bloknina et al., 2003). According to Jadhav et al. (1996), lipid oxidation is the reaction of oxygen with unsaturated fatty acids. In the initial stages free radicals form molecules susceptible to attacks from atmospheric oxygen O_2, by removal of allylic hydrogen from fatty acid molecular carbons. These free radicals act as propagators of the reaction, and are converted to peroxides and hydro-peroxides (also radicals), which are the primary products of lipid oxidation. In the end, the new radicals combine to form stable and secondary products of oxidation by splitting and rearrangement, to form volatile and non-volatile epoxide compounds.

In recent years, substantial evidence has accumulated and indicated key roles for reactive oxygen species and other oxidants in causing numerous disorders and diseases. The evidence has brought the attention of scientists and the general public to an appreciation of antioxidants for prevention and treatment of diseases, and maintenance of human health (Halliwell & Gutteridge, 2007).

Antioxidants stabilize or deactivate free radicals, often before they attack targets in biological cells. Although almost all organisms possess antioxidant defense and repair systems to protect against oxidative damage, they cannot prevent the damage entirely.

Interest in naturally occurring antioxidants has considerably increased for use in food, cosmetic and pharmaceutical products, replacing synthetic antioxidants which are often restricted due to carcinogenic effects (Djeridane et al., 2006; Wannes et al., 2010). Aromatic and medicinal plants source natural antioxidants like polyphenols and essential oils which are secondary metabolites.

The purpose of this chapter is to review antioxidant classes, and methods for *in vitro* assessment of the antioxidant activity of natural products. We do not pretend to do a comprehensive review of the literature, but rather to present introductory information on the subject. In this chapter there is a list of some Brazilian medicinal plants with antioxidant activity.

2. Natural products and antioxidant activity

In this section we present the main classes (natural and synthetic) of antioxidant compounds, as well as important methods for assessment of *in vitro* antioxidant activity of natural products and plant extracts. Antioxidant activity is an important and fundamental function in life systems. Many other biological functions such as the anti-mutagenic, anti-carcinogenic, and anti-aging responses, originate from this property.

2.1 The main classes of antioxidant compounds

Antioxidants inhibit or delay the oxidation of other molecules by limiting either the initiation, or the propagation of oxidizing chain reactions. The natural antioxidants are phenolic compounds (tocopherols, flavonoids, phenolic acids), nitrogen compounds (alkaloids, chlorophyll derivatives, amino acids, and amines), carotenoids or ascorbic acid. Synthetic antioxidants are phenolic structures with various degrees of alkyl substitution (Velioglu et al., 1998).

In general, antioxidants are substances present in low concentrations (compared to the oxidizable substrate), which significantly delay or inhibit oxidation. The radicals formed from antioxidants do not propagate the lipid oxidative chain reaction mentioned above, but are neutralized by reaction with other radicals to form stable products, or recycled by other antioxidants. The chemical structures of natural and synthetic antioxidants most commonly used are shown in Table 1. Table 2 presents some Brazilian medicinal plants having antioxidant activity.

2.1.1 Synthetic antioxidants

Synthetic antioxidants such as butylated hydroxyanisole (BHA), and butylated hydroxytoluene (BHT), have been used as antioxidants since the beginning of this century.

Antioxidant	Chemical structure	Synthetic or Natural?
Ascorbic acid		Synthetic or natural
Butylated hydroxyanisole (BHA)		Synthetic
Butylated hydroxytoluene (BHT)		Synthetic
Gallic acid		Natural
Propyl gallate		Synthetic
Quercetin		Natural
Tertiary butylhydroquinone (TBHQ)		Synthetic
α-Tocoferol		Natural
Trolox®		Synthetic

Table 1. Chemical structures of natural and synthetic antioxidants commonly used. (Adapted from Alves et al., 2010).

Plant name	Chemical content	Reference
Acacia podallyriifolia	Phenolic compounds	Andrade et al., 2007
Anacardium occidentale	Hydroalcoholic extract	Broinizi et al., 2008
Anadenanthera peregrina	Ethanol extract and partitions	Mensor et al., 2001
Anaxagorea dolichocarpa	Ethanol extract and partitions	Almeida et al., 2011
Apuleia leiocarpa	Ethanol extract and partitions	Mensor et al., 2001
Baccharis articulata	Flavonoids	Borgo et al., 2010
Baccharis trimera	Methanol extract	Morais et al., 2009
Brillantaisia palisatii	Ethanol extract and partitions	Mensor et al., 2001
Brosimum guianense	Ethanol extract and partitions	Mensor et al., 2001
Camelia sinensis	Methanol extract	Morais et al., 2009
Cenostigma macrophyllum	Phenolic compounds	Sousa et al., 2007
Copernicia cerifera	Phenolic compounds	Sousa et al., 2007
Croton argyropphylloides	Essential oil	Morais et al., 2006
Croton nepetaefolius	Essential oil	Morais et al., 2006
Croton zenhtneri	Essential oil	Morais et al., 2006
Cymbopogon citratus	Methanol extract	Morais et al., 2009
Duguetia chrysocarpa	Ethanol extract and partitions	Almeida et al., 2011
Encholirium spectabile	Ethanol extract	Carvalho et al., 2010
Hyptis elegans	Ethanol extract and partitions	Mensor et al., 2001
Hyptis tetracephala	Ethanol extract and partitions	Mensor et al., 2001
Jacaranda puberula	Ethanol extract	Santos et al., 2010
Lantana camara	Ethanol extract and partitions	Mensor et al., 2001
Lantana trifolia	Ethanol extract and partitions	Mensor et al., 2001
Laurencia dendroidea	Sesquiterpenes	Gressler et al., 2011
Lippia alba	Methanol extract	Morais et al., 2009
Lonchocarpus filipes	Flavonoids	Santos et al., 2009
Marsypianthes chamaedrys	Ethanol extract and partitions	Mensor et al., 2001
Matricaria recutita	Methanol extract	Morais et al., 2009
Mentha arvensis	Methanol extract	Morais et al., 2009
Palicourea rigida	Flavonoids	Rosa et al., 2010
Platypodium elegans	Ethanol extract and partitions	Mensor et al., 2001
Pseudopiptadenia contorta	Ethanol extract and partitions	Mensor et al., 2001
Punica granatum	Etheric, alcoholic and aqueous extracts	Jardini & Mancini-Filho, 2007
Pyrus malus	Methanol extract	Morais et al., 2009
Qualea grandiflora	Phenolic compounds	Sousa et al., 2007
Raphiodon echinus	Ethanol extract and partitions	Mensor et al., 2001
Terminalia brasiliensis	Phenolic compounds	Sousa et al., 2007
Terminalia fagifolia	Phenolic compounds	Sousa et al., 2007
Turnera ulmifolia	Phenolic compounds	Nascimento et al., 2006
Verbena litoralis	Ethanol extract and partitions	Mensor et al., 2001
Vitex cymosa	Ethanol extract and partitions	Mensor et al., 2001
Vitex polygama	Ethanol extract and partitions	Mensor et al., 2001

Table 2. Some Brazilian plants having antioxidant activity.

They are commonly used to preserve food. Restrictions on the use of these compounds are being imposed because of their carcinogenicity. Thus, the interest in natural antioxidants has increased considerably (Velioglu et al., 1998). The replacement of synthetic with natural antioxidants (because of implications for human health) may be advantageous.

Although synthetic antioxidants, such as BHA, BHT and propyl gallate, have been commonly added to food products to retard lipid oxidation, the demand for natural antioxidants has increased because of the negative perception consumers have about the long-term safety of synthetic antioxidants. Yet, regular consumption of fruit and vegetables containing natural antioxidants is correlated with decreased risks for diseases such as cancer and cardiovascular diseases (Jang et al., 2010).

In the food industry, synthetic antioxidants such as ascorbic acid and BHT have been widely used as additives to preserve and stabilize foods and animal feed products for freshness, nutritive value, flavour, and colour. Yet, at least one study has shown BHT to be potentially toxic, especially in high doses, making it important to consider health risks associated with long-term dietary intake of BHT (Oliveira et al., 2009a).

In recent years, while the toxicity of synthetic chemical antioxidants has been criticized, studies have begun to investigate the potential of plant products to serve as antioxidants for protection against free radicals. Phenolics, flavonoids, tannins, proanthocyanidins, and various plant and herbal extracts have been reported to be radical scavengers that inhibit lipid peroxidation.

Synthetic antioxidants Trolox®, and TBHQ (tertiary butylhydroquinone) are widely used. TBHQ is a derivative of hydroquinone, substituted with a *tert*-butyl group. It is a highly effective antioxidant used in foods as a preservative for unsaturated vegetable oils and many edible animal fats. The *tert*-butyl substituents in TBHQ, BHA and BHT function mainly to increase the lipid solubility.

2.1.2 Natural antioxidants

2.1.2.1 Ascorbic acid

Ascorbic acid (vitamin C) is widely known for its antioxidant activity and is therefore used in cosmetics and degenerative disease treatments. Vitamin C has many physiological functions, among them a highly antioxidant power to recycle vitamin E in membrane and lipoprotein lipid peroxidation. Paradoxically, however, it should also be noted that, *in vitro*, vitamin C is also capable of pro-oxidant activity. It has long been known that the combination of ascorbate and ferrous ions generates hydroxyl radicals, which induces lipid peroxidation (Haslam, 1996). Vitamin C is a potent antioxidant for hydrophilic radicals, but poor against lipophilic radicals.

Ascorbic acid

2.1.2.2 Tocopherols

Tocopherols and tocotrienols are widely distributed in nature. Vitamin E is the common name given to a group of lipid-soluble compounds of which α-tocopherol is the most familiar. It is found in lipoproteins and membranes, and acts to block the chain reaction of lipid peroxidation by scavenging intermediate peroxyl radicals being generated. The highly steric (hindered) α-tocopheryl radical is much less reactive in attacking fatty acid side chains and converts back to its parent phenol thru ascorbic acid, thus breaking the chain reaction (Haslam, 1996).

α-Tocopherol

Tocotrienol analogue

2.1.2.3 Carotenoids

Carotenoids protect lipids against peroxidative damage by inactivating singlet oxygen (without degradation) reacting with hydroxyl, superoxide, and peroxyl radicals. Relative to phenolics and other antioxidants, carotenoids are not particularly good quenchers of peroxyl radicals, but they are exceptional at quenching singlet oxygen, at which most other phenolics and antioxidants are relatively ineffective. The antioxidant activity of carotenoids is due to the ability to delocalize unpaired electrons through their structure of conjugated double bonds. Three proposed mechanisms for free radical reactions involving carotenoids are reported in the literature. Much of our present knowledge comes from epidemiological studies and indicates that the incidence of some forms of cancer and cardiovascular disease appear to be lower in populations with large relative intakes of antioxidant nutrients such as vitamins C, and E, and the various carotenoids (Haslam, 1996).

The β-carotene is the most abundant of the carotenoids and widely used in therapies. It is almost completely insoluble in water but readily soluble in hydrophobic environments, and slightly polar solvents. β-carotene is highly reactive with electrophiles and oxidants. While many studies have shown β-carotene inhibition of lipid auto-oxidation in biological tissues and food, few details of the kinetics or mechanism of these reactions have been revealed (Alves et al., 2010). Lycopene is also well known for its antioxidant activity.

β-Carotene

Lycopene

2.1.2.4 Phenolic compounds

Phenolic compounds are commonly found in both edible and non-edible plants, and they have been reported to have multiple biological effects, including antioxidant activity. Crude extracts of fruits, herbs, vegetables, cereals, and other plant materials rich in phenolics are increasingly being used in the food industry because they retard oxidative degradation of lipids and improve the quality and nutritional value of food. The antioxidant constituents of plants are also raising interest among scientists, food manufacturers, and consumers as the trend of the future is toward functional food with specific health effects for the maintenance of health, protection from coronary heart disease, and cancer (Kähkönen et al., 1999).

Phenolic compounds are considered secondary metabolites and are synthesized by plants during normal development, and in response to infections, wounding, UV radiation, and insects. These phytochemical compounds derived from phenylalanine and tyrosine occur ubiquitously in plants and are very diversified (Naczk & Shahidi, 2004).

Phenolic plant compounds fall into several categories; simple phenolics, phenolic acids (derivatives of cinnamic and benzoic acids), coumarins, flavonoids, stilbenes, tannins, lignans and lignins (Figure 1). Chief among these are the flavonoids which have potent antioxidant activities.

2.1.2.5 Flavonoids

Flavonoids are naturally occurring in plants and are thought to have positive effects on human health. Studies on flavonoidic derivatives have shown a wide range of antibacterial, antiviral, anti-inflammatory, anticancer, and anti-allergic activities (Di Carlo et al., 1999; Montoro et al., 2005). With their biological activity, flavonoids are important components of the human diet, although they are generally considered as non-nutrients. Sources of flavonoids are foods, beverages, different herbal drugs, and related phytomedicines (Montoro et al., 2005).

Flavonoids are an important class of phenolic compounds, and have potent antioxidant activity. The antioxidant property of flavonoids was the first mechanism of action studied with regard to their protective effect against cardiovascular diseases. Flavonoids have been shown to be highly effective scavengers of most oxidizing molecules, including singlet oxygen, and various free radicals (Bravo, 1998) implicated in several diseases.

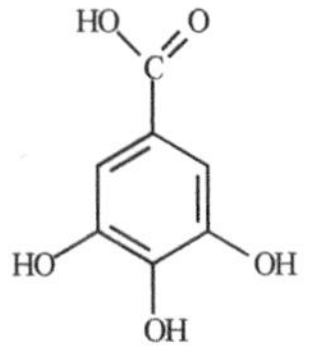

Gallic acid (Hydroxybenzoic acid)

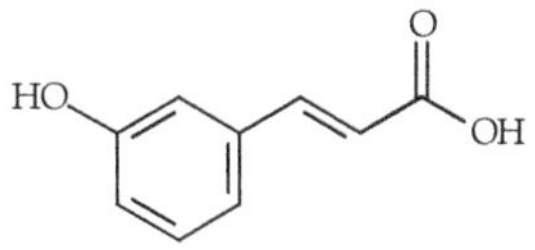

Coumaric acid (Hydroxycinnamic acid)

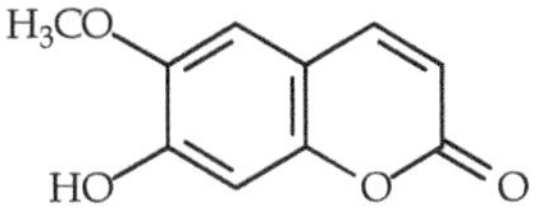

Escopoletin (Coumarin)

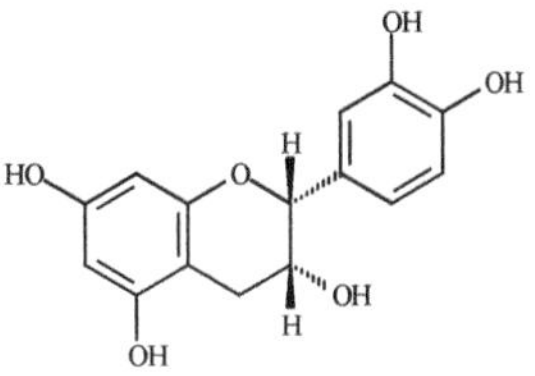

Epicatechin (Flavonoid)

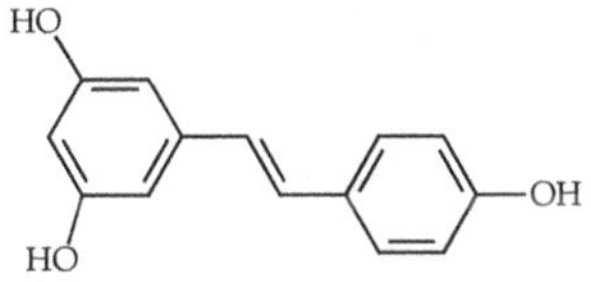

Resveratrol (Stilbene)

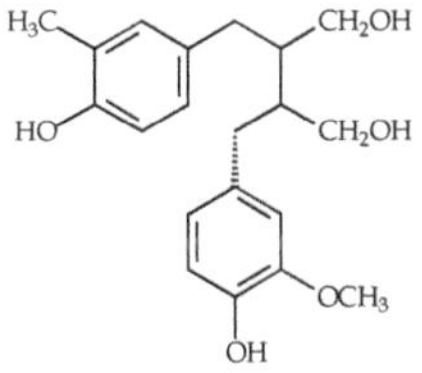

Secoisolariciresinol (Lignan)

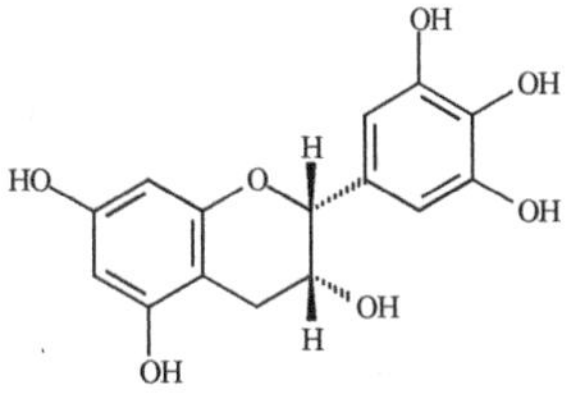

Epigalocatechin (Flavonoid)

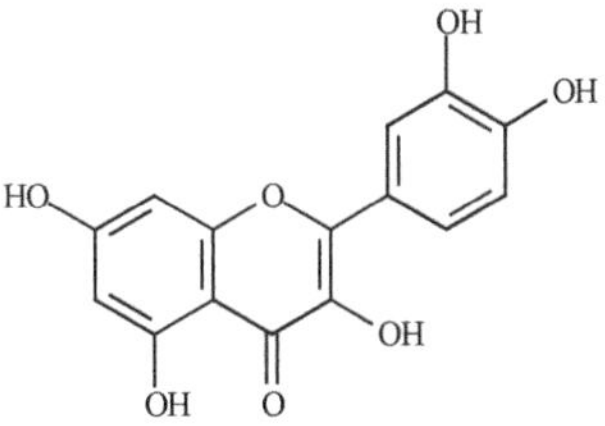

Quercetin (Flavonoid)

Fig. 1. Chemical structures of some phenolic compounds.

The antioxidant mechanism involves suppressing reactive oxygen formation, by inhibiting enzymes, chelating trace elements involved in free-radical production, scavenging reactive species, and up-regulating and protecting antioxidant defences (van Acker et al., 1996).

More than 4000 flavonoids have been identified, and the number is still growing. Flavonoids can be further divided into chalcones, anthocyanins, flavones, isoflavones, flavanones, flavononols and flavanols (Ignat et al., 2011). The chemical structures of the main classes of flavonoids are shown in Figure 2.

Anthocyanins are probably the largest group of phenolic compounds in the human diet, and their strong antioxidant activities suggest their importance in maintaining health (Velioglu et al., 1998). When consumed regularly, by humans, these flavonoids have been associated with a reduction in the incidence of diseases, such as cancer and heart disease.

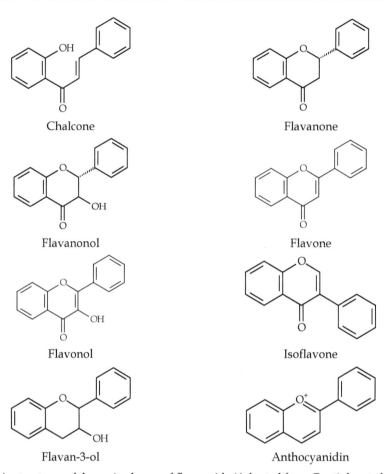

Fig. 2. Basic structures of the main classes of flavonoids (Adapted from Coutinho et al., 2009).

2.1.2.6 Essential oils

Essential oils also called volatile or ethereal oils are aromatic compounds, oily liquids obtained from different plant parts, and widely used as food flavours. Essential oils are complex mixtures comprised of many single compounds. Chemically they are derived from terpenes, and their oxygenated compounds. Essential oils have been useful in food preservation, aromatherapy and the fragrance industry (Bakkali et al., 2008).

In nature, essential oils have an important role in protecting plants. They serve as antibacterial agents, antivirals, antifungals, and insecticides, and also against the action of herbivores. They sometimes attract insects to help the spread of pollen or repel other unwanted insects. They are liquid, volatile, transparent, rarely coloured, soluble in organic solvents, and have lower densities than that of water. Synthesized by all organs of the plant, such as buds, flowers, leaves, stems, seeds, fruits, roots and bark, they are stored in secretor cells, cavities, channels, epidermal cells, and glandular trichomes (Bakkali et al., 2008).

Terpenoids form a large and structurally diverse family of natural products derived from isoprenoid units C_5. These compounds have carbon skeletons being multiples of n (C_5), and are classified as hemiterpenes (C_5), monoterpenes (C_{10}), sesquiterpenes (C_{15}), diterpenes (C_{20}), sesterpenes (C_{25}), triterpenes (C_{30}) and tetraterpenes (C_{40}) (Dewick, 2002). Monoterpenes are primary components of essential oils, and the effects of many medicinal herbs have been attributed to them. Among various monoterpenes that have antioxidant activity are carvacrol, thymol, γ-terpinene and terpinolene, linalool, and isopulegol, among others (Figure 3).

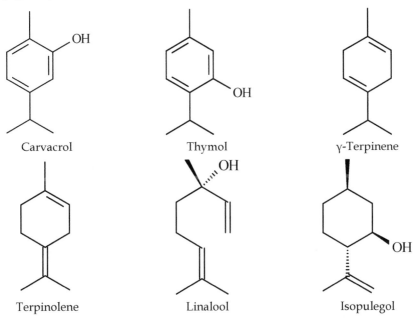

Fig. 3. Chemical structures of monoterpenes with antioxidant activity.

2.2 Methods of antioxidant activity assessment for natural products

Studies on free radicals and the development of new methods for evaluation of antioxidant activity (AA) have increased considerably in recent years. The noted deleterious effect of free radicals on cells in relation to certain diseases has encouraged the search for new substances that can prevent or minimize oxidative damage. Due to the different types of free radicals and their different forms of action in living organisms, it is unlikely that a single, simple and accurate universal method by which antioxidant activity can be measured will ever be developed. However, the search for faster and more efficient testing has generated a large number of methods to assess the activity of natural antioxidants, and they use a variety of systems to generate free radicals (Alves et al., 2010).

Several techniques have been used to determine the antioxidant activity *in vitro* in order to allow rapid screening of substances and/or mixtures of potential interest in the prevention of chronic degenerative diseases. These studies are extremely important, since substances that have low antioxidant activity *in vitro*, will probably show little activity *in vivo*. What follow are some methods for antioxidant activity evaluation and their main applications.

2.2.1 DPPH assay

DPPH reactivity is one popular method of screening for free radical-scavenging ability in compounds, and has been used extensively for antioxidants in fruits and vegetables. This method was first described by Blois in 1958, and was later modified slightly by numerous researchers. DPPH is a stable free radical that reacts with compounds that can donate a hydrogen atom. The method is based on scavenging of DPPH through the addition of a radical species or antioxidant that decolourises the DPPH solution (Figure 4). The degree of colour change is proportional to the concentration and potency of the antioxidants. Antioxidant activity is then measured by the decrease in absorption at 517 nm. A large decrease in the absorbance of the reaction mixture indicates significant free radical scavenging activity of the compound under test (Krishnaiah et al., 2011). This method is considered, from a methodological point of view, one of the easiest, most accurate and productive for evaluation of antioxidant activity in fruit juices, plant extracts and pure substances like flavonoids and terpenoids (Alves et al., 2010). The method is influenced by the solvent and the pH of the reactions. The antioxidants BHA, BHT and Trolox® can be used as references in the experiments.

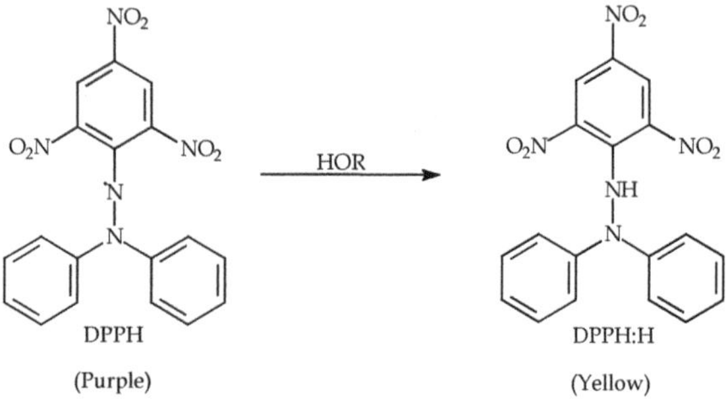

Fig. 4. Radical and non-radical forms of DPPH.

The electron donation ability of natural products can be measured by 2,2-diphenyl-1-picrylhydrazyl radical (DPPH) purple-coloured solution bleaching. The anti-radical activity (three replicates per treatment) is expressed as IC_{50} ($\mu g/ml$), the concentration required to cause a 50% DPPH inhibition. The presence of the phenolic hydroxyls appears essential for scavenger properties.

2.2.2 β-carotene bleaching test

The β-carotene/linoleic acid oxidation method evaluates the inhibitory activity of free radicals generated during the peroxidation of linoleic acid. The method is based on spectrophotometric discoloration measurements or (oxidation) of β-carotene-induced oxidative degradation products of linoleic acid. This method is suitable for plant samples.

The β-carotene bleaching method is based on the loss of β-carotene's yellow colour due to its reaction with radicals formed by linoleic acid oxidation when in an emulsion. The rate of the β-carotene bleaching can be slowed in the presence of antioxidants (Kulisic et al., 2004). The reaction can be monitored by spectrophotometer, β-carotene loss of staining at 470 nm, with intervals of 15 min for a total time of 2 h. The results are expressed as IC_{50} ($\mu g/ml$), the concentration required to cause a 50% β-carotene bleaching inhibition. Tests are realized in triplicate. The results can be compared with synthetic standards such as BHA, BHT and Trolox®, or natural, such as gallic acid and quercetin (Alves et al., 2010).

2.2.3 ABTS method

The 2,2′-azinobis(3-ethylbenzthiazoline-6-sulphonic acid), commonly called ABTS, radical scavenging method was developed by Rice-Evans and Miller and was then modified by Re et al. in 1990. The modification is based on the activation of metmyoglobin with hydrogen peroxide in the presence of ABTS·+ to produce a radical cation. The improved method generates a blue/green ABTS·+ chromophore via the reaction of ABTS and potassium persulfate. It is now widely used. Along with the DPPH method, the ABTS radical scavenging method is one of the most extensively used antioxidant assays for plant samples. The ABTS radical cation is generated by the oxidation of ABTS with potassium persulfate, its reduction in the presence of hydrogen-donating antioxidants is measured spectrophotometrically at 734 nm. Decolourisation assays measure the total antioxidant capacity in both lipophilic and hydrophilic substances. The effects of oxidant concentration and inhibition duration, of the radical cation's absorption are taken into account when the antioxidant activity is determined. Trolox is used as a positive control. The activity is expressed in terms of Trolox-equivalent antioxidant capacity for the extract or substance (TEAC/mg) (Krishnaiah et al., 2011).

2.2.4 ORAC assay

The peroxyl radical is an oxidant commonly found in biological substrates. It is less reactive than OH• having a half-life from seconds to nanoseconds (Alves et al., 2010). The ORAC (oxygen radical absorbance capacity) assay uses beta-phycoerythrin (PE) as an oxidizable protein substrate, and 2,2′-azobis(2-amidinopropane)dihydrochloride (AAPH), as a peroxyl radical generator, or a Cu^{2+}-H_2O_2 system as a hydroxyl radical generator. To date, it is the only method that takes the free radical reaction to completion, and uses an area-under-the curve (AUC) technique for quantification, combining both the inhibition percentage and the length of inhibition time for free radical action into a single quantity. The assay has been widely used in many recent studies of plants (Krishnaiah et al., 2011). Trolox is used as a standard antioxidant.

2.2.5 Reducing power assay

In this assay, the yellow colour of the test solution changes to green depending on the reducing power of the test specimen. The presence of the reductants in the solution causes the reduction of the Fe^{3+}/ferricyanide complex to the ferrous form. Therefore, Fe^{2+} can be monitored by absorbance measurement at 700 nm.

In the reducing power method, the sample is mixed in 1 ml of methanol with a phosphate buffer (5 ml, 0.2 M, pH 6.6) and potassium ferricyanide (5 ml, 1%). The mixture is incubated at 50 ºC for 20 min. Next, 5 ml of trichloroacetic acid (10%) are added to the reaction mixture, which is then centrifuged at 3000 RPM for 10 min. The upper layer of the solution (5 ml) is mixed with distilled water (5 ml), and ferric chloride (1 ml, 1%), and the absorbance is measured at 700 nm. A stronger absorbance indicates increased reducing power (Krishnaiah et al., 2011).

2.2.6 NBT assay or the superoxide anion scavenging activity assay

Xanthine oxidase (XO) is the enzyme responsible for conversion of xanthine into uric acid, resulting in the production of hydrogen peroxide and superoxide (Figure 5). It is considered a major biological source of reactive oxygen species. It is possible that inhibition of this enzymatic process by compounds that exhibit antioxidant properties may have therapeutic use (Alves et al., 2010).

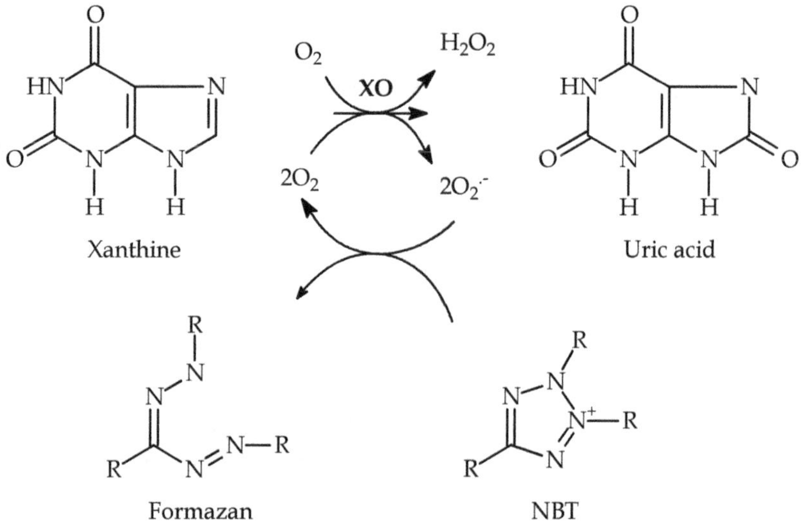

Fig. 5. Formation of formazan from NBT (Adapted from Alves et al., 2010).

The scavenging potential for superoxide radicals is analysed with a hypoxanthine/xanthine oxidase-generating system coupled with nitroblue tetrazolium (NBT) reduction (measured spectrophotometrically). The reaction mixture contains 125 µl of buffer (50 mM KH_2PO_4/KOH, pH 7.4), 20 µl of a 15 mM Na_2EDTA solution in buffer, 30 µl of a 3 mM hypoxanthine solution in buffer, 50 µl of a 0.6 mM NBT solution in buffer, 50 µl of xanthine oxidase in buffer (1 unit per 10 ml buffer), and 25 µl of the plant extract in buffer (a diluted, sonicated solution of 10 µg per 250 µl buffer). Microplates (96 wells) are read at 450 nm 2.5 min after the addition of the xanthine oxidase using a series 7500 Microplate Reader. Superoxide scavenger activity is expressed as percent inhibition compared to the blank, in which buffer is used in place of the extract. When using this system, any inhibition by tannins in the plant extracts must be due to their antioxidant activity and any action upon the enzyme must be excluded as a possibility (Krishnaiah et al., 2011).

2.2.7 Chelating effect on ferrous ions

Chelating activity of samples can be determined by the ferrozine assay. Ferrozine quantitatively forms complexes with Fe^{2+}. In the presence of other chelating agents, the complex formation is disrupted with a resulting decrease in the red colour of the complex. Measurement of the rate of colour reduction allows estimation of the chelating activity of the coexistent chelator (Yamaguchi et al., 2000; Wannes et al., 2010).

2.2.8 Determination of phenol content by Folin-Ciocalteu method

Folin-Ciocalteu phenol reagent consists of a mixture of the hetero-poly phosphomolybdic and phoshotungstic acids in which the molybdenum and tungsten are in the 6+ state. On reduction with certain reducing agents, molybdenum blue and tungsten blue are formed, in which the mean oxidation state of the metals is between 5 and 6. It is known that Folin-Ciocalteu reagent reacts not only with phenols but also with a variety of other compounds. The total phenolic content measured by the Folin-Ciocalteu procedure does not give a full picture of the quantity, or quality of the phenolic constituents in the extracts. In addition, there may also be interference arising from other chemical components present in the extract, such as sugars or ascorbic acid (Singleton & Rossi, 1965). Gallic acid is used as a standard for the calibration curve. The total phenolic content is expressed as mg of gallic acid equivalent (GAE). Figure 6 show the reaction of gallic acid with molybdenum, a component of the Folin-Ciocalteu reagent.

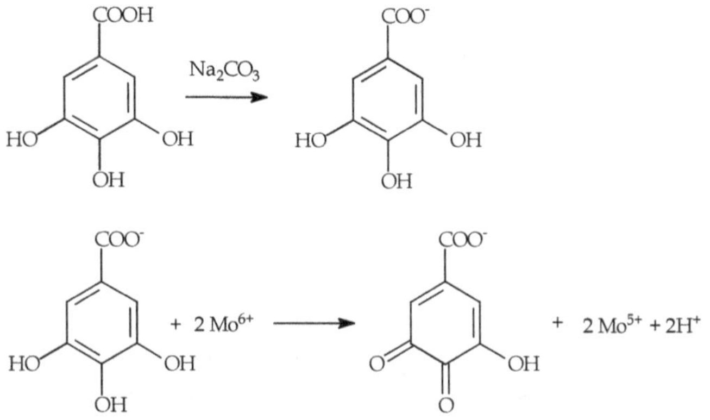

Fig. 6. Reaction of gallic acid with molybdenum, a component of the Folin-Ciocalteu reagent (Adapted from Oliveira et al., 2009b).

2.2.9 Total flavonoid content

Total flavonoid content is determined by using a colorimetric method described previously (Dewanto et al., 2002). Briefly, 0.30 mL of the EtOH and AcOEt extracts or (+)-catechin standard solution is mixed with 1.50 mL of distilled water in a test tube followed by addition of 90 µL of a 5% $NaNO_2$ solution. After 6 min, 180 µL of a 10% $AlCl_3.6H_2O$ solution is added and allowed to stand for another 5 min before 0.6 mL of 1 M NaOH is added. The mixture is brought to 330 µL with distilled water and mixed well. The absorbance is measured immediately against the blank at 510 nm using a spectrophotometer in comparison with the standards prepared similarly with known (+)-catechin concentrations. The results are expressed as mg of catechin equivalents per gram of extract (mg CE/g) through a calibration curve with catechin.

3. Conclusion

Oxidative stress is involved in the development of various diseases and their symptoms, especially degenerative diseases. Scientific knowledge of the antioxidant activity of natural products, along with state of the art *in vitro* methods for evaluation has been increasing over time. *In vitro* testing has become an important tool in the search for bioactive substances, and for raw material selection studies as well. These tests have demonstrated the importance of diets rich in fruits and vegetables by confirming the presence of antioxidants that help fight free radicals, and which in moderate consumption are beneficial to human health.

4. Acknowledegments

The authors are grateful to the *Conselho Nacional de Desenvolvimento Científico e Tecnológico (CNPq)*, and the *Fundação de Amparo à Ciência e Tecnologia do Estado de Pernambuco (FACEPE)* for financial support.

5. References

Almeida, J. R. G. S.; Oliveira, M. R.; Guimarães, A. L.; Oliveira, A. P.; Ribeiro, L. A. A.; Lúcio, A. S. S. C.; Quintans-Júnior, L. J. (2011). Phenolic quantification and antioxidant activity of *Anaxagorea dolichocarpa* and *Duguetia chrysocarpa* (Annonaceae). *International Journal of Pharma and Bio Sciences*, Vol.2, No.4, (October 2011), pp. 367-374, ISSN 0975-6299.

Alves, C.Q.; David, J.M.; David, J.P.; Bahia, M.V.; Aguiar, R.M. (2010). Methods for determination of *in vitro* antioxidant activity for extracts and organic compounds. *Química Nova*, Vol.33, No.10, (October 2010), pp. 2202-2210, ISSN 0100-4042.

Andrade, C. A.; Costa, C. K.; Bora, K.; Miguel, M. D.; Miguel, O. G.; Kerber, V. A. (2007). Determination of the phenolic content and evaluation of the antioxidant activity of *Acacia podalyriifolia* A. Cunn. ex G. Don, Leguminosae-Mimosoideae. *Brazilian Journal of Pharmacognosy*, Vol.17, No.2, (April 2007), pp. 231-235, ISSN 0102-695X.

Bakkali, F.; Averbeck, S.; Averbeck, D.; Idaomar, M. (2008). Biological effects of essential oils – a review. *Food and Chemical Toxicology*, Vol.46, No.2, (February 2008), pp. 446-475, ISSN 0278-6915.

Barreiros, A.L.B.S.; David, J.M. (2006). Estresse oxidativo: relação entre geração de espécies reativas e defesa do organismo. *Química Nova*, Vol.29, No.1, (February 2006), pp. 113-123, ISSN 0100-4042.

Blois, M.S. (1958). Antioxidant determinations by the use of a stable free radical. *Nature*, Vol.181, (April 1958), pp. 1199-1200, ISSN 0028-0836.

Bloknina, O.; Virolainen, E.; Fagerstedt, K.V. (2003). Antioxidants, oxidative damage and oxygen deprivation stress: a review. *Annals of Botany*, Vol.91, pp. 179-194, ISSN 0305-7364.

Borgo, J.; Xavier, C. A. G.; Moura, D. J. ; Richter, M. F. ; Suyenaga, E. S. (2010). The Influence of drying processes on flavonoid level and the antioxidant activity of *Baccharis articulata* (Lam.) extracts. *Brazilian Journal of Pharmacognosy*, Vol.20, No.1, (March 2010), pp. 12-17, ISSN 0102-695X.

Bravo, L. (1998). Polyphenols: chemistry, dietary sources, metabolism and nutritional significance. Nutrition Reviews, Vol.56, No.11, (November 1998), pp. 317–333, ISSN 0229-6643.

Broinizi, P. R. B.; Andrade-Wartha, E. R. S.; Silva, A. M. O.; Torres, R. P.; Azeredo, H. M. C.; Alves, R. E.; Mancini-Filho, J. (2008). Antioxidant properties in cashew Apple byproduct (*Anacardium occidentale* L.): effect on lipoperoxidation and the polyunsaturated fatty acids profile in rats. *Brazilian Journal of Pharmaceutical Sciences*, Vol.44, No.4, (October 2008), pp. 773-781, ISSN 1984-8250.

Carvalho, K. I. M.; Fernandes, H. B.; Machado, F. D. F.; Oliveira, I. S.; Oliveira, F. A.; Nunes, P. H. M.; Lima, J. T.; Almeida, J. R. G. S.; Oliveira, R. C. M. (2010). Antiulcer activity of ethanolic extract of *Encholirium spectabile* Mart. ex Schult & Schult f. (Bromeliaceae) in rodents. *Biological Research*, Vol.43, (November 2010), pp. 459-465, ISSN 0716-9760.

Coutinho, M.A.S.; Muzitano, M.F.; Costa, S.S. (2009). Flavonóides: potenciais agentes terapêuticos para o processo inflamatório. *Revista Virtual de Quimica*, Vol.1, No.3, (June 2009), pp. 241-256, ISSN 1984-6835.

Dewanto, V.; Wu, X.; Adom, K.; Liu, R.H. (2002). Thermal Processing Enhances the Nutritional Value of Tomatoes by Increasing Total Antioxidant Activity. *Journal of Agricultural and Food Chemistry*, Vol.50, No.10, (April 2002), pp. 3010-3014, ISSN 0021-8561.

Dewick, P.M. (2002). *The mevalonate pathway: terpenoids and steroids.* In: Dewick, P.M. *Medicinal Natural Products: a biosynthetic approach.* Jonh Wiley & Sons, 2nd edition, ISBN 9780470741672.

Di Carlo, G.; Mascolo, N.; Izzo, A.A.; Capasso, F. (1999). Flavonoids: old and new aspects of a class of natural therapeutic drugs. *Life Sciences*, Vol.65, No.4, (June 1999), pp. 337-353, ISSN 0024-3205.

Djeridane, A.; Yousfi, M.; Nadjemi, B.; Boutassouna, D.; Stocker, P.; Vidal, N. (2006). Antioxidant activity of some algerian medicinal plants extracts containing phenolic compounds. *Food Chemistry*, Vol.97, No.4, (August 2006), pp. 654-660, ISSN 0308-8146.

Gressler, V.; Stein, E. M.; Dorr, F.; Fujii, M. T.; Colepicolo, P.; Pinto, E. (2011). Sesquiterpenes from the essential oil of *Laurencia dendroidea* (Ceramiales, Rhodophyta): isolation, biological activities and distribution among seaweeds. *Brazilian Journal of Pharmacognosy*, Vol.21, No.2, (March 2011), pp. 248-254, ISSN 0102-695X.

Gupta, V. K. & Verma, A. K. (2010). *Comprehensive Bioactive Natural Products.* Vol 4. Stadium Press LCC, ISBN 1-933699-54-X, Houston, USA.

Halliwell, B. & Gutteridge, J.M.C. (2007). *Free Radicals in Biology and Medicine.* 4th edition. Clarendon, ISBN 9780198500445, Oxford, UK.

Haslam, E. (1996). Natural polyphenols (vegetable tannins) as drugs: possible modes of action. *Journal of Natural Products*, Vol.59, No.2, (February 1996), pp. 205-215, ISSN 0163-3864.

Ignat, I.; Volf, I.; Popa, V.I. (2011). A critical review of methods for characterization of polyphenolic compounds in fruits and vegetables. *Food Chemistry*, Vol.126, No.4, (June 2011), pp. 1821–1835, ISSN 0308-8146.

Jadhav, S.J.; Nimbalkar, S.S.; Kulkarni, A.D.; Madhavi, D.L. (1996). *Lipid oxidation in biological and food systems.* In: Madhavi, D.L.; Deshpande, S.S.; Salunkhe, D.K. *Food antioxidants: technological, toxicological and health perspectives.* Marcel Dekker, ISBN 082479351X, pp. 5-63, New York, USA.

Jang, I.C.; Jo, E.K.; Bae, M.S.; Lee, H.J.; Jeon, G.I.; Park, E.; Yuk, H.G.; Ahn, G.H.; Lee, S.C. (2010). Antioxidant and antigenotoxic activities of different parts of persimmon (*Diospyros kaki* cv. Fuyu) fruit. *Journal of Medicinal Plants Research*, Vol.4, No.2, (January 2010), pp. 155-160, ISSN 1996-0875.

Jardini, F. A.; Mancini-Filho, J. (2007). Antioxidant activity evaluation of different polarities extracts by pulp and seeds of pomegranate (*Punica granatum*, L.). *Brazilian Journal of Pharmaceutical Sciences*, Vol.43, No.1, (January 2007), pp. 137-147, ISSN 1984-8250.

Kähkönen, M.P.; Hopia, A.I.; Vuorela, H.J.; Rauha,J.P.; Pihlaja, K.; Kujala, T.S.; Heinonen, M. (1999). Antioxidant activity of plant extracts containing phenolic compounds. *Journal of Agricultural and Food Chemistry.* Vol. 47, No.10, (September 1999), ISSN 3954-3962.

Krishnaiah, D.; Sarbatly, R.; Nithyanandam, R. (2011). A review of the antioxidant potential of medicinal plant species. *Food and Bioproducts Processing*, Vol.89, No.3, (July 2011), pp. 217-233, ISSN 0960-3085.

Kulisic, T.; Radonic, A.; Katalinic, V.; Milos, M. (2004). Use of different methods for testing antioxidative activity of oregano essential oil. *Food Chemistry*, Vol.85, No.4, (May 2004), pp. 633-640, ISSN 0308-8146.

Magder, S. (2006). Reactive oxygen species: toxic molecules or spark life? *Critical Care*, Vol.10, No.1, (February 2006), pp. 1-8, ISSN 1466-609X.

Mensor, L. L.; Menezes, F. S.; Leitão, G. G.; Reis, A. S.; Santos, T. C.; Coube, C. S.; Leitão, S. G. (2001). Screening of Brazilian plant extracts for antioxidant activity by the use of DPPH free radical method. *Phytotherapy Research*, Vol.15, pp. 127-130, ISSN 0951-418X.

Montoro, P.; Braca, A.; Pizza, C.; De Tommasi, N. (2005). Structure–antioxidant activity relationships of flavonoids isolated from different plant species. *Food Chemistry*, Vol.92, No.2, (September 2005), pp. 349-355, ISSN 0308-8146.

Morais, S. M.; Cavalcanti, E. S. B.; Costa, S. M. O.; Aguiar, L. A. (2009). Antioxidant action of teas and seasonings more consumed in Brazil. *Brazilian Journal of Pharmacognosy*, Vol.19, No.1B, (January 2009), pp. 315-320, ISSN 0102-695X.

Morais, S. M.; Catunda-Júnior, F. E. A.; Silva, A. R. A.; Martins-Neto, J. S.; Rondina, D.; Cardoso, J. H. L. (2006). Antioxidant activity of essential oils from Northeastern Brazilian *Croton* species. *Química Nova*, Vol.29, No.5, (May 2006), pp. 907-910, ISSN 0100-4042.

Naczk, M. & Shahidi, F. (2004). Extraction and analysis of phenolics in food. *Journal of Chromatography A*, Vol.1054, No.1-2, (October 2004), pp. 95–111, ISSN 0021-9673.

Nascimento, M. A.; Silva, A. K.; França, L. C. B.; Quignard, E. L. J.; López, J. A.; Almeida, M. G. (2006). *Turnera ulmifolia* L. (Turneraceae): Preliminary study of its antioxidant activity. *Bioresource Technology*, Vol.97, pp. 1387-1391, ISSN 0960-8524.

Oliveira, A.C.; Valentim, I.B.; Silva, C.A.; Bechara, E.J.H.; Barros, M.P.; Mano, C.M.; Goulart, M.O.F. (2009a). Total phenolic content and free radical scavenging activities of methanolic extract powders of tropical fruit residues. *Food Chemistry*, Vol.115, No.2, (July 2009), pp. 469-475, ISSN 0308-8146.

Oliveira, A.C.; Valentim, I.B.; Goulart, M.O.F.; Silva, C.A.; Bechara, E.J.H.; Trevisan, M.T.S. (2009). Fontes vegetais naturais de antioxidantes. *Química Nova*, Vol.32, No.3, (April 2009), pp. 689-702, ISSN 0100-4042.

Rosa, E. A.; Silva, B. C.; Silva, F. M.; Tanaka, C. M. A.; Peralta, R. M.; Oliveira, C. M. A.; Kato, L.; Ferreira, H. D.; Silva, C. C. (2010). Flavonoids and antioxidant activity in *Palicourea rigida* Kunth, Rubiaceae. *Brazilian Journal of Pharmacognosy*, Vol.20, No.4, (September 2010), pp. 484-488, ISSN 0102-695X.

Sanchez, G. M.; Hernandez, R. D.; Garrido, G. G.; Garcia, M. G.; Rivera, D. G.; Betancourt, E. P.; Selles, A. J. N. (2003). *Mitos y Realidades de la Terapia Antioxidante*. Vimang: Nuevo Producto Natural Antioxidante. Center of Pharmaceutical Chemistry: Havana, pp. 88.

Santos, P. M. L.; Japp, A. S.; Lima, L. G.; Schripsema, J.; Menezes, F. S.; Kuster, R. M. (2010). Antioxidant activity from the leaf extracts of *Jacaranda puberula* Cham., Bignoniaceae, a Brazilian medicinal plant used for blood depuration. *Brazilian Journal of Pharmacognosy*, Vol.20, No.2, (May 2010), pp. 147-153, ISSN 0102-695X.

Santos, E. L.; Costa, E. V.; Marques, F. A.; Vaz, N. P.; Maia, B. H. L. N.; Magalhães, E. G.; Tozzi, A. M. A. (2009). Toxicity and antioxidant activity of flavonoids from *Lonchocarpus filipes*. *Química Nova*, Vol.32, No.9, (November 2009), pp. 2255-2258, ISSN 0100-4042.

Singleton, V.L. & Rossi, J.A. (1965). Colorimetry of total phenolics with phosphomolybdic-phosphotungstic acid reagents. *American Journal of Enology and Viticulture*, Vol.16, No.3, pp. 144-158, ISSN 002-9254.

Sousa, C. M. M.; Silva, H. R. S.; Vieira-Júnior, G. M.; Ayres, M. C. C.; Costa, C. L. S.; Araújo, D. S.; Cavalcante, L. C. D.; Barros, E. D. S.: Araújo, P. B. M.; Brandão, M. S.; Chaves, M. H. (2007). Total phenolics and antioxidant activity of five medicinal plants. *Química Nova*, Vol.30, No.2, (January 2007), pp. 351-355, 2007, ISSN 0100-4042.

van Acker, S.A.B.E.; van den Berg, D.J.; Tromp, M.N.J.L.; Griffioen, D.H.; van Bennekom, W.P.; van der Vijgh, W.J.F.; Bast, A. (1996). Structural aspects of antioxidant activity of flavonoids. *Free Radical Biology and Medicine*, Vol.20, No.3, (May 1996), pp. 331-432, ISSN 0891-5849.

Velioglu, Y.S.; Mazza, G.; Gao, L.; Oomah, B.D. (1998). Antioxidant activity and total phenolics in selected fruits, vegetables and grain products. *Journal of Agricultural and Food Chemistry*, Vol.46, No.10, (August 1998), pp. 4113-4117, ISSN 0021-8561.

Yamaguchi, F.; Ariga, T.; Yoshimira, Y.; Nakazawa, H. (2000). Antioxidant and anti-glycation of carbinol from *Garcinia indica*. *Journal of Agricultural and Food Chemistry*, Vol.48, No.2, (January 2000), pp. 180-185, ISSN 0021-8561.

Wannes, W. A.; Mhamdi, B.; Sriti, J.; Jemia, M. B.; Ouchikh, O.; Hamdaoui, G.; Kchouk, M. E.; Marzouk, B. (2010). Antioxidant activities of the essential oil and methanol extracts from myrtle (*Myrtus communis* var. *italica* L.) leaf, stem and flower. *Food and Chemical Toxicology*, Vol.48, No.5, (May 2010), pp. 1362-1370, ISSN 0278-6915.

Antiadhesive Effect
of Plant Compounds in Bacteria

Orlando A. Abreu[1] and Guillermo Barreto[2]
[1]Faculty of Chemistry, University of Camagüey,
[2]Faculty of Veterinary Scienses, University of Camagüey,
Cuba

1. Introduction

Bacteria have been evolving in our planet for 3 500 – 4 000 million years; thus, based on chemical signals microbial communities have developed different systems to interact with their own colonies and with other species, even with host like plants or animals. Antibiotics release is one of the most outstanding microorganism behaviour. Microbial interaction in nature shows an unexpected performance, sublethal concentrations of antibiotics can modulate dynamic among microorganisms and it can achieve the activation of cooperation, self defence or motility mechanisms among microorganisms (Ratcliff & Denison, 2011).

Notwithstanding the arsenal of antibiotic drugs developed in last decades and, socioeconomic background of outbreaks or epidemic level of colibacilosis, tuberculosis, or cholera in Developing Countries, an underlying problem is challenging ahead: the eclosion of more virulent and resistant microbes. This is an unreliable phenomenon that stresses health care systems in countries and regions (von Baum & Reinhard Marre, 2005; Marcusson et al., 2009; Mediavilla et al., 2005; Wagenlehner & Naber, 2004).

One of the ways by which microbes avoid antibiotic products is by biofilm formation, a usually lipospolisacaride based microorganism aggregates that confer protection, it is a selective advantage for persistence under hostile environmental conditions; biofilm also promotes host colonization. Few decades ago there was a common misunderstanding of the microcosm, since 99% microbes in nature live in communities as biofilms and not in planktonic forms as they were usually cultured and studied (Barreto & Rodríguez, 2009, 2010).

Microorganism biofilm are systems that behave as a whole, determining what, when, and how to interact with the environment (physical or biological). This is mediated by the so called quorum-sensing (QS), a cell-to-cell communication mechanism in which the expression of certain genes in response to the presence of small signal molecules is coordinated (Defoirdt et al., 2011, Dobrindt & Hacker, 2008).

Urinary tract infections (UTIs) are a worldwide health problem, second only to infections of the respiratory tract. Sexual active women are the most susceptible population to UTI, but it is also frequent in elder people and catheterized patients. *Escherichia coli* is the prevalent etiological agent isolated in UTI (Johnson, 1997; 2003; Scholes et al., 2000; Svanborg &

Godaly, 1997; Zhang & Foxman, 2003). Chemotherapy is the main UTI conventional therapy, but antibioresistant strains are continuously emerging, for this reason, antibiotics therapy is sometimes inefficient, specially for β_lactamics, trimethoprim-sulfamethoxazole, and more recent drugs like fluoroquinolones (von Baum & Reinhard Marre, 2005; Drekonja & Johnson, 2008; Gupta et al.,1999; Hooton, 2003; Jadhav et al., 2011; Mediavilla et al., 2005; Storby, 2004; Wagenlehner & Naber, 2004).

In this never ending cycle, there is a race to develop different kinds of vaccines and effective new generation drugs. But it seems that immunologicals or antibiotics are not an exclusive criterion to deal with bacteria, some other subtle ways can be even more promising. If microorganism advantage adaptations are interfered, host abilities to overcome infection and restore itself will be increased.

This review deals with microbiological sciences related to the search of new antibacterial mechanisms, fimbriae as a virulence factor target, and the possibilities of using plant origin compounds as antiadhesive in bacterial attachment, particularly exposed by studies on uropathogenic *Escherichia coli*.

2. Uropathogenic *Escherichia coli* and virulence factors

Escherichia coli (Escherich, 1885 - *Enterobacteriaceae*) is a versatile bacteria that has become the most thoroughly studied organism in the planet (Barreto, 2007), it is a human and warm-blooded animal enteric comensal but, as a result of genetic fluidity of pathogenicity encoding genes, it could have different pathogenic behaviours (Dobrindt, 2005; Ahmed et al., 2008; Schubert et al., 2009); therefore, *E. coli* can become in a virulent bacteria adapted to different niches. Beside gastroenteritis, it can cause urinary tract infection, abdominal sepsis, septicaemia, and meningitis.

Eight virulence factors (VFs) armed pathovars have been described and classified as either diarrheagenic *E. coli*, enteropathogenic *E. coli* (EPEC), enterohemorrhagic *E. coli* (EHEC), enterotoxigenic *E. coli* (ETEC), enteroinvasive *E. coli* (EIEC) including Shigella, enteroaggregative *E. coli* (EAEC), and diffusely adherent *E. coli* (DAEC); or extraintestinal *E. coli* (ExPEC), uropathogenic *E. coli* (UPEC); and neonatal meningitis *E. coli* (NMEC) (Sasakawa & Hacker, 2006; Croxen & Finlay, 2010).

Uropathogenic *E. coli* is a facultative enteric bacterium, but if carrying some VFs, it can reach the lower urinary tract and cause cystitis or, travel further into the kidneys and cause pyelonephritis (Croxen & Finlay, 2010; Dobrindt & Hacker, 2008; Zhang & Foxman, 2003). UTI it is much more common in young women than men and female anatomy is determinant. It is estimated that 11 percent of women in U.S.A. are diagnosed for UTI every year, about half of all women have a UTI by their late twenties, 20-30 percent will have two or more infections, and 5 percent will suffer from recurrent UTI (Foxman et al., 2000; Zhang & Foxman, 2003).

It is a fact that comensal enteric bacteria must carry a subset of VFs, required in a hostile environment like the urinary tract, to be an ExPEC, and explore niches outside the gastrointestinal tract. Virulence factors provide mechanism by which bacteria survive at least for a period of time needed for each step of infection. Tropism in UPEC is remarkable; once it reaches the uroepithelium, it attaches to its surfaces impeding urinary mechanical clearance and starting colonization; then, it travels to the bladder and kidneys; haeminic iron could be a gold medal in nephrones. However, UPEC needs a toolbox of VFs like: adhesins, alpha-haemolysin, cytotoxic necrotizing factor, and iron acquisition systems, to cause cystitis and pyelonephritis, which are associated with a number of symptoms such as: inflammation, haematuria, urohaemolitic syndrome, and renal scars; while subvert host unspecific immunity, provoke epithelial exfoliation and invade deeper cells (Gal-Mor & Finlay, 2006; Johnson, 1997, 2003; Kaper et al., 2004; Wiles et al., 2008).

Genetic expressions of VFs are coordinated by QS as a way to be effective in colonization and surviving at least of a reduct of bacterial cell in each infection step. In a recent review, Wu et al. (2008) classified VFs as follows:

- Membrane proteins, which play roles in adhesion, colonization, and invasions; promote adherence to host cell surfaces, are also responsible for resistance to antibiotics, and intercellular communication
- Polysaccharide capsules that surround the bacterial cell and have antiphagocytic properties
- Secretory proteins, such as toxin which can modify the host cell environment and are responsible for some host cell–bacteria interactions
- Cell wall and outer membrane components, such as lipopolysaccharide (LPS or endotoxin) and lipoteichoic acids
- Other virulence factors, such as biofilm forming proteins and siderophores

Virulence factors play a key role in adaptation and evolution. According to Jain et al. (2010), microbes either communal or individual ones provoke chronic or persistent infections, which are largely associated with populations of microbes, and have individual bacterial virulence traits associated with acute infections. VFs are encoded in large continuous blocks of virulence in genome, named pathogenicity associated islands (PAIs), and their expression can be regulated by the host and by environmental signals (Bergsten et al., 2005; Gal-Mor & Finlay, 2006; Johnson, 1997). Horizontal DNA transfer is mediated by plasmids, phages, and PAIs; this is one of the processes that generate bacterial and host genome evolution (Ahmed et al., 2008; Beauregard-Racine et al., 2011; Schubert et al., 2009; Tettelin et al., 2008; Zaneveld et al., 2008).

In *E. coli* pathotypes, several VFs are associated and could be expressed at the same time or not. In the last two decades, VFs research in molecular biology has advanced enough to explain different mechanisms of UPEC pathogenesis, and modern "omics" are focussed in relation to PAIs and UTI epidemiology; thus, aetiology of UTI is better understood, different purposes to disrupt VFs are supported, therapeutic guidelines can be much more successful, and new approaches on antimicrobials research are rendered (Ahmed et al., 2008; Dobrindt, 2005; Henderson et al., 2009; Johnson, 1997; Johnson & Russo, 2006; Westerlund-Wikström & Korhonen 2005; Zhang & Foxman, 2003). A lethal battery of VFs is responsible for the human food borne virulent *E. coli* 0157:H7 and the European recent lethal *E. coli* O104:H4, both strains produce hemolytic uremic syndrome.

2.1 Uropathogenic *E. coli* and fimbriae

Pili or fimbriae are hair-like polymeric (assembled from multiple subunits) proteinaceous appendages expressed on the outer surface of bacteria that enable pathogens to recognize host receptors, anchor, and begin infection; adhesion is produced by a bacterial adhesin located at the tip of a pilus structure (Dodson et al., 2001; Johnson, 1997, 2003; Niemann et al., 2004). Fimbriae are determinant in early steps of colonization of most *E coli* pathovars. In UPEC are significant, they avoid lavage by the host, attaching to the urinary tract mucosa and triggering signals to start the disease process. This VF is associated to invasion, biofilm formation, cell motility, and transport of proteins and DNA across membranes (Gal- Mor & Finlay, 2006; Johnson, 2003; Kaper et al., 2004; Wiles et al., 2008).

If fimbriae-receptor interaction is not well established, UTI symptoms never occur; when bacterial persist in this condition the patient will have an asymptomatic bacteriuria (ABU). Adhesins have been termed as the most important determinant of pathogenicity (Le Bouguénec, 2005; Croxen & Finlay, 2010; Mulvey, 2002; Niemann et al., 2004; Sauer et al., 2000). The process of a UTI is viewed by Schilling et al. (2001) as a number of measures and counter-measures taken by the host and UPEC. The disease is triggered by fimbriae, inducing the host and bacterial cells signal pathways that involve different mutual responses. In the "two-step" model of UTI pathogenesis described by Bergsten et al. (2005), the first step is the activation of the innate response, and the second one is the effector phase involved in bacterial clearance, which depends on neutrophils and their ability to remove lingering inflammatory cells and bacteria. Electron microscopy shows hat this immunological response could be advantageous to bacteria, because it allow them to internalized and survive at the underlying bladder epithelium and creating a reservoir protected from immune surveillance and antibiotics. They remain in a quiescent state for several weeks before reemerging and provoking a recurrent acute infection (Caper et al., 2004; Lane & Mobley, 2007; Mulley et al., 2001; Mulley, 2002).

Uropathogenic *E. coli* type 1 fimbriae and type P fimbriae, are molecularly and epidemiologically well characterized. Both types of fimbriae are assembled in cell bacteria by a highly conserved periplasmatic chaperone and outer membrane usher proteins (Le Bouguénec, 2005; Waksman and Hultgren, 2009). Type 1 fimbriae are so far, the most common adhesin in non complicated low UTI (cystitis); while P fimbriae, encoded by *E. coli* pap (pyelonephritis-associated pilus) operon, adhere to kidney uroepithelium (Croxen and Finlay, 2010; Verger et al., 2007). Fimbriae can be classified according to their receptor-binding specific traits. Type 1 fimbriae mediate mannose-sensitive haemagglutination (MSHA), but P fimbriae are cause of mannose-resistant haemagglutination (MRHA) (Abraham et al. 1998; Johnson, 2003; Westerlund-Wikström and Korhonen, 2005).

Haemagglutination is an *E. coli* visual test to detect types 1 and P bacterial fimbriae, since some red blood cells (RBC) have carbohydrate residue receptors similar to adhesin uroepithelial receptors. When the adhesin of a bacterial cell suspension contacts the receptor of a RBC suspension, a surface reaction occurs and the RBC aggregate like macroscopic glomerules. Uroepithelial cells and oral cells can lead to an agglutination reaction too. Designation of P fimbriae is for the ability of these *E. coli* strains to agglutinate P blood antigens erythrocytes (Johnson, 1991).

Type 1 fimbriae consist in a 7 nm thick helical rod with a tip structure containing the adhesin FimH and two adaptor proteins, FimF and FimG. About 70 % of isolated UPEC encoded a variant of FimF adhesin that binds to monomannose residues. In addition to trimannose receptors, this affinity to monomannose receptors leads to tropism within uroepithelial cells (Johnson, 2003; Mulvey, 2002; Niemann et al., 2004; Verger et al., 2007). P fimbria is a 6.8 nm rod composed of repeating PapA subunits arranged in a right- handed helical cylinder, with a distally located adhesin PapG on its tip. Receptors of P pili are globoseries of membrane glycolipids with a disaccharide galabiose (Gal-α (1-4)-Gal). There are three PapG alleles (I-III) which bind to different isoreceptors that differ in carbohydrate residues to the common Gal-α (1-4)-Gal core. PapG II binds mainly to globotetrasyl ceramide (GbO4) and it is associated with pyelonephritis symptoms like inflammation and uroepithelial exfoliation (Dodson et al., 2001; Johnson, 2003; Mulvey, 2002; Niemann et al., 2004; Westerlund-Wikström & Korhonen, 2005; Wullt, 2003;). It was demonstrated that class II adhesin is a prerequisite for acute pyelonephritis in primates; besides, in induced mixed infection with P fimbriated *E. coli* and not fimbriated strains it gives a competitive advantage to colonize bladder (Winberg et al., 1995).

The role of fimbriae as virulent factor in UTI pathogenesis has been thoroughly studied in the last thirty years, also confirming the special pathogenesis theory by means of modern methods (Beached, 1981; Johnson, 2001, 2003; Kaper et al., 2004; Verger et al., 2007; Wiles et al., 2008; Zhang & Foxman, 2003). See most of the review articles cited in this subchapter for details and graphics of VFs effects and UTI steps.

3. Experiences against fimbrial adhesion

Interference of VFs is an attractive approach to manage diseases due to bacterial infection. In the case of UPEC, fimbriae are an important target to prematurely neutralize them, before they spread within urinary tract, and if is not timely flushed out become in an asymptomatic bacteriruria. Beside UTI overcome, if this purpose is clinically effective, it is expected in these conditions that possibility of generating antibioresistance will be remote.

Fimbriae have been studied from different perspectives. Regarding enteropathogenic and uropathogenic *E. coli*, Barreto et al. (2001a) reviewed the following experimental attempts:

a. sublethal antibiotic concentrations: fimbrial adhesive ability of *E. coli* to attach to uroepithelium, enterocytes, and some erythrocytes could be decreased by a previous exposition to sublethal antibiotic concentrations of amphicillin, gentamycin, sulfonamides, trimethropim, and tetracycline, however, nalidixic acid can increase adhesion (Barreto et al., 1994; Hales & Aymes, 1985; Johnson, 1991; Padilla et al., 1991; Stenquist et al., 1987; Vosbeck et al., 1982). Sublethal amounts of gentamycin, chloramphenicol and kanamycin tested in *E. coli* G7 inhibit adhesiveness in this strain at 95%, 85%, 80% y 75%, respectively (Barreto et al., 1994). It was found that, in general, those antibiotics that inhibit protein synthesis also inhibit fimbrial expression at sublethal concentrations of either P fimbriae, or K88 and K99 fimbriae (Padilla et al., 1991; Barreto et al., 1994), without culture media influence (Barreto et al., 1995a, 1995b). But this is not the best option in therapy as it has the limitation of antibioresistance emergence (Barreto et al., 2000).

b. immunological methods (antifimbrial vaccines, monoclonal antibodies): Search for a vaccine that blocks *E. coli* fimbriae has been performed since the 1980´ and many results have been obtained, mainly in veterinary medicine. Several methods have been applied to obtain this products, attenuated strains, semipure antigenic extracts, and recombinant technology (Barreto et al., 2001a; Ofek et al., 2003; Campal et al. 2007, 2008). Fimbrial subunits vaccines are more efficient than conventional ones, since other non-protective cell components, or endotoxins that induce shock, vascular permeability, and abortion in swine are not present (Kaper & Levine, 1988; Levine et al., 1993; Wong et al., 1995). In Cuba, the administration of VACOLI® vaccine to swine protect piglet by suckling in a 93 %, and in 98 % post-weaning (Wong et al., 1995).

A vaccine that induces an antibody response against FimH was tested in humans proving its effectiveness against an UPEC strain in mouse cystitis model (Langermann et al., 1997; Langermann & Ballou, 2003). A high level of protection against P fimbriae has been developed too in a primate model (Soderhall et al., 1997). Molecular microbiology of bacterial pathogenesis and new technologies show favorable expectations concerning discoveries of new vaccines against bacterial infectious diseases (Moingeon et al., 2003; Sasakawa & Hacker, 2006; Westerlund-Wikström & Korhonen, 2005). The wide fimbriae diversity encoded by enteric E. coli, and the selective pressure exerted by vaccination usually make bacteria population change toward fimbrial fenotypes not covered by the vaccine. On the other hand, adhesin diversity of enteropathogenic E coli is higher in human beings than in animals; antigenic diversity is the principal disadvantage for an UPEC P fimbriae vaccine (Barreto, 2007; Barreto & Campal, 2001; Barreto et al., 2001b).

c.   medicinal plant extracts: it is exposing in next epigraph.

Some of these items were coincident with the strategies for UTI management mentioned by Reid (1999): prophylaxis by antibiotics, including natural peptides; vaccines, probiotics and others like avoiding spermicide and keeping a proper hygiene. In a review about anti-adhesion therapy for different bacterial germs, Ofek et al. (2003), referred to receptor analogs and adhesin analogs as anti-adhesive agents, dietary inhibitors of adhesion, adhesin-based vaccines, and host-derived anti-adhesins in innate immunity.

4. Medicinal plants extracts and virulence factors

In the last years, attention to medicinal plant research related to VFs inhibition as a target activity is increasing; several bioassays to evaluate VFs have been develop for several microorganisms, mainly bacteria and yeast. This is a valuable source of compounds to investigate new anti-virulence factors mechanisms of pathogenic microbes.

Different medicinal plant metabolites have antimicrobial activity (Cowan, 1999; Mahady, 2005). In traditional medicine systems of diverse cultures and regions, plants to treat urinary tract diseases are well known. Usually the same species are used for different purposes or medical conditions related to urinary system, i.e. as diuretic (most common), antilithic, and agents for cystitis or pyelonephritis treatment. However common people call all of them as "kidney diseases" or "urinary complaints".

Researches focused on adhesin-receptor medicinal plants interference are recent, since few studies have reported this action in plants, except those related in vitro, in vivo, and clinical trial of UPEC antiadhesion effects of cranberry fruit (Vaccinium macrocarpon Ait., Ericaceae). This is the only one commercial herbal product or food claimed as an antiadherent for UTI treatment. Besides, cranberry was among the top ten marketed herbal products in U.S. in the 1990´ (Siciliano, 1998).

In Cuba, first reports about plant extracts against fimbrial adhesion are those of Eucabev, an antidiarrheic drug for veterinary use, manufactured from Eucaliptus spp. (Myrtaceae) bark.

After using a decoction of *Eucaliptus* spp. bark to treat diarrheic syndrome in different animal species (Velázquez et al., 1991), and confirming no bactericide or bacteriostatic effect on ETEC at several concentrations (Barreto et al., 1993a), an antiadhesive mechanism of this plant was explored as antidiarrheic. Enteropathogenic *E. coli* strains G7 (08 K87, K88ab) and B44 (09 K30, K99) were tested as fimbrial antiadhesives by MSHA assay (Blanco & Blanco, 1993) or monoclonal antibodies assays. After exposure of each strain in media cultures with decoction, infusion, and water extract of *Eucaliptus saligna* and *E. citriodora*, fimbriae inhibition was found significant, 83,3% and 100%, respectively (Barreto et al., 1993b, 1993c; 1995a, 1995b; Barreto & Campal, 2001).

Similar experiments were carried out to screen P fimbriae-receptor interference in UPEC strains of medicinal plants traditionally used for urinary diseases. Wild *E coli* P+ strains cultured or not with *Lepidium virginicum* (*Apiaceae*) and *Achyranthes aspera* (*Amaranthaceae*) extracts were tested by MRHA assay (Guerra et al., 1995; Prieto et al., 1995). Then, plant antiadhesin activity was determined by MRHA and anti-PapA monoclonal antiserum assays in *E. coli* ATCC 25922 to screen extracts of *A. aspera*, *L. virginicum*, *Ageratum conyzoides* (*Asteraceae*), *Zingiber officinale* (*Zingiberaceae*), *Curcuma longa* (*Zingiberaceae*) and *Costus speciosus* (*Costaceae*). Antiadhesive effect was detected in all plant species except *C. longa* extracts (Barreto et al., 2001). Besides, based on a previous study on K99 adhesin, effect of plant extracts on erythrocytes receptors was evaluated (Barreto et al., 1993b), finding activity in all plant species. Results of antiadhesin effect and Gal-Gal receptors are summarized in Table 1.

Plant	Extracts	Effect on fimbriae	Effect on receptors
A. aspera	ethanol 90%	-	-
	ethanol 20%	-	-
	decoction	-	+
L. virginicum	ethanol 90%	+	+
	ethanol 20%	-	-
	decoction	-	-
A. conyzoides	ethanol 90%	-	-
	ethanol 20%	-	-
	decoction	-	-
Z. officinale	ethanol 90%	-	-
	ethanol 20%	-	+
	decoction	-	-
C. longa	ethanol 90%	+	+
	ethanol 20%	+	+
	decoction	+	-
C. speciosus	ethanol 90%	+	+
	ethanol 20%	-	+
	decoction	+	-

Table 1. Effect of plant extracts on fimbrial expression and fimbrial receptors, from Barreto et al., (2001). (+ = positive adhesion - unaltered fimbriae or receptors; - = no adhesion -no expression of fimbriae or altered receptors).

Source	Microorganism	Effects on Virulence Factor	Reference
Vaccinium macrocarpon (Ericaceae)	See epigraph below		
Berberis aristata (Berberidaceae) berberine sulfate	UPEC	inhibit adhesion	Sun et al., 1988a
B. aristata berberine sulfate	*Streptococcus pyogenes*	inhibit adhesion to epithelial cells, fibronectin, and hexadecane	Sun et al., 1988b
Arctostophylos uva-ursi (Ericaceae) Vaccinium vitis-idaea	*E. coli*	enhance aggregation	Türi et al., 1999
Matricaria recutita (Asteraceae) M. matricarioides		block aggregation	
Psidium guajava (Myrtaceae) galactose-specific lectin	*E. coli* 0157:H7	inhibit adhesion to red cells	Coutiño et al., 2001
Azadirachta indica (Meliaceae)	*Streptococcus sanguis*	inhibit adhesion	Ofek et al., 2003
Camelia sinensis (Theacae) (green tea) (-) epicatechin gallate, (-) gallocatechin gallate	*P. gingivalis*		
(oolong tea) polyphenol	*S. mutans, S. sobranus*		
Galanthus nivalis (Amaryllidaceae) mannose-sensitive lectin	*E. coli*		
Gloipeltis furcata and *Gigartina teldi* (seaweeds) sulfated polysaccharides	*S. sobrinus*		
Humulus lupulus (Urticaceae) bract polyphenols	*S. mutans*		
Melaphis chinensis gallotannin	*S. sanguis*		
Persea americana (Lauraceae) tannins	*S. mutans*		
Andrographis paniculata (Acanthaceae)	*S. mutans*	inhibit adhesion	Limsong et al., 2004
Senna alata (Cassia alata) (Caesalpinaeae)			
C. sinensis			
Harrisonia perforata (Simaroubaceae)			
Punica granatum (Punicaceae)	*Staphylococcus aureus*	Staphylococcal enterotoxin A	Braga et al., 2005
Streblus asper (Moraceae) leaf	*Candida albicans*	inhibit adhesion to denture acrylic	Taweechaisupapong et al., 2006
Resveratrol (found in grapes seeds-*Vitis vinifera) (Vitaceae)*	*Proteus mirabilis*	Swarming, flagella, haemolysin and urease	Wang et al. 2006
Conocarpus erectus (Combretaceae)	*Chromobacterium violaceum* and *Agrobacterium tumefaciens*	quorum sensing-disrupting (QS-D)	Adonizio et al., 2006
Chamaecyce hypericifolia (Euphorbiaceae)			
Callistemon viminalis (Myrtaceae)			
Bucida burceras (Combretaceae),			
Tetrazygia bicolor (Melastomataceae)			
Quercus virginiana (Fagaceae).			
V. macrocarpon	*C. violaceum*	QS-D	Vattem et al., 2007
V. angustifolium			

Rubus idaeus (*Ericaceae*)			
R. eubatus			
Fragaria sp. (*Rosaceae*)			
Vitis sp.			
Origanum vulgare (*Lamiaceae*)			
Rosemarinus officinalis (*Lamiaceae*)			
Ocimum basilicum (*Lamiaceae*)			
Thymus sp. (*Lamiaceae*)			
Brassica oleracea (*Brassicaceae*)			
Curcuma longa (*Zingiberaceae*)			
Zingiber officinale (*Zingiberaceae*)			
Galla chinensis	*E. coli* (ETEC)	heat-labile enterotoxin	Chen et al., 2006
Z. officinale	*E. coli* (ETEC)	heat-labile enterotoxin	Chen et al., 2007a
Chaenomeles speciosa fruit (*Rosaceae*)	*E. coli* (ETEC)	heat-labile enterotoxin	Chen et al., 2007b
Pelargonium sidoides (*Geraniaceae*)	*Helicobacter pylori*	inhibit adhesion to intact human stomach tissue	Wittschier et al., 2007
P. sidoides (*Geraniaceae*)	*Streptococcus pyogenes*	HEp-2 cells and buccal epithelial cells	Conrad et al., 2007
V. angustifolium or *V. corymbosum* *V. myrtillus* *V. ovalifolium, V. ovatum, V. parvifolium*	*H. pylori* and *Streptococcus* spp.	adhesion	Yarnell & Abascal, 2008
C. sinensis	*S. mutans*		
Galla chinensis[1] methyl gallate (MG) and gallic acid (GA)	*S. mutans*	antibiofilm	Kang et al., 2008
Holarrhena antidysenterica (*Apocynaceae*)	EPEC	inhibit adhesion to enteric epithelial cells	Kavitha & Niranjali 2009
Glycyrrhiza glabra (*Fabaceae*)	*Porphyromonas gingivalis*	adhesion	Wittschier et al., 2009
G. glabra glycyrrhizin	*E. coli* (ETEC)	Heat-labile enterotoxin	Chen et al., 2009
Ibicella lutea (*Martyniaceae*) aereal part	*Proteus mirabilis*	swarming differentiation, hemagglutination and biofilm formation	Sosa, & Zunino et al., 2009
Dodonaea viscosa var. angustifolia (*Sapindaceae*)	*C. albicans*	adherence to oral epithelial cells	Patel et al., 2009
Aegle marmelos (*Rutaceae*) unripe fruit decoction	*E. coli* (EPEC), *E. coli* (EIEC) and *Shigella flexneri*	Adhesion to HEp-2 cell line, decrease production of heat labile toxin and its binding to ganglioside monosialic acid	Brijesh et al., 2009
P. guajava decoction	*E. coli* (EPEC), *E. coli* (EIEC) and *S. flexneri*	idem.	Birdi et al., 2010
P. sidoides root extract specific proanthocyanidins	*S. pyogenes*	anti-adhesion	Janecki et al., 2011

[1] Gall caused by aphids on *Rhus* spp. (*Anacardiaceae*)

Piper bredemeyeri (Piperacae) P. brachypodom P. bogotence	C. violaceum	QS-D	Olivero et al., 2011
Terminalia catappa (Combretaceae) Tannin-rich fraction	C. violaceum and Pseudomonas aeruginosa	QS-D antibiofilm and LasA staphylolytic activity	Taganna et al., 2011
Delisea pulchra (red marine alga) Halogenated furanones	bacteria	QS-D	Defoirdt et al., 2011
Halobacillus salinus isolated from sea grass, phenetylamide metabolites	bacteria including Vibryo harveyi		
Compounds bacteria isolated from a marine alga Colpomenia sinuosa	bacteria		
Chamaecrista desvauxii (Fabaceae) Fruits	Staphylococcus epidermidis	antibiofilm	Trentin et al., 2011
Commiphora leptophloeos (Burseraceae) Stem bark			
Dioclea grandiflora (Fabaceae) Fruits			
Eugenia brejoensis (Myrtaceae) Leaves			
Libidibia ferrea var ferrea (Caesalpinaeae) Fruits			
Melocactus zehntneri (Cactaceae) Roots, Cephalium			
Myracrodruoun urundeuva (Anacardiaceae) Leaves, Branches, Stem bark			
Myroxylon peruiferum (Fabaceae) Leaves			
Parkinsonia aculeata (Caesalpinaeae) Leaves			
Piptadenia viridiflora (Mimosoideae) Branches, Fruits			
Pityrocarpa moniliformis (Mimosoideae) Leaves			
Polygala boliviensis (Polygalaceae) Leaves, Branches			
P. violacea Leaves, Roots			
Senna macranthera (Caesalpinaeae) Fruits			
S. splendida Branches			
Sida galheirensis (Caesalpinaeae) Leaves, Branches			
Euphorbia trigona (Euphorbiaceae) latex extracts	P. mirabilis and P.aeruginosa	swarming, antibiofilm rhamnolipid production inhibition of urease	Nashikkar et al., 2011
Lactuca indica (Asteraceae)	E. coli	inhibit effect on focus adhesin kinasa phosphorylation	Lüthjea et al., 2011

Table 2. Effect of natural products on microorganism virulence factor.

There is an increasing evidence that plant metabolites can inhibit different VFs expressions allowing host defense to overcome an infection; for instance, fimbrial adhesin interference in UTI, that is fundamental to avoid bacterial colonization, invasion, and then disease first symptoms. Results show this is a plausible mechanism by which maybe underestimated non-bacteriostatic/bactericides medicinal plants, traditionally used in treating "urinary complaints" are worthy.

Some studies of medicinal plants, food plants and seaweeds against different VFs on several Gram positive bacteria, Gram negative bacteria, and against *Candida albicans* are compiled in Table 2. Referring more than 60 plant species from diverse families, but there really are few species considering the potential of the world flora. Of particular interest is the evidence of activity of edible plants or seasoning plants like: *Camellia sinensis* (*Theacae*), *Psidium guajava* (*Myrtaceae*), *Vitas vinifera* (*Vitaceae*) and *Zingiber officinale* (*Zingiberaceae*), since daily ingestion as food of such plants could prevent infections. Ginger and *Curcuma* with antifimbrial UPEC activity (Table 1) are reported too as anti quorum sensing-disrupting. Most of summarized plants have traditional renown in microbial gastrointestinal disorders or urinary complaints treatment (Roig, 1974).

E. coli references are related to antiadhesion activity, or inhibition of toxins of enteric pathotypes; and in an early reference of Sun et al. (1988a), it is described the antiadhesive effects of berberine alkaloids inhibiting the expression of fimbrial subunits on UPEC. There are also studies on antiadhesion properties of certain plant extracts against oral and dental plaque forming bacteria.

In some studies, modern technology search for non-conventional antimicrobials is based on folk medicine (Birdi et al., 2010; Brijesh et al., 2009; Chen et al., 2007a, 2007b, 2009; Coutiño et al., 2001; Kavitha & Niranjali 2009;). In recent years, the increase in number of articles including new trends in VFs research, like biofilm inhibition or quorum sensing-disrupting is noticeable. Screening is reported for quorum sensing-disrupting in dietary plant (food or seasoning plant) (Vattem et al., 2007), in which all species were active. Taking into account ethnobotanic criteria, a quorum sensing-disrupting and antibiofilm effects of plants from Florida, USA, and Caatinga plants from Brazil, respectively, were screened (Adonizio et al., 2006; Trentin et al., 2011).

Several VFs can be neutralized by plant compounds. A broad field of research on this subject is ahead; science advances in phytochemistry, molecular microbiology, *in silico* designs, and "omics" providing new features that will end in VFs based new therapy strategies. Another point is that, like in other biological activities, ethnomedical knowledge-based criteria can afford success in the search for antivirulence factor novel drugs or herbal medicine (Abreu & Cuéllar, 2008).

4.1 Cranberry (*Vaccinium macrocarpon*) antiadhesive therapy leader

Cranberry is a fruit currently use widely as food and as medicine mainly for women in prophylaxis of ITU because of its antibacterial properties. Herein are present a bulk of information that allows stating that cranberry can be consider as a leader in the bacterial antiadhesive therapy.

4.2 Botany

Taxonomy: *Ericaceae* family, *Vaccinioideae* Subfamily, *Vaccinieae* Tribe; the genus comprises 450 species (Berazaín, 1992). Among the most common species used as medicine and food are *V. mirtillus* (blueberry), and *V. corymbosum* (highbush), *V. ashei* (rabbiteye) and *V. angustifolium* (lowbush). Description: *V. macrocarpon* is an evergreen trailing shrub, rhizomatous habits when young; pink, simple, axilar flowers. Ovary has four locules. Wind or insects are needed for pollination. Fruit is a shining red epigynous berry, ripening occurs 60-120 days after pollination. Distribution: east bogs in North America, from Newfoundland to Manitoba, south of Virginia, Ohio and north of Illinois.

4.3 Traditional use

Native people from North America cranberry use fruit as food in meat dishes and as medicine for erysipelas, tonsilitis, scarlatina sore throat, ulcers, pleuresy (leaves) (Moerman (2004); cancer and scurvy (Duke, 2007), and to treat cystitis and prevent UTI (Farnsworth, 2003).

4.4 Phytochemistry

V. macrocarpon is among the most phytochemically studied *Vaccinium* species (Abreu et al., 2008). Cranberry fruit mainly contains organic acids such as: citric, chlorogenic, malic, quinic and shiquimic acids (Duke, 1992; Jensen 2002); and polyphenols like flavonoids, and anthocyanic pigment glycosides of cyanidin and paeonidin (Abreu et al., 2008; Duke 1992). Polyphenolic compounds have been the most researched in *Vaccinium* spp. because of its antioxidant and anti-UTI activity, mainly in *V. macrocarpon* and *V. mirtillus* fruits.

Trimeric type A proanthocyanidines characterized in cranberry by Foo et al. (2000a), is of particular interest, since authors demonstrated it is the active compound in UPEC P fimbriae interference.

4.5 *In vitro* and *in vivo* antimicrobial activity

Almost all biological effects of cranberry fruit so far evaluated are antimicrobial activity. There are references of antivirus activity (Konowalchuk & Speirs, 1978), antifungal activity (Cipollini & Stiles, 1992; Marwan & Nagel, 1986) and antibacterial activity (Lee et al., 2000; Leitão et al. 2005; Marwan & Nagel, 1986). The last author reports no activity of cranberry juice (pH- 3, 5 and 6, 9) and cranberry proanthocyanidin-rich fractions against *E. coli* and other bacteria. Thus, cranberry use in UTI prevention or treatment is not due to bacteriostatic/bactericide activity; however, there is a great number of *in* vitro and *in vivo* research related to the antiadhesive effect of cranberry on UPEC P+. Besides, there are reports of cranberry as a fimbrial antiadhesive in other bacteria (Moerman et al., 2003).

At the beginning of 20th century, antimicrobial cranberry studies were based on the possibility of acidification of urine or by excretion of hypoxic acid, a potent bacteriostatic associated to the fruit ingestion (Blatherwick, 1923; Moen, 1962); but other results questioned this mechanism (Fellers, 1933; Nickey, 1975). It is in the 1980' that research on bacterial adhesion began to be considered as a mechanism of action of cranberry in UTI (Schmidt & Sabot, 1989; Sabot, 1984; Safire et al., 1989); since then, dozen of articles have been reporting *in vitro*, *ex vivo*, and *in vivo* experiences of its antiadhesion activity. Among models used were HARM and HASR in guinea pigs and human erythrocytes; uroepithelial cells, bladder cultured cell lines and laboratory animal models (Nowak & Schmitt, 2008). Using micro plate technology and turbidity assessment for testing the adherence of *Escherichia coli* P+ to human uroepithelial cell line T24, Turner et al. (2005), developed a high-throughput assay to study *V. macrocarpon* extracts. A bioassay like this could also be use in the screening of extracts of plants used traditionally in urinary tract system diseases.

Certainty on cranberry antifimbrial effect was achieved by Ahuja et al. (1998) by means of electronic microscopy, no fimbrial expression or loose of them, and change in *E. coli* morphology were clear. More recently, isolated cranberry proanthocyanidins (PACs) at 60 μm/ml were tested on UPEC P+ resulting in a potent antiadhesive activity (Foo et al., 2000a, 2000b, Howel et al., 2005).

Ex vivo studies on exposed UPEC strains in urine from healthy volunteers under different cranberry administration schedules, and several researches on humans have validated cranberry for UTI prevention. Prospective clinical trial in young women with recurrent UTI has demonstrated a protective effect. In a metaanalysis of human clinical trials, Jepson & Craig (2008) conclude that:

"There is some evidence that cranberry juice may decrease the number of symptomatic UTIs over a 12 month period, particularly for women with recurrent UTIs. Its effectiveness for other groups is less certain. (...) The evidence is inconclusive as to whether it is effective in older people (both men and women), and current evidence suggest that it is not effective in people with a neuropathic bladder. (...) Further properly designed studies with relevant outcomes are needed."

4.6 Proanthocyanidins

Proanthocyanidins (condensed tannins) are oligomeric and polymeric end products of the flavonoid biosynthetic pathway. They are present in the fruits, bark, leaves and seeds of many plants, where they provide protection against predation. They are charactehrized by their flavor and astringency in beverages like wine, tea, and fruit juices; and they have been used as leather tanning agents for a long time. An important property of this kind of tannins is their ability to bind proteins; hence they can inhibit enzymes and reduce protein availability in animal nutrition (Dixon et al., 2005; Miranda & Cuéllar, 2001). Like other plant polyphenol compounds, in recent years PACs have been biologically studied, mainly for their antioxidand activity (King et al., 2007). In general, their bioavailability is poor, since PACs high molecular weight difficult absorption, but this could be beneficial for gut health due to their effects on lipid oxidation, inflammation, immunity, and pathogenic bacterial adhesion (Reed & Howell, 2008).

Unusual A-type proanthocyanidins (B-type linkage is more common in plant kingdom), consisting primarily of epicatechin tetramers and pentamers (Fig. 1), with at least one A-type linkage has been elucidated in UPEC antiadhesive active fractions of cranberry. It is structurally characterized by a linkage between C2 of the upper unit (C ring), and the oxygen at C7 of the starter unit (A-ring), in addition to the linkage between C4 of the upper unit and positions 6 or 8 of the lower unit (Dixon et al., 2005; Foo et al., 2000b;. Howell et al., 2005). A-type linkage is a structural prerequisite for antiadhesion effects, since Howell et al., (2008) compared cranberry PACs with other B-type proanthocyanidins from commercial foods and not found *in vitro* or *ex vivo* activity.

Cranberry PACs decreases bacterial adhesion forces in UPEC (Pinzón-Arango et al, 2009) and influences *Streptococcus mutans* biofilms on saliva-coated apatitic surface and on dental caries development *in vivo* (Koo et al, 2010). Besides, cranberry PACs perform a cytotoxic activity in different cell lines (Singh et al., 2009).

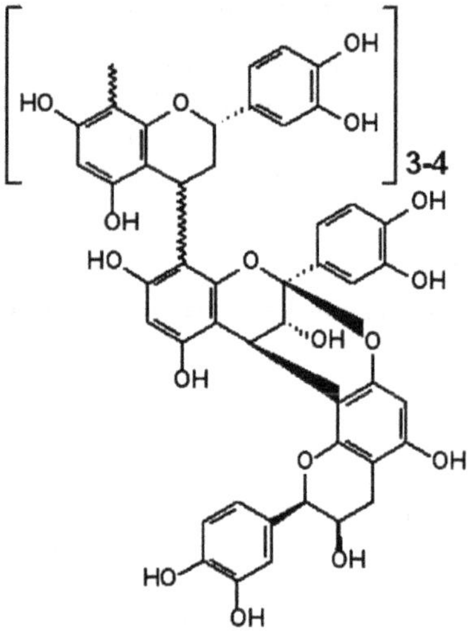

Fig. 1. Cranberry A-type proanthocyanidin.

5. Possible mechanism of plant antiadhesion effects

Chemical signal interactions between host and pathological microorganisms, or innocuous microorganisms have been recently understood, and seem to be very common in nature; in such magnitude, that plant origin product by host consumed could compete with microbes for specific receptors. These interactions are mediate by a complex dynamics of physico-chemical and biological parameters, in which time can also be a prominent variable. Quorum sensing coordinated the infection steps recognizing each critical moment of the process by biofilm bacterial density.

Mechanism of fimbrial adhesin inhibition can be related to different effects of plant metabolites such as: delection of genes encoding fimbrial subunits, enzymes or proteins associated to its transportation and allocation at the cell surface and cell receptor analogues that binds to adhesin subunits or nearby, impeding their interaction with receptors.

Antifimbrial activity at genetic level is similar to some antibiotics mechanism proposed at sublethal concentrations (Barreto et al., 1994; Padilla et al., 1991); besides *V. macrocarpon*, this mechanism had been proposed for berberine alkaloid (Sum et al., 1988).

Results on plant extracts blockade of adhesin-receptor interaction in RBC, suggest it can be mediated by glycoprotein (like lectins) with pectidic sequences similar to Pap G or Pap G-Pap F, or by compounds that subvert spatial configuration of Gal-Gal receptors. In both cases, structural analogues of adhesin-receptor interaction could also be interfered due to esteric constraints.

Thermodynamic approach of fimbriae interaction is another point of view, in which Liu et al. (2008), calculate the Gibbs free energy of adhesion changes by interfacial tensions on human kidney uroepithelial cells and fimbriated or not fimbriated *E. coli* strains treated three hours with cranberry juice extracts.

Interference of plant compounds in adhesin-receptor interaction should not promote microorganism antibioresistance, since at sublethal concentrations selection pressure is not established. Therefore, as effect is only exerted over pathogen VFs, it is not expected deleterious side effects on comensal microbiota as in chemotherapy usually occurs (candidiasis, colon disbacteriosis).

Synergy it is known among plant metabolites, in this case for instance, some plant species reported in table 1 and table 2, besides antiadhesion effects, have activity on further VFs, thus, the sum of those effects help to avoid or suppress infection. In UPEC, is traditionally reported diuretic effect in those plants (Roig, 1974), this activity can synergized too as anti-infective in UTI, increasing bacterial clearance.

6. Approach from nature in antibacterial research

Science development has explained several host-bacteria interactions and ways to rationally manage them. However, there is too much knowledge to acquire in this sense, but certainly these natural signalling mechanisms among microbes and their environment, including hosts, is rendering new clinical strategies and drug candidates. It is noteworthy how this kind of interaction is present in newborn mammals and during their span life. Food is something more than a mere matrix containing nutrients; starting from microbiota, human feeding has also coevolved with diverse biological niches.

Antiadhesive properties of human milk oligosaccharides in relation to pathogenic bacteria are remarkable. They show to be effective inhibitors of adhesion of gastric and uroepithelial bacterial pathogens *in vitro* and *in vivo*, and prevent diarrhoea in infants (Bavington & Page, 2005; Mårild et al., 2004; Ofek et al., 2003).

Carbohydrate compounds are usual in food stuff, but they are not only important to supply energy; recently, it is known that in several ways they are involved in a microorganism molecular mechanism of adhesion, invasion, and infection. Glycoproteins (lectins) and a broad range of non-nutrient components of food plants (phytochemicals) can also be active in this way.

Before vertebrates appeared, microorganisms and plants were part of the whole system of Nature. Plant phytochemicals are part of the pool of signals in food plant that deal with the microbe world. Plants that act against pathogens by a non-cidal mechanism are selected by Nature; but also culturally, humans have selected them as safe food plants, medicinal plants, or both at once. In the last decades, borders between food and medicine are disappearing, i.e. functional food. It is not surprising that most of them were always there, but now they are new products. Gastrointestinal tract and genito-urinary system are plenty of microorganism receptors and plant origin compounds receptors, thus dietary patterns or herbal products can probably promote a first barrier defence avoiding pathogen virulence factors like QS, fimbriae, or toxins.

Ethnobotany of antimicrobial food or medicinal plants can be corroborated by new antivirulence factor target techniques and other modern bioassays. Novel antimicrobial activities like antiadhesion effect could provide tools to eliminate or decrease virulence of infections that, in spite of quemotherapy advances, seem to become more inflexible microorganisms.

7. Acknowledgment

To Professor Marisel Boleiro for manuscript language revision.

8. References

Abraham, S.N., Jonssontt, A-B. & Normarkts, S. (1998). Fimbriae-mediated host-pathogen cross-talk. *Current Opinion in Microbiology*, 1:75-81.

Abreu, O.A. & Cuéllar, A. (2008). Criterios de selección de plantas medicinales para ser investigadas. *Revista Cubana de Plantas Medicinales,*13(3).

Abreu, O.A., Cuéllar, A. & Prieto, S. (2008). Fitoquímica del género *Vaccinium* (*Ericaceae*). *Revista Cubana de Plantas Medicinales*, 13(3).

Adonizio, A.L., Downum, K., Bennett, B.C. & Mathee, K. (2006). Anti-quorum sensing activity of medicinal plants in southern Florida. *Journal of Ethnopharmacology,*105(3): 427-435.

Ahmed, N., Dobrindt, U., Hacker, J. & Hasnain, S.E. (2008). Genomic fluidity and pathogenic bacteria: applications in diagnostics, epidemiology and intervention. *Nature reviews microbiology*, 6,387- 394.

Ahuja, S., Kaack, B. & Roberts, A. (1998). Loss of fimbrial adhesion with the addition of *Vaccinum macrocarpon* to the growth medium of P-fimbriated *Escherichia coli. J. Urol.*, 159 (2): 559-62.

Barreto, G., Ramos, O., Lezcano, Y., Velásquez, B., Moreno, M. & Pardo G. (1993a). Efecto bactericida o bacteriostático de un medicamento a base de eucalipto (Eucabev). *Rev. Prod. Anim.*, 7 (1 y 2): 69-71.

Barreto, G., Lezcano, Y., Ramos, O., Velásquez, B., Moreno, M. & Pardo, G. (1993b). Efecto de un medicamento a base de eucalipto (EUCABEV) sobre la producción de los factores de colonización F4 y F5 de *E. coli* enterotoxigénica (ETEC). *Rev. Prod. Anim.*, 7(1 y 2):73-76.

Barreto, G., Velásquez, B., Moreno, M., Ramos, O., Lezcano, Y. & Rodríguez, H. (1993c). Efecto de un medicamento a base de eucalipto (Eucabev) sobre los receptores para F5 de *E. coli* enterotoxigénica (ETEC). *Rev. Prod. Animal*, 7(3): 135-136.

Barreto, G., Martín, M., Pardo, G. & Pazos, M. (1994). Efecto de concentraciones subletales de antibióticos en la expresión del factor de colonización F4. *Rev. Prod. Anim.*, 8 (1): 61-3.

Barreto, G., Pazos, M., Pardo, G., Martín, M., Díaz, S. & Velásquez, B. (1995a). Acción de extractos de *E. saligna* y *E. citriodora* sobre el factor de colonización F4. *Rev. Prod. Anim.*, 9 (1): 71-74.

Barreto, G., Jiménez, O., Prieto, M., Guerra, A. & Guevara, G. (1995b). Expresión fimbrial (F4 y P) de *E. coli* en medios convencionales. *Rev. Prod. Anim.*, 9: 83-87.

Barreto, G., Sedrés, M., Ortíz, A. & Ricardo M. (1999). Esquema para el diagnóstico de *E. coli* enterohemorrágico y otras categorías enteropatógenas a partir de alimentos. *Rev. Prod. Anim.*, 11 (annuary): 39-43.

Barreto, G., Campal, A.C., Abreu, O. & Velásquez, B. (2001a). El bloqueo de la adhesión fimbrial como opción terapéutica. *Rev. Prod. Anim.*, 13 (1): 71-82.

Barreto, G., Hernández, R.I., Ortíz, A. & Santiago Y. (2001b). Presencia de *E. coli* enteropatógenas en pacientes con diarrea aguda. *Archivo Médico de Camagüey*, 5(2).

Barreto, G. & Campal, A. (2001). Efecto de extractos de *Eucalyptus saligna* y *Eucalyptus citriodora* sobre la viabilidad y expresión fimbrial (K88y CFA/I) de *E coli* enterotoxigénica. *Rev. Prod. Anim.*, 13,(2): 67-75.

Barreto, G., Reynoso, A. & Campal, A. (2002). Elementos para el tamizaje aplantas que evalúe su acción sobre la adhesividad fimbrial bacteriana. *Rev. Prod. Anim.*, 14 (2): 47-51.

Barreto, G. (2007). *Escherichia coli*, últimos 122 años. *Rev. Prod. Anim.* (special issue): 55-67.

Barreto, G. & Rodríguez, H. (2009). La cápsula, algo más que una estructura no esencial (Revisión). *Rev. Prod. Anim.*, 20 (1): 69-80.

Barreto, G. & Rodríguez, H. (2010). Biofilms bacterianos versus antimicrobianos; nutracéuticos, una opción promisoria. *Rev. Prod. Anim.*, 22 (2).

Bavington, C. & Page, C. (2005). Stopping bacterial adhesion: A novel approach to treating infections. *Respiration*, 72 (4) 335-344.

Baum von, H. & Marre, R. (2005). Antimicrobial resistance of *Escherichia coli* and therapeutic implications. *International Journal of Medical Microbiology*, 295 503-511.

Beachey, E.H. (1981). Bacterial adherence: adhesi-receptor interacytion mediating the attachment of bacteria to mucosal surface. *Journal of Infectious Disease*. 143. 325-345.

Beauregard-Racine, J., Bicep, C., Schliep, K., Lopez, P., Lapointe, F-J. & Bapteste, E. (2011). Of Woods and Webs: Possible alternatives to the tree of life for studying genomic fluidity in *E. coli*. *Biology Direct*, 6:39.

Berazaín, R. (1992). *Ericaceae*. Flora de la República de Cuba. *Fontqueria*, 35:21-77.

Bergsten, G., Wullt, B. & Svanborg, C. (2005). *Escherichia coli*, fimbriae, bacterial persistence and host response induction in the human urinary tract. *International Journal of Medical Microbiology*, 295, 487-502.

Birdi, T., Daswani, P., Brijesh, S., Tetali, P., Natu, A. & Antia, N. (2010). Newer insights into the mechanism of action of *Psidium guajava* L. leaves in infectious diarrhoea. *BMC Complementary and Alternative Medicine*, Vol 10.

Blanco, J. & Blanco, M. (1993). ETEC, NCEC y VTEC de origen humano y bovino. Patogénesis, epidemiología y diagnóstico microbiológico. Servicio de Publicaciones Diputación Provincial San marcos. p. 35-48, 71-77, 104-107, 115-120, 173-176, 207-209, 235-239, 306-308, 310-316. Galicia.

Blatherwick ND Long ML. (1923). Studies of urinary acidity - The increased acidity by eating prunes and cranberries. *Journal of Biological Chemistry*; 57: 815-818.

Braga, L.C., Shupp, J.W., Cummings, C., NET, M., Takahashi, J.A., Carmo, L.S, Chartone-Souza, E. & Nascimento, A.M.A. (2005). Pomegranate extract inhibits *Staphylococcus aureus* growth and subsequent enterotoxin production. *Journal of Ethnopharmacology*, 96(1-2): 335-339.

Brijesh, S., Daswani, P., Tetali, P., Antia, N. & Birdi, T. (2009). Studies on the antidiarrhoeal activity of Aegle marmelos unripe fruit: Validating its traditional usage. *BMC Complementary and Alternative Medicine*, 9:47.

Bouguénec Le, Ch. (2005). Adhesins and invasins of pathogenic *Escherichia coli*. *International Journal of Medical Microbiology*, 295 471-478.

Campal, A., Junco, J., Casas, S., Arteaga, N., Castro, M., Fuentes, F., León, L., Barreto, G., Pardo, G. (2007). Anticuerpos monoclonales que reconocen epítopes conformacionales de la fimbria F41 de la *E. coli* enterotoxigénicas *REDVET*, 8(8).

Campal, A., Junco, J.A., Arteaga, N.O., Castro, MD., Casas, S., León, L., Barreto, G., Pardo, G. (2008). Procedimiento general para purificar a pequeña escala las fimbrias expresadas por cepas porcinas de *Escherichia coli* enterotoxigénicas. *Rev. Colomb. Biotecnol*, 10(1): 119-128.

Chen, J-C., Hob, T-Y., Chan, Y-S., Wu, S-L. & Hsian, C-Y. (2006). Anti-diarrheal effect of *Galla chinensis* on the *Escherichia coli* heat-labile enterotoxin and ganglioside interaction. *Journal of Ethnopharmacology*, 103 (3): 385-391.

Chen, J.C., Huang, L.J., Wu, S.L., Kuo, S.C., Ho, T.Y., Hsiang, C.Y., 2007b. Ginger and its bioactive component inhibit enterotoxigenic *Escherichia coli* heat-labileenterotoxin-induced diarrhea in mice. *Journal of Agricultural and Food Chemistry*, 55, 8390-8397.

Chen, J-C., Chan, Y-S., Wu, S-L., Chao, D-C., Chan C-S., Li, C-C., Ho, T-Y., & Hsian, C-Y. (2007a). Inhibition of *Escherichia coli* heat-labile enterotoxin-induced diarrhea by *Chaenomeles speciosa*. *Journal of Ethnopharmacology*, 113 (2): 233-239.

Chen, J-C., Ho, T-Y., Chan, Y-S., Wu, S-L., Li, C-C., & Hsian, C-Y. (2009). Identification of *Escherichia coli* enterotoxin inhibitors from traditional medicinal herbs by *in silico, in vitro*, and *in vivo* analyses. *Journal of Ethnopharmacology*, 121 (3): 372-378.

Cipollini, M.L. & Stiles, E.W. (1992). Antifungal activity of ripe ericaceous fruits: phenolic-acid interactions and palatability for dispersers. *Biochem Syst Ecol*, 20 6: 501-514.

Conrad, A., Jung I., Tioua G., Lallemand C., Carrapatoso F., Engels I., Daschner, F.D. & Frank U. (2007). Extract of *Pelargonium sidoides* (EPs® 7630) inhibits the interactions of group A-streptococci and host epithelia *in vitro*. *Phytomedicine*, 14, Supplement 1, 52-59.

Coutiño, R.R., Hernández, C.P. & Giles, R.H. (2001). Lectins in fruits having gastrointestinal activity: their participation in the hemagglutinating property of *Escherichia coli* O157:H7. *Archives of Medical Research*, 32, 251-257.

Cowan, M.M. (1999). Plant Products as Antimicrobial Agents. *Clinical Microbiology Reviews*, 12(4): 564-582.

Croxen, M.A. & Finlay, B.B. (2010) Molecular mechanisms of *Escherichia coli* pathogenicity. *Nature Reviews Microbiology* 8, 26-38.

Defoirdt, T., Sorgeloos, P. & Bossier, P. (2011). Alternatives to antibiotics for the control of bacterial disease in aquaculture. *Current Opinion in Microbiology*, 14:251-258.

Dixon, R.A., Xie, D-Y. & Sharma, S.B. (2005). Proanthocyanidins – a final frontier in flavonoid research? *New Phytologist*,165 : 9-28.

Dobrindt, U. & Hacker, J. (2008). Targeting virulence traits: potential strategies to combat extraintestinal pathogenic *E. coli* infections. *Current Opinion in Microbiology*, 11:409-413.

Dobrindt, U. (2005). (Patho-)Genomics of *Escherichia coli*. *International Journal of Medical Microbiology*, 295 357-371.

Dodson, KW, Pinkner, J.S., Rose, T., Magnusson, G., Hultgren, S.J. & Waksman, G. (2001). Structural Basis of the Interaction of the Pyelonephritic *E. coli* Adhesin to Its Human Kidney Receptor. *Cell*, 105, 733-743.

Drekonja, D.M. & Johnson, J.R. (2008). Urinary tract infections. *Prim Care*, 35(2):345-67.

Duke, J. (2007). *Vaccinium*. In: *Phytochemical & Ethnobotanical Database*, 2007, Available from: http://www.ars-grin.gov/duke/

Farnsworth, N.R. (2003). *Vaccinium*. In: *The NAPRALERT Database*, 2003), Available from: http://pcog8.pmmp.uic.edu/mcp/MCP.html

Fellers CR, Redmon BC, Parrott EM. Effects of cranberries on urinary acidity and blood alkali reserve. J. Nutr. 1933; 6:455-463.

Foo, L.Y., Lu, Y., Howell, A.B. & Vorsa, N. (2000a). A-type proanthocyanidin trimers from cranberry that inhibit adherence of uropathogenic P-fimbriated *Escherichia coli*. *J. Nat. Prod.*, 63, 1225–1228.

Foo, L.Y., Lu, Y., Howell, A.B. & Vorsa, N. (2000b). The structure of cranberry proanthocyanidins which inhibit adherence of uropathogenic P-fimbriated *Escherichia coli* in vitro. *Phytochemistry*, 54, 173–181.

Foxman, B., Barlow, R., D'Arcy, H, Gillespie, B & Sobel, JD. (2000). Urinary tract infection: estimated incidence adn associated cost. *J. Clin Epidem.* 10, 509-515.

Gal-Mor, O. & Finlay, B.B. (2006). Pathogenicity islands: a molecular toolbox for bacterial virulence. *Cellular Microbiology*,8(11), 1707–1719.

Guerra, A., Pérez, S., Barreto, G., Pardo, G. & González, G. Caracterización de cepas uropatógenas y entéricas: acción de extractos de *Achyranthes aspera*. *Trabajo de Diploma*. Facultad Química-Farmacia. Universidad de Camagüey, 1995.

Gupta, G., Hootom, T., Wobbe, C.L. & Stamm, W.E. (1999). The prevalence of antimicrobial resistance among uropathogens causing acute uncomplicated cystitis in young women. *International Journal of Antimicrobial Agents*; 11 305-308.

Hales, BA. & Amyes, SGB. (1985). The effect of a range of antimicrobial drugs on the haemagglutination of two clinical isolates from urinary tract infection. *J. Antimicrob. Chemother.*,16: 671-674.

Henderson, J.P., Crowley, J.R., Pinkner, J.S., Walker, J.N., Tsukayama, P., et al. (2009). Quantitative Metabolomics Reveals an Epigenetic Blueprint for Iron Acquisition in Uropathogenic *Escherichia coli*. *PLoS Pathog*, 5(2).

Hooton, T.M. (2003). The current management strategies for community-acquired urinary tract infection. *Infect Dis Clin North* Am, 17: 303-32.

Howell, A.B., Reed, J D., Krueger, C.G., Winterbottom, R., Cunningham, D.G., & Leahy M. (2005). A-type cranberry proanthocyanidins and uropathogenic bacterial anti-adhesion activity. *Phytochemistry*, 66 2281–2291.

Jain, R., Kosta, S. & Tiwari, A. (2010). Bacterial virulence traits: A potential area of study for drug development. *J Pharm Bioall Sci*,2:376.

Jadhav, S. Hussain, A., Devi, S., Kumar A., Parveen S., Gandham N., Wieler, L.H., Ewers C. & Ahmed, N. (2011). Virulence Characteristics and Genetic Affinities of Multiple Drug Resistant Uropathogenic *Escherichia coli* from a Semi Urban Locality in India. *PLoS One.*,; 6(3);

Janecki, A., Conrad, A., Engels, I., Frank, U. & Kolodziej, H. (2011). Evaluation of an aqueous-ethanolic extract from *Pelargonium sidoides* (EPs® 7630) for its activity against group A-streptococci adhesion to human HEp-2 epithelial cells. *Journal of Ethnopharmacology*, 133(1): 147-152.

Jepson, R.G. & Craig, J.C. (2008). Cranberries for preventing urinary tract infections. Cochrane Database of Systematic Reviews. In: *The Cochrane Library*, Issue 04, Art. No. CD001321.

Jepson, R.G., Mihaljevic, L. & Craig, J.C. (2008). Cranberries for treating urinary tract infections. Cochrane Database of Systematic Reviews. In: *The Cochrane Library*, Issue 04, Art. No. CD001322.

Johnson, JR. (1991). Virulence factors in *Escherichia coli* urinary tract infection. *Clinical Microbiology Reviews*, 4: 80-128.

Johnson, JR. & T. Berggren. (1994). Pigeon and dove eggwhite protect mice against renal enfections due to P fimbriated *E. coli*. *Am. J. Med.Sci.s*, 307: 335-339.

Johnson, J.R. (1997). Urinary Tract Infection. En: *Escherichia coli: Mechanism of Virulence*. Max Sussman Ed., Cambridge University Press. 495-549.

Johnson, J.R. (2003). Microbial virulence determinants and the pathogenesis of urinary tract infection. *Infect Dis Clin North Am*, 17: 261-78.

Johnson, J.R. & Russo T.A. (2005). Molecular epidemiology of extraintestinal pathogenic (uropathogenic) *Escherichia coli*. *Int. J. Med. Microb.*, 295 383–404.

Kaack, M.B., Svenson, L., Baskin, S., Steele, G. & Roberts J. (1993). Protective anti-idiotype antibodies in the primate model of pyelonephritis. *Infect. Immun.*, 61: 2289-2295.

Kang, M-S., Oh, J-S., Kang, I-C., Hong. S.J. & Choi C-H. (2008). Inhibitory effect of methyl gallate and gallic acid on oral bacteria. *The Journal of Microbiology*, 46 (6):744-750.

Kaper J.B. & Levine M. (1988). Progress toward a vaccine against ECET. *Vaccine* 6: 197-199.

Kaper, J.B., Nataro, J.P. & Mobley, H.L.T. (2004). Pathogenic *Escherichia coli*. *Nature Reviews Microbiology*, 2: 123-140.

Kavitha, D. & Niranjali, S. (2009). Inhibition of Enteropathogenic *Escherichia coli* Adhesion on Host Epithelial Cells by *Holarrhena antidysenterica* (L.) WALL. *Phytother. Res.*, 23, 1229–1236.

King, M., Chatelain K., Farris D., Jensen D., Pickup, J., Swapp, A., O'Malley, S. & Kingsley, K. (2007). Oral squamous cell carcinoma proliferative phenotype is modulated by proanthocyanidins: a potential prevention and treatment alternative for oral cancer. *BMC Complementary and Alternative Medicine*, 7:22.

Konowalchuk, J. & Speirs, J.I. (1978). Antiviral effect of commercial juices and beverages. *Appl Environ Microbiol*, 35 : 1219.

Koo, H., Duarte, S., Murata, R.M., Scott-Anne, K., Gregoire, S., Watson, G.E., Singh, A.P., Vorsa, N. (2010). Influence of cranberry proanthocyanidins on formation of biofilms by *Streptococcus mutans* on saliva-coated apatitic surface and on dental caries development in vivo. *Caries Research*, 44(2): 116-126.

Lane, M.C., Mobley, H.L., 2007. Role of P-fimbrial-mediated adherence in pyelonephritis and persistence of uropathogenic *Escherichia coli* (UPEC) in the mammalian kidney. *Kidney Int,*. 72, 19–25.

Langermann, S., Palaszynski, S., Barnhart, M., Auguste, G., Pinkner, J.S., Burlein, J., Barren, P., Koenig, S., Leath, S., Jones, C.H. & Hultgren, S.J. (1997). Prevention of mucosal *Escherichia coli* infection by FimHadhesin-based systemic vaccination. *Science*, 276:607-611.

Langermann, S. & Ballou, W.R., (2003). Development of a recombinant FimCH vaccine for urinary tract infections. *Adv. Exp. Med. Biol.*, 539, 635–648.

Lee, Y.L., Owens, J., Thrupp, I. & Cesario, T,C. (2000). Does cranberry juice have antibacterial activity? *J Amer Med Ass*, 28 (13): 1691.

Leitão, D.P.S., Polizello, A.C.M., Ito, I.Y. & Spadaro, A.C.C. (2005). Antibacterial Screening of Anthocyanic and Proanthocyanic Fractions from Cranberry Juice. *J Med Food*, 8 (1), 36–40.

Levine, M., Kaper, J., Black, R. & Clemments M. (1993). New knowledge of pathognesis of bacterial enteric infection as applied to vaccine development. *Microbiol. Rev.*, 47 510-520.

Limsong, J., Benjavongkulchai, E. & Kuvatanasuchati, J. (2004). Inhibitory effect of some herbal extracts on adherence of *Streptococcus mutans*. *Journal of Ethnopharmacology*, 92(2-3): 281-289.

Liu Y., Gallardo-Moreno A.M., Pinzon-Arango P.A., Reynolds Y., Rodriguez G., Camesano, T.A. (2008). Cranberry changes the physicochemical surface properties of E. coli and adhesion with uroepithelial cells. *Colloids and Surfaces B: Biointerfaces*,65 35-42

Lüthjea, P., Dzunga, D. & Brauner A. (2011). *Lactuca indica* extract interferes with uroepithelial infection by *E. coli*. *Journal of Ethnopharmacology*, 135 (3):672-677.

Mahady, G.B. (2005). Medicinal Plants for the Prevention and Treatment of Bacterial Infections. *Current Pharmaceutical Design*, 11, 2405-2427.

Marcusson, L.L., Frimodt-Møller, N., Hughes D. (2009). Interplay in the Selection of Fluoroquinolone Resistance and Bacterial Fitness. *PLoS Pathog*, 5(8).

Mårild, S., Hanson, S., Jodal, U., Odén, A. & Svedverg K. (2004). Protective effect of breastfeeding against urinary tract infection. *Acta Paediatr.*, 93, 164-168.

Marwan, A. & Nagel, C.M. (1986). Microbial inhibitors of cranberries. *J Food Sci* 51 4: 1009-1013.

Miranda, M. & Cuellar, A. (2001). Farmacognosia y Química de los Productos Naturales. Ed. Félix Varela, 354-356 La Habana.

Mediavilla, A., Florez, J. & Gacía_Lobo, J.M. (2005). Farmacología de las enfermedades infecciosas: principios generales, selección y asociación de antibióticos. En: *Farmacología Humana*. J. Florez, J.A. Armijo & A. Mediavilla (Dir.) Ed. Masson S.A., Barcelona, 1084-1086.

Moerman, D. (2004). *Vaccinium*. In: *Native American Ethnobotany Database*, 2004, Available from: http://www.umic.edu

Moen DV. (1962). Observations on the effectiveness of cranberry juice in urinary infections. *Wisconsin Med. J.*, 61: 282-283.

Mulvey, M.A., Schilling, J.D. & Hultgren J.H. 2001. Establishment of a persistent *Escherichia coli* reservoir during the acute phase of a bladder infection. *Infect. Immun.*, 69, 4572-4579.

Mulvey, M.A. (2002). Adhesion and entry of uropathogenic *Escherichia coli*. *Cell Microb.*, 4(5):257-271.

Moingeon, P., Almond, J. & de Wilde, M. (2003). Therapeutic vaccines against infectious diseases. *Current Opinion in Microbiology*, 6:462-471.

Niemann H.H., Schubert W-D. & Heinz D.W. (2004). Adhesins and invasins of pathogenic bacteria: a structural view. *Microbes and Infection* 6 101-112.

Nickey KE. (1975). Urine pH: effect of prescribed regimen of cranberry juice and ascorbic acid. *Arch. Phys. Med. Rehab.*, 56: 556.

Nowack, R. & Schmitt, W. (2008). Cranberry juice for prophylaxis of urinary tract infections – Conclusions from clinical experience and research. *Phytomedicine*, 15, 653-667.

Ofek, I., Hasty, D.L. & Sharon, N. (2003). Anti-adhesion therapy of bacterial diseases: prospects and problems. *FEMS Immunology and Medical Microbiology*, 38, 181-191.

Olivero, J.T.V., Pájaro, N.P.C. & Stashenko, E. (2011). Actividad antiquórum sensing de aceites esenciales aislados de diferentes especies del género *Piper*. *Vitae*, 18, 1, 77-82.

Padilla, C., Vázquez, M. & Faundéz, O. (1991). Effects of minimun inhibitory concentrations of three antimicrobians on the growth cell and fimbriation of uropathogenic *E. coli*. *Rev. Lat-Amer. Microbiol.*, 33: 105-108.

Patel, M., Gulube, Z., & Dutton, M. (2009). The effect of *Dodonaea viscosa var. angustifolia* on *Candida albicans* proteinase and phospholipase production and adherence to oral epithelial cells. *Journal of Ethnopharmacology,* 124(3): 562-565.

Pinzón-Arango, P.A., Liu, Y. & Camesano, T.A. (2009). Role of Cranberry on Bacterial Adhesion Forces and Implications for *Escherichia coli*–Uroepithelial Cell Attachment. *J Med Food,* 12 (2), 259-270.

Prieto, M., Jiménez, O., Barreto, G., Pazos, M. & Pardo, G. (1995). Estudio de cepas uropatógenas: comportamiento fisiológico, efecto de extractos de *Lepidium virginicum* L. *Trabajo de Diploma.* Universidad de Camagüey.

Ratcliff, W.C. & Denison, R. (2011). Alternative Actions for Antibiotics. *Science,* 332, 547-548.

Reed, J.D. & Howell, A.B. (2008). Biological Activity of Cranberry Proanthocyanidins: Effects on Oxidation, Microbial Adhesion, Infl ammation, and Health. In: *Botanical Medicine: From Bench to Bedside.* Edited by R. Cooper & F. Kronenberg

Roig, J.T. (1974). Plantas medicinales, aromáticas o venenosas de Cuba. Editorial Ciencia y Técnica. p. 365-368. La Habana.

Sasakawa, C. & Hacker, J. (2006). Host-microbe interaction: bacteria Editorial Overview. *Current Opinion in Microbiology,* 9:1–4.

Sauer FG, Mulvey MA, Schilling JD, Martínez JJ and Hultgren SJ. (2000). Bacterial pili: molecular mechanisms of pathogenesis *Current Opinion in Microbiology,* 3:65–72.

Schmidt, D.R, Sobota, A.E. (1989). An examination of the anti-adherence activity of cranberry juice on urinary and non-urinary bacterial isolates. *Microbios;* 55, 173-81.

Scholes, D., Hootom, T., Roberts, P.L., Stapleton, A.E., Gupta, G. & Stamm, W.E. (2000). Risk factor for recurrent Urinary Tract Infection in young women. *The Journal Inf Dis,* 182, 1177-1182.

Schubert, S., Darlu, P., Clermont, O., Wieser, A. & Magistro, G.(2009) Role of Intraspecies Recombination in the Spread of Pathogenicity Islands within the *Escherichia coli* Species. *PLoS Pathog,* 5(1).

Singh, A.P., Singh, R.K., Kim, K.K., Satyan, K.S., Nussbaum, R., Torres, M., Brard, L. & Vorsa, N. (2009). Cranberry Proanthocyanidins are Cytotoxic to Human Cancer Cells and Sensitize Platinum- Resistant Ovarian Cancer Cells to Paraplatin *Phytother. Res,.* 23, 1066-1074.

Siciliano AA. Cranberry. The Journal of the American Botanical Council and the Herb Research Foundation 1998; 38.

Soderhall, M., Normark, S., lshikawa, K., Karlsson, K., Teneberg, S., Winberg, J. & Mollby, R. (1997) Induction of protective immunity after *Escherichis coli* ladder infection in primates. Dependence of the globoside-specific P-fimbrial tip adhesin and its cognate receptor *J Clin West,* 100:364-372.

Sosa, V. & Zunino, P. (2009). Effect of *Ibicella lutea* on uropathogenic *Proteus mirabilis* growth, virulence, and biofilm formation. *J Infect Dev Ctries,* 3(10):762-770.

Sobota, A. E. (1984). Inhibition of bacterial adherence by cranbrrry juice: potential use for the treatment of urinary tract infection. *J.Urol.,* 131: 1013-6.

Stenquist, K., Sandberg, T., Ahlstedt, S., Korhonen, T.K. & Svanborg Eden, C. (1987). Effects of subinhibitory concentrations of antibiotics and antibodies on the of *Escherichia coli* to human uroepithelial cells in vitro. *Scand. J. Infect. Dis.,* 33: 104-107.

Storby, K.A., Österlund, A. & Kahlmeter, G. (2004). Antimicrobial resistance in *Escherichia coli* in urine samples from children and adults: a 12 year analysis. *Acta Paediatr,* 93, 487-491.

Sun, D., Abraham, S.N. & Beachey, E.H. (1988a). Influence of berberine sulfate on synthesis and expression of Pap fimbrial adhesin in uropathogenic *Escherichia coli*. *Antimicrob. Agents Chemother.* 32 (8), 1274–1277.

Sun, D., Courtney, H.S. & Beachey, E.H. (1988b). Berberine sulfate blocks adherence of *Streptococcus pyogenes* to epithelial cells, fibronectin, and hexadecane. *Antimicrob Agents Chemother,* 32:1370-1374.

Svanborg Eden, C. & Godaly, G. (1997). Bacterial virulence in urinary tract infection. *Infect. Dis. Clin. N. Amer.,* 11, 513–525.

Taganna, J.C., Quanico, J.P., Perono, R.M.G., Amor, E.C. & Rivera, W.L. (2011). Tannin-rich fraction from *Terminalia catappa* inhibits quorum sensing (QS) in Chromobacterium violaceum and the QS-controlled biofilm maturation and LasA staphylolytic activity in *Pseudomonas aeruginosa. Journal of Ethnopharmacology,* 134 (3): 865-871.

Taweechaisupapong, S., Klanrit, P., Singhara, S., Pitiphat, W. & Wongkham, S. (2006). Inhibitory effect of *Streblus asper* leaf-extract on adhesion of *Candida albicans* to denture acrylic. *Journal of Ethnopharmacology,*106(3): 414-417.

Tettelin, H., Riley D., Cattut, C. & Medini D. (2008). Comparative genomics: the bacterial pan-genome. *Current Opinion in Microbiology,* 12:472–477.

Trentin, D.S., Giordani, R.B., Zimmer, K.R., da Silva, A.G., da Silva, M.V., Correia, M.T.S., Baumvol, I.J.R. & Macedo A.J. (2011). Potential of medicinal plants from the Brazilian semi-arid region (Caatinga) against *Staphylococcus epidermidis* planktonic and biofilm lifestyles. *Journal of Ethnopharmacology,* in Press,doi:10.1016/j.jep.2011.05.030

Türi, E., Türi, M., Annuk, H. & Arak, E. (1999). Action of aqueous extracts of bearberry and cowberry leaves and wild camomile and pineapple-weed flowers on *Escherichia coli* surface structures. *Pharmaceutical Biology,* 37 (2): 127–133.

Turner, A., Chen, S-N., Joike, M.K., Pendland, S.L., Pauli, G.F. & Farnsworth, N.R. (2005). Inhibition of Uropathogenic *Escherichia coli* by Cranberry Juice: A New Antiadherence Assay. *J. Agric. Food Chem.,* 53, 8940-8947.

Vattem, D.A., Mihalik, K., Crixell, S.H. & McLean, R.J.C. (2007). Dietary phytochemicals as quorum sensing inhibitors. *Fitoterapia* 78, 4, 302-310.

Velázquez, B., Barreto, G., Vidal, I. & N. Izquierdo (1991). Diagnóstico y tratamiento de la colibacilosis porcina. *Rev. Prod. Animal,* 6(2): 139-141.

Verger, D., Bullitt, E., Hultgren, S.J. & Waksman, G. (2007). Crystal Structure of the P Pilus Rod Subunit PapA. *PLoS Pathog,* 3(5).

Vosbeck, K., Mett, K., Huber, U., Bohn, J. & Petignat, M. (1982). Effects of low concentrations of antibiotics *Escherichia coli* adhesion. *Antimicrobial Agents and Chemotherapy,* 21: 864-869.

Waksman G. & Hultgren, S.J. (2009). Structural biology of the chaperone–usher pathway of pilus biogenesis. *Nature Reviews Microbiology,* 7, 765-774.

Wagenlehner, F.M.E. & Naber, K.G. (2004). Antibiotic treatment for urinary tract infections: pharmacokinetic/ pharmacodynamic principles. *Expert Rev. Anti Infect. Ther.,* 2(6).

Wang, W-B., Lai H-C., Hsueh, P-R., Chiou, R.Y-Y., Lin, S-B. & Liaw, S-J. (2006). Inhibition of swarming and virulence factor expression in *Proteus mirabilis* by resveratrol. *Journal of Medical Microbiology,* 55, 1313–1321.

Westerlund-Wikström, B. & Korhonen, T.K. (2005). Molecular structure of adhesin domains in *Escherichia coli* fimbriae. *International Journal of Medical Microbiology,* 295 479–486.

Wiles, T.J, Kulesus, R.R. & Mulvey ,M.A. (2008). Origins and virulence mechanisms of uropathogenic *Escherichia coli*. *Experimental and Molecular Pathology*, 85 11–19.

Winberg, J., Mollby, R., Bergstrom, J., Karlsson, K-A., Leonardsson, I., Milh, MA., Teneberg, S., Haslam D., Marklund, B-I. & Normark, S. (1995). The PapG-Adhesin at the tip of P-fimbriae provides *Escherichia coli* with a competitiveedge in experimental bladder infection in cynomolgus monkeys. *J. Exp. Med.*, 182, 1695-1702.

Wittschier, N., Faller, G. & Hensel, A. (2007). An extract of *Pelargonium sidoides* (EPs 7630) inhibits in situ adhesion of *Helicobacter pylori* to human stomach *Phytomedicine*, 14(4): 285-288.

Wittschier, N., Faller, G. & Hensel, A. (2009). Aqueous extracts and polysaccharides from Liquorice roots (*Glycyrrhiza glabra* L.) inhibit adhesion of *Helicobacter pylori* to human gastric mucosa. *Journal of Ethnopharmacology*, 125 (2): 218-223.

Wong, I., Moreno, M., Molino, M., Valderrama, J., Jogler, M., Horrach, M., Bover, E., Borroto, A., Basulto, R., Calzado, I., Hernández, R., Herrera, L., Silva, R., & de la Fuente J. (1995). Immunity and protection elicited by recombinant vaccine against ECET. *Biotecnología Aplicada*,12 (1): 9-15.

Wullt B. (2003). The role of P fimbriae for *Escherichia coli* establishment and mucosal inflammation in the human urinary tract. *Int J Antimicrob Agents.*, 21(6):605-21.

Yarnell, E. & Abascal, K. Antiadhesion Herbs. (2008). *Alternative and Complementary Therapies*, 14(3): 139-144.

Zafriri, D., Ofek, I., Adar, R., Pocino, M., Sharon, N. (1989). Inhibitory activity of cranberry juice on adherence of type 1 and type P fimbriated *Escherichia coli* to eucaryotic cells. *Antimicrob Agents Chemother*, 33: 92-98.

Zaneveld, J, Turnbaugh, P.J., Lozupone, C., Ley R.E., Hamady M., Gordon J.I & Knight R. (2008). Host-bacterial coevolution and the search for new drug targets. *Curr Opin Chem Biol*, 12, 1, 109-114.

Zhang, L. & Foxman, B. (2003). Molecular epidemiology of *Escherichia coli* mediated urinary tract. *Frontiers in Bioscience*, 8, 235-244.

3

Improved Fertility Potential and Antimicrobial Activities of Sesame Leaves Phytochemicals

Lukeman Adelaja Joseph Shittu[1,2] and Remilekun Keji Mary Shittu[2]
[1]*Department of Anatomy, Benue State University College of Medicine*
[2]*Medical Microbiology Unit, Jireh International Foundation Laboratories,*
Abuja, Gwagwalada,
Nigeria

1. Introduction

Broadly speaking, reproductive infertility is defined as the involuntary absence of conception in a couple after a general period of at least one year of regular unprotected sexual intercourse (Shittu et al., 2005; WHO, 1991).

The rapid advancement in the field of human reproductive biology (*in-vitro* fertilization-IVF etc) in this era has attracted a lot of interest amongst scientists such as andrologists, gynaecologists, biologists and epidemiologists worldwide (Schwartz, 1980; Shittu et al., 2005; Shittu et al., 2006a).

In view of the fact that any methodology that is empirical in infertility study ultimately determine the overall result quality with lots of consequence on the potential treatment options and other prevention programmes available (Thonneau & Spira, 1990), makes it necessary for clarification of some confusing terms often used in infertility studies amongst the readers. Such that a couple is said to be a fertile if they have conceived in the past and infertile if they have not conceived after at least one year of unprotected sexual intercourse as the case may be. While, a fecund couple is one who can conceive and an infecund couple is one that is impossible to conceive for whatever reason (Leridon, 1977; Thonneau & Spira, 1990).

In addition, primary infertility is defined as the absence of conception and secondary infertility is seen as the inability of obtaining any further (second or other) conception (WHO, 1991). While, the incidence of infertility also defined as the number of new infertile couples who started consulting within a given period of time (usually 1 year) and in a given place in proportion to the total number of non-infertile couples in the same place at the beginning of the same period of time.

Infertility is a medical condition considered to be a public health problem based on its global impact on the socio-economic status and the quality of health life of the society at large and with a prevalence of over 80 million couples affected worldwide (Shittu et al., 2005; Shittu et al., 2006a; WHO, 1991). Such that approximately 15% of couples suffered from infertility worldwide (Nishimune & Tanaka, 2006; Norris, 2001) as compared to about 8% and 8.5% of couples affected in the US (Leke et al., 1993) and Canada (Norris, 2001) respectively.

Worldwide, infertility is more prevalence in the women than men with a traceable male factor accounting for 40–50% of infertile couples (De Kretser & Baker, 1999; Shittu et al., 2005; Shittu et al., 2006a; Nishimune & Tanaka, 2006; WHO, 1987). However, in developing nations of the world like Africa for example, where there are more infertile cases with limited or no treatment options especially assisted reproductive technology available for the management of this medical condition (Shittu et al., 2005, Shittu et al., 2006a; WHO, 1987), there is a higher prevalence rate of about 30–40% (Leke et al., 1993; Shittu et al., 2005, Shittu et al., 2006a) with male factor accounting for 30% of cases seen (Leke et al., 1993). Other previous studies have also shown that the infertility risk for older women aged 35-44 years appeared to be twice as high as that of young woman of 30-34 years and that the infertility risk for a black woman is also 1.5-times higher than the whites (Thonneau & Spira, 1990).

Hence, male fertility and subfertility have also attracted a lot of considerable interest amongst basic medical scientists and clinicians alike over the past few years now (Skakkebaek, 2003; Shittu, 2006, 2010; Shittu et al., 2005, Shittu et al., 2006a).

In addition, there is a rising prevalence of male factor infertility worldwide, as a result of exposure to environmental toxicants/endocrine disruptors and the infiltration of biogenetically engineered western diets and lifestyles among other factors into the developing worlds especially (Izegbu et al., 2005; Shittu, 2006, 2010; Shittu et al., 2007a, Shittu et al., 2008a). Such that more alarming is the decreasing sperm quality of human and wildlife species due to environmental exposures to these endocrine disruptor pollutants and chemicals that are believed to cause gene mutations as expressed over the past few years now (Duty et al., 2003, Sharpe & Irvine, 2004; Sharpe & Shakkebeak, 1993; Shittu, 2006, 2010; Shittu et al., 2008a; Vos et al., 2000; Zuping et al., 2006).

The major risk factors responsible for the increase in prevalence of infertility in the 20-24 year age group of women include STDs (sexually transmitted diseases) and their tubal consequences (Mosher & Aral, 1985; WHO, 1991).

The fact that microbial infections/STD (such as gonorrhea, syphilis, Chlamydia, Candidiasis) is one of the leading causes of infertility in both male and females couples especially in this part of the world (WHO, 1987; WHO, 1991) and with the associated problems of numerous unwanted effects of the synthetic chemical/hormonal agents (antibiotics and steroids etc) available as treatment options have both raised cause for concern in recent times (Shittu, 2006, 2010; Shittu et al., 2009).

Incidentally, the last decade have witnessed increasing intensive study on isolates and other active phytochemicals been extracted from plant species used in folkloric medicine for over thousands of years now (Bankole et al., 2007; Hanilyn, 1998; Nascimento et al., 2000; Shittu, 2010; Shittu et al., 2006b; Shittu et al., 2007b). Moreover, these agents are equally recognized by the World Health organization to have proven potential of treating microbial infections, diabetes, cancers and infertility/ subfertility among other known chronic medical conditions (Bankole et al., 2007; Shittu, 2010; Shittu et al., 2006b; Shittu et al., 2007a; Shittu et al., 2008a; Shittu et al., 2009).

In addition, in this era of ours, natural resources have been used to produce various bioactive compounds such as alkaloids, ethanol, organic acids, immunomodulator, vitamins and polysaccharides etc that are of medicinal values in food, medical, chemical and biochemical industries (Hanilyn, 1998; Shittu, 2006, 2010).

Hence, expressed worldwide is the search for an ideal folkloric phyto-chemical medicinal agent with a broad spectrum and proven potential of treating infertility/ subfertility conditions including microbial infection among the other causes of infertility with minimal or no side effects as compared to their synthetic counterparts (Bankole et al, 2007; Shittu, 2006, 2010; Shittu et al, 2006b; Shittu et al, 2007, 2007b, 2007c; Shittu et al, 2008a, Shittu et al, 2009; Shittu et al, 2010).

The phytoestrogens appeared to be one of such natural estrogenic agents that have attracted so much attention in the last decade in view of their reported health benefits and they include four broad classes of phytochemicals namely the lignans (sesame seed and flaxseed), isoflavonoids (soybeans), stillbenes and coumestrol (Adlercreutz et al., 1986; Murkies, 1998; Shittu, 2006, 2010). These agents mimic endogenous estrogens and depending on their concentrations, they either act agonistically or antagonistically by displaying the endogenous estrogens from the binding sites on the estrogens receptors (α and β) among its other mechanisms of actions (Kuiper et al, 1997; Shittu, 2006, 2010).

Based on the fact that they are consumed in large amounts in the diet, the metabolic effects noticed are usually that of antiestrogenic, thus, compete with the much more potent endogenous estradiol for the estrogens receptor (ER1 & ER2) binding sites and ultimately blocked their estrogenic activity (Martin et al., 1978; Whitten & Naftolin, 1991).

In addition, sesame plant is one of the richest food sources of phytoestrogenic lignans, a valuable phytochemical known to man since the dawn of civilization (Thompson et al, 1991) and is now increasingly being incorporated into human diet worldwide because of their reported health benefits (Shittu, 2006, 2010).

The plant is rich in trce elements/minerals such as calcium, iron, magnesium, zinc, copper and phosphorus (Obiajunwa et al, 2005; Shittu, 2006, 2010; Shittu et al., 2006b, Shittu et al, 2009).

All parts of the sesame plant such as the seed, oil and leaves are also useful and are locally consumed as a staple food by subsistence farmers in the Northern, South-west and Middle - belt regions of Nigeria and celebrated also in folkloric medicine in Asia and Africa (Akpan – Iwo et al, 2006; Shittu et al, 2006b; Shittu, 2010). Thus, this may account for the high fecundity among the adult male population in these particular areas (Shittu, 2006; Shittu, 2010). The local names of the plants depend on the source areas of cultivations in the world, such as ekuku–gogoro (Yoruba- Sesamum radiatum), yanmoti (Yoruba-S. indicum), ridi (Hausa) and beni (Tiv/Idoma and English) or gingelly (English) (Gill, 1992; Shittu, 2006, 2010; Shittu et al, 2009).

Recent study on bioavailability of sesame plants consumption in humans have shown that the lignans usually undergo extensive metabolism in the intestine depending on the characteristics of the individual intestinal microflora to produce mammalian lignans-enterolactone especially (Penalvo et al., 2005; Shittu et al, 2009). Moreover, plasma lignans concentrations showed a linear correlation with urinary excretion of lignans (Penalvo et al., 2005; Shittu et al, 2009).

Once, spermatozoa are released from the testis, they enter into the epididymis, which is a steroid-dependent organ for storage and then undergo another physiological maturation (capacitation) process involving other various morphological and biochemical changes with the resultant initiation of progressive motility and acquisition of fertilizing ability by the matured epididymal spermatozoa (Shittu, 2006, 2010; Shittu et al, 2007a).

The epididymal sperm cells are also susceptible to oxidative damage from reactive oxygen species due to their lack of proper cytoplasm and fragile membrane nature (Aitken & Fisher,1994; Shittu, 2006, 2010; Shittu et al, 2006a; Shittu et al, 2007a). No doubt, the acquisition of sperm motility is seen as an integral part of the whole epididymal sperm maturation process (Orgebin-Crist, 1967), which occurs in the micro-environment provided by the epididymal secretory products and its antioxidant enzymes such as sialic acid, acetyl carnitine, glyceryl-phosphoryl choline (GPC) among others. These epididymal secretions helped to maintain the basic osmolarity of the epididymal luminal fluid (Wales et al,, 1966), which is steroid regulated (Schwaab et al, 1998) and assist in stability of the spermatozoal membranes (Scott et al, 1963; Zini & Schlegel 1997; Shittu, 2006, 2010). All these activities are important in the metabolism of spermatozoa after capacitation (Mitra & Chowdhury, 1994; Shittu, 2006, 2010).

In addition, most of the testicular fluid (about 96%) is reabsorbed by the non-ciliated cells in the efferent ductules (Clulow et al., 1998) and without this fluid re-absorption, the sperm will remain over diluted and incapable of maturation within the epididymis and as such, any blockage or interference in normal functioning of the estrogen receptors or estrogens may result in infertility (Oliveira et al, 2000; Shittu, 2006, 2010)..

1.1 Aims and objective

As a result of paucity of knowledge and folkloric claim on the *Sesamum radiatum* leaves effectiveness in treating infertility and infections, our aims and objectives are to determine the following:

i.   The antimicrobial activity of the aqueous crude extract of *Sesamum radiatum* leaves phytochemicals (essential oils and phytoestrogenic lignans) on some selected microorganisms

ii.   The histomorphometric and stereological evidence of fertility potential of sesame leaves phytochemicals on adult male Sprague Dawley (SD) ratss` epididymal tubules.

2. Material and methods

2.1 Collection of plant materials

Sesame radiatum plants (Schum and Thonn - Pedaliacaea family) were purchased from a vendor in Agege market, Lagos after being identified by Dr. Shittu in May 2011. However, the plant was initially authenticated by the herbarium section of Forestry Institute of Research (FRIN) with FHI # 107513 on the 5th of August, 2005 (Shittu, 2006; Shittu *et al.*, 2006). In addition, voucher specimens were deposited in Botany Departments of University of Ibadan and Lagos State University, respectively.

2.2 Preparation of aqueous crude extracts

The leaves having been separated from the rest of the plants were air dried for 2 weeks and later grounded into a powdery form using a grinder. 100g of the powdered leaves were added to 1.0 litre of distilled water at a ratio of 1:10 in a clean dried beaker and allowed to boil to boiling temperature after intermittent stirring on a hotplate for one hour. The decoction was filtered into another clean beaker using a white sieve clothing material and the filtrate evaporated at 50 °C to dryness in a desiccator to produce a black shinning crystal residue form with a yield of 83% w/w of the extract. The crude extract was kept in the refrigerator (4°C) before being reconstituted and later used for the in-vivo study.

2.2.1 Preparation of aqueous, ethanolic and methanolic extraction of sesame leaves

Aqueous, ethanolic and methanolic extraction of Sesame leaves using modified Okogun, (2000) method of extraction was adopted in the process (Shittu et al, 2007c) for the present antimicrobial studies. Such that the diluents used were absolute methanol, ethanol and sterile distilled water respectively. 1g of the raw air-dried and grinded Sesame leaves was added to 10ml of each diluent in a 20ml screw cap bottle. The modification was in the extraction time, which was for 5 days (120 hours) and the storage of the solution took place in the refrigerator at 4oC. The extracts obtained were regarded as the full concentration. Methanolic, ethanolic and aqueous extracts of *Sesamum radiatum* leaves were studied for their *in-vitro* antimicrobial activity against both gram positive and gram negative micro-organisms and yeast using Agar diffusion method.

2.3 Phytochemical screening using gas chromatography-mass spectral

Crude methanolic extracts of Sesame leaves were analyzed by GC/MS. GC analyses were performed using a Hewlett Packard gas chromatograph (model 6890) equipped with a flame ionization detector and injector MS transfer line temperature of 230°C respectively. A fused silica capillary column HP-InnoWax (30 in x 0.25 mm, film thickness 0.25 (mu)m) was used. The oven temperature was held at 50 °C for 5 min holding time and the temperature was raised, from 50-230°C at a rate of 2 °C /min. Helium was the carrier gas at a flow rate of 22cm/sec. One millilitre of extract mixed with methanol (80%), at a split ratio of 1:30 was injected (Shittu et al, 2006b; Shittu et al, 2007b).

GC/MS analyses were carried out on a Agilent Technologies Network mass spectrometer (model 5973) coupled to H.P. gas chromatograph (model 6890) equipped with NBS 75K Library Software data. The capillary column and GC conditions were as described above. Helium was the carrier gas, with a flow rate of 22cm/s. Mass spectra were recorded at 70 eV/200°C. The scanning rate of 1scan/sec and the run time was 90 minutes as described in our previous study (Shittu et al., 2007b).

Compound identification was accomplished by comparing the GC relative retention times and mass spectra to those of authentic substances analyzed under the same conditions, by their retention indices (RI) and by comparison to reference compound (Shittu et al., 2007b).

2.4 Selection of micro-organisms

Staphylococcus aureus (clinical), *Streptococcus pneumonia* (clinical) and *Candida albicans* (clinical) were the microorganisms used for this study and they were obtained from the Microbiology Laboratory of the Lagos State University Teaching Hospital (LASUTH). These microorganisms were identified and confirmed at the Microbiology department of the Drug

Quality Control Laboratory, LASUTH, Ikeja, Lagos. In addition, standard strain of *Staphylococcus aureus* (ATCC 29213) of oxoid Culti-loop (Oxoid Ltd., Hampshire, England) was also used. The choice for the selection of these organisms was based on their high resistance to common available antibiotics and their implication in pelvic inflammatory disease, one of the leading causes of infertility.

2.4.1 Preparation of 24 hours pure culture

A loop full of each of the selected *microorganisms* was suspended in about 10ml of physiological saline in a Roux bottle. Each of these was streaked on to the appropriate culture slants and was incubated at 37°C for 24 hours except for *Candida albicans* that was incubated at 25°C for 24-48 hours.

2.4.2 Standardization of micro-organisms

Each of the 24 hour old pure cultures was suspended in a Roux bottle containing 5ml of physiological saline. Each suspension of *microorganisms* was standardized to 25% transmittance at 560nm using an Ultraviolet (UV) -visible spectrophotometer.

2.5 Standard antibiotics used for study comparison

The primary standard of Cloxacillin obtained from Sigma-Aldrich (St Louis, MO, USA) was used for this study. However, the secondary standards with antibacterial and antifungal activity used for comparison with the various crude extract of sesame were obtained from local manufacturers in the Nigeria.

2.5.1 Antimicrobial screening

The modified Collin et al (1995) agar-well diffusion method was employed to determine the antimicrobial activities for the various crude extracts. Various concentrations of each of the aqueous, ethanolic and methanolic extracts respectively was made by diluting 1ml of each reconstituted extract in 2ml, 4ml, 6ml and 8ml of sterile distilled water respectively.

2.5.2 The Mean Inhibitory Concentration (MIC)

The MIC of the various crude extracts of sesame leaves against the tested *micro-organisms* was obtained. Agar-well diffusion method using Modified Collins et al (1995) was employed; approximately 10ml of sterile Muller-Hinton Agar (MHA) was poured into sterile culture plates and allowed to set. About 10ml of the antibiotic medium No 2 seeded with 0.5ml of 24 hours old culture of bacteria isolates was layered onto the MHA and allowed to set. The seed medium was then allowed to dry at room temperature for about 30 minutes. In the case of *Candida albicans*, Sabouraud Dextrose Agar (SDA) seeded with a 24 hours old *Candida albicans* was layered on the MHA. With the aid of a sterile cork borer, wells of about 8mm in diameter were punched on the plates. About 0.5ml of each dilution of the extracts was dispensed into the wells and the plates were incubated at 37°C for 24 hours except for the plates seeded with *Candida albicans*, which were already incubated at 25°C for 24-48 hours. At the end of the period, inhibition zones formed on the medium were evaluated in mm.

2.5.3 Measurement of Zone of Inhibition (ZI)

The zones of inhibition of the tested *microorganisms* by the various crude sesame extracts were measured using a Fisher-Lilly antibiotic zone reader model 290 (USA). The diameter sizes in mm of the zone of inhibition are shown in the respective tables below.

2.5.4 Minimum Inhibitory Concentration (MIC) of each extract

The MIC for each selected *microorganism* used was determined using microdilution method previously described (Bankole et al, 2007; Eloff ,1998; Shittu et al, 2006b;Shittu et al, 2007b)) as the last dilution of the extract that inhibited the growth of the tested pathogenic *microorganisms*. The various MIC are shown in the respective tables below.

2.6 Animal

Thirty matured and healthy adult male Sprague Dawley rats weighing 120 to 216g were procured from Ladoke Akintola University, College of Medicine, Ogbomosho and housed in a well ventilated wire-wooden cages in the departmental animal house. They were maintained under controlled light schedule (12 hours Light: 12 hours Dark) at room temperature (28°C) and with constant humidity (40-50%). The animals were allowed to acclimatize for a period of 7 days before treatment during the experiments. During this period they were fed with standard rat chows/pellets supplied by Pfizer Nigeria Ltd and water *ad-libitum*. Individual identification of the animal was made by ear tags (Shittu et al, 2007a, Shittu et al, 2008, Shittu, 2010).

2.6.1 Experimental procedure

The rats were randomly divided into three groups (A to C) comprising of ten rats each. The group A served as the control while B and C constituted the treated groups.

The animals in group A received equal volume of 0.9% (w/v) normal saline daily while group B received aqueous extract of sesame leaves at 14.0mg/kg body weight /day.

The animals in group C were given aqueous extract of sesame at 28.0mg/kg body weight /day (twice the group B dose). All the doses were given via gastric gavage (oro-gastric intubation) daily for a period of 6 weeks. All procedures involving animals in this study conformed to the guiding principles for research involving animals as recommended by the Declaration of Helsinki and the Guiding Principles in the Care and Use of Animals (American Physiological Society, 2002) and were approved by the Departmental Committee on the Use and Care of Animals.

All animals were observed for clinical signs of drug toxicity (such as tremors, weakness, lethargy, refusal of feeds, weight loss, hair-loss, coma and death) throughout the duration of the experiment.

2.6.2 Animal sacrifice

The rats were anaesthetized at the time of sacrifice by being placed in a sealed cotton wool soaked chloroform inhalation jar between 0900 and 1100 hours done the following day after the termination of the experiment after post over night fasting of the animals. The weights of the animals were taken weekly and before the sacrifice (Shittu et al, 2007a, Shittu et al, 2008, Shittu, 2010).

2.7 Organ harvest and tissue processing for light microscopy

The Epididymes were carefully dissected out, trimmed of all fat and blotted dry to remove any blood. Their weights were noted and volume measured by water displacement with the aid of a 10ml measuring cylinder. Later, the sizes (length and width) were recorded by use of a sliding gauge (d= 0.1) before being fixed in freshly prepared 10% formol saline solution. The fixed tissues were transferred into graded alcohol and then processed for 17.5 hours in an automated Shandon processor after which were passed through a mixture of equal concentration of xylene. Following clearance in xylene the sections were then infiltrated and embedded in molten paraffin wax. Prior to embedding, it was ensured that the mounted sections to be cut by the rotary microtone were orientated perpendicular to the long axes of the epididymes. These sections were designated "vertical sections". Serial sections of 5µm thickness were cut , floated onto clean slides coated with Mayer's egg albumin for proper cementing of the sections to the slides and were then stained with Haematoxylin and eosin stains. (Adelman and Cahill, 1989; Shittu, 2006, 2010; Shittu et al, 2007a).

2.8 Determination of morphometric parameters

Epididymal volume and weight estimations were done as stated above. Parameters of the two epididymes from each rat were measured and the average value obtained was regarded as one observation. However, for each epididymis, seven vertical sections from the polar and the equatorial regions were taken by systematic random sample method to ensure fair distribution between the polar and equatorial regions of each epididymis (Shittu, 2006, 2010).

The following morphometric parameters namely the volume and weight; diameter and cross-sectional area of the epididymal tubules were determined.

The diameter (D) of epididymal tubules with profiles that were round or nearly round for each animal was estimated. A mean diameter "D", was taken as the average of two diameters, D1 and D2 (where D1 is the short axis while D2 is the long axis; both D1 and D2 are perpendicular to each other). D1 and D2 were considered only when the ratio of D1:D2 or D1/D2 > 0.85 (Form factor) (Shittu, 2006, 2010; Shittu et al., 2006b; Shittu et al, 2009).

The cross-sectional areas (AC) of the epididymal tubules were determined from the formula $AC = \Pi D2/4$, (where Π is equivalent to 3.142 and D = the mean diameter of the epididymal tubules (Shittu, 2006, 2010; Shittu et al., 2006b; Shittu et al, 2009).

2.8.1 Determination of stereological parameters

Serial transverse sections of 5 µm of the H and E-stained specimens prepared were subjected to un-biased stereological techniques modified from previous report (Mouton, 2002; Shittu et al., 2006, 2010; Shittu et al, 2006c). Each image of the epididymal tubules at a magnification of 400 X was projected and drawn on a 16-point grid, completely counted in six different fields to make a total of 96 point-test grid for each of the systemic randomly selected section such that 5 sections/rat were taken from each group. Manual point intercept counting methods consist of a counting grid made up of a series of crosses in a regular and uniform square array. The density of crosses was such that one cross represented an area of 4 cm2 on the counting grid. The total number of crosses (circled or otherwise) falling on each structure per each section of specimen was counted and then added-up to get the final estimated result. Using this procedure, the volume density of the stroma, epithelia lining and tubular lumen of epididymal tubules were estimated as previously described (Weibel & Gomez, 1962; Shittu, 2006, 2010; Shittu et al, 2008b; 2009). The percentage volume density was determined by multiplying the volume density by 100.

2.9 Statistical analysis

The weight data were expressed in Mean $\pm$ S.D (Standard deviation) while other data were expressed as Mean $\pm$ S.E.M (standard error of mean). Comparisons between groups were done using the student's t-test, ANOVA and non-parametric Mann-Whitney U test with input into SPSS 12 software Microsoft computer (SPSS, Chicago, Illinois). Statistical significance was considered at P≤0.05 as used in previous studies (Shittu, 2006, 2010; Shittu et al, 2007a; Shittu et al, 2008).

3. Result

No obvious signs of toxicity such as weakness, lethargy, tremors, refusal of feeds, weight loss, hair-loss, coma and death were seen in any of the animals. Moreover, most of the animals exhibited calmness; improve appetite for food and water and general sense of well-being, all through the duration of the study as reflected in the increase in their body weight through the study duration.

The GC-MS showed that the methanolic extract of *sesamum radiatum* leaves contained mainly essential oils such as aromatic phenolic compounds- sesamol, sesaminol, sesamin, phosphorus, calcium, vitamin C, carboxylic acids and other classes of compounds including fatty acids like palmitic acids, arachidonic/arachidic acid, stearic acid, myristic acid, oleic acid, linoleic acids, thiazole, pyrroles, disulphide and aldehyde. In addition, it confirmed the presence of trace minerals, vitamins and steroids such as adrostenedione among others in the leaves of *sesamum radiatum* plant.

Combination of both methanolic and ethanolic extracts of sesamum radiatum leaves would have a broad spectrum antimicrobial effect against all the tested clinical micro-*organisms* except for the aqueous extract that has mild inhibitory activities on *Candida albican* only as shown in table 1.

The results obtained in table 1 showed that the methanolic extract demonstrated a mild antimicrobial activity against S*taphylococcus aureus* at both the full concentration and 1:2 dilution of the extract without any inhibitory effect on either the tested S*treptococcus pneumoniae* or *Candida albicans*. While, the ethanolic extract had a very strong antimicrobial effect against S*treptococcus pneumoniae* at full concentration including a strong and mild antimicrobial effect on *Candida albicans* at both full and 1:2 dilution of the extracts respectively. However, ethanolic extract has no inhibitory effects on tested S*taphylococcus aureus*. *Candida albicans growth on the culture plates* was also mildly inhibited by the aqueous extract at full concentration, 1:2; 1:4 and 1:6 dilutions of the extracts and with no other antimicrobial effects observed against the tested S*treptococcus pneumoniae and Staphylococcus aureus*.

Microorganisms	Crude Extract	Sensitivity				
		Full	1:2	1:4	1:6	1:8
S. aureus	Methanolic	+	+	-	-	-
	Ethanolic	-	-	-	-	-
	Aqueous	-	-	-	-	-
S.pneumoniae	Methanolic	-	-	-	-	-
	Ethanolic	+++	-	-	-	-
	Aqueous	-	-	-	-	-
C. albicans	Methanolic	-	-	-	-	-
	Ethanolic	++	+			
	Aqueous	+	+	+	+	-

(+) susceptibility (inhibition zone ≥ 10 mm)
(-) absence of susceptibility

Table 1. Showed the sensitivity of 3 tested micro-organisms to the different crude extracts of Sesamum radiatum leaves

Microorganisms	Crude Extract	Full	1:2	1.4	1:6	1: 8
	Methanolic		39.3			
	Ethanolic					
S. aureus	Aqueous					
	Methanolic					
	Ethanolic	76.2				
S.pneumoniae	Aqueous					
	Methanolic					
	Ethanolic		28.2			
C. albicans	Aqueous					31.0

The MICs is measured in μg/ml of the crude extracts on tested microorganisms

Table 2. Showed the minimum inhibitory concentrations (MICs) of different crude extracts of Sesamum radiatum leaves against the tested microorganisms.

Name of antibiotic/ antifungal	Zone diameter of tested Microorganisms			Concentration Used (μg/ml)
	Staph. aureus	Strept pneumoniae	Candida albicans	
Fluconazole tablet 500mg (2o standard)	-	-	40mm	100
Clotrimazole Vaginal tablet (2o standard)	-	-	35.5mm	100
Ampiclox tablet 500mg (2o standard)	30.5mm	-	-	100
Amoxycillin (2o standard)	15.5mm	11.5mm	-	100
Cloxacillin tablet(1o standard)	30 mm	-	-	100

Table 3. Antimicrobial effect of primary (1o) standard(Cloxacillin) and secondary (2o) standard antibiotics (Amoxycillin tablet, Ampiclox tablet, 500mg) and antifungal (Clotrimazole vaginal tablet 200mg and Fluconazole tablet, 500mg) on tested pathogenic microrganisms.

We observed a significant (P< 0.05) body weight gain using one-way ANOVA in all the treated animals. There was significant weight gain in both raw weight and relative weight of the epididymis per 100g body weight in a dose dependent manner as seen in Table 6.

Weight	A(Control)	B (High dose)	C (Low dose)
Initial (pre-experiment) (g)	127.3 ± 5.55	206.2 ± 6.45	186.3 ± 1.99
Final (post- experiment) (g)	185.2 ± 11.05*	248.2 ± 14.40*	219.8± 4.47*
weight gain (g)	58.5 ± 5.50*	42.0 ± 7.95*	33.4± 2. 48*

Values are mean ± S.D. *P < 0.05 was considered significant.

Table 4.a) Average weekly body weight of animal.

Group	Raw weight (g)	Epididymo-somatic weight (wt/100 g bwt)
Group A (control)	0.55 ± 0.03	–
Group B (high dose)	0.75 ± 0.01*	0.30 ± 0.00*
Group C (low dose)	0.57 ± 0.01*	0.26 ± 0.01*

Values are mean ± S.D.
*P < 0.05 was considered significant.

Table 4.b) Summary of weight (g) of epididymis.

The mean epididymal diameter and volume density of the tubular lumen significantly (P< 0.05) increased by 65% and 71% respectively in low dose sesame as compared to the control group. Similar findings in high dose sesame were also observed.

Group	N	Mean ± S.E.M
A(control)	10	3.4 ± 0.4
B (high dose)	10	1.6 ± 0.26*
C (low dose)	10	0.8 ± 02 *

The epididymal tubular profile of group C is the lowest of all the groups. Group B is 2.0 times higher than group C. This also correspond to the epididymal weight per 100g body weight of the animals
Values are mean ± S.E.M.
*P < 0.05 was considered significant.

Table 5.a) Summary of epididymal tubular profile

Group	N	Mean ± S.E.M
A	18	217.8 ± 8.9
B	9	242.6 ± 32.4*
C	4	358.4 ± 21.0 *

Group C has the largest tubular diameter of all the groups.
Values are mean ± S.E.M.
*P < 0.05 was considered significant.

Table 5.b) Summary of epididymal tubular diameter

Group	N	interstitium	surface epithelia	tubular lumen
A	10	4.6 + 0.4*	7.0 + 0.6*	.3.8 + 0.7*
B	10	4.0 + 0.5*	3.2 + 0.9*	8.0 + 0.7*
C	10	4.0 + 1.1*	4.2 + 1.0*	6.6 + 0.8*

Group B and C have the same significant interstitial activity; Group A has the highest epithelial activity. While, B is 1.3 times more than A in epithelial activity. Group B has the highest significant luminal activity with 1.3 times more than B group in its luminal activity.
Values are mean ± S.E.M.
*P < 0.05 was considered significant.

Table 5.c) Summary of volume fractions of Epididymal tissue profile

Group	N	Mean ± S.E.M
A	10	0.21 ± 0.02
B	10	0.1 ± 0.02*
C	10	0.06 ± 0.01 *

Group C has the lowest significant epididymal density of the groups; B group is twice C group in their density.
Values are mean ± S.E.M.
*P < 0.05 was considered significant.

Table 5.d) Summary of Numerical density (Nv) of epididymal tubular profile

Also, the high dose group showed evidence of matured spermatozoa fullness within the varying tubular lumens of the different sizes epididymal tubules seen in the photomicrographs fig 2 and 3.in the X100 magnifications. Hence, the epididymal lumen appeared wider and fuller with matured spermatozoa when compared to the control as seen in figure 1-3.

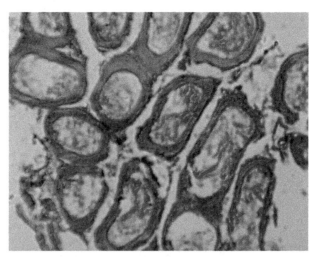

Group A micrograph showed normal sized and sparsely fullness of the epididymal tubules with spermatozoa.as compared to the treated animal groups. Group A X 100 magnification.

Fig. 1. Micrographs of the epididymes of the animals in group A

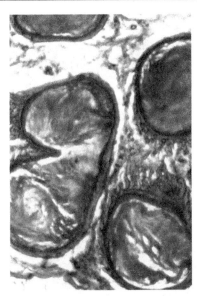

Group B micrograph showed widening and fullness of the epididymal tubules with matured spermatozoa. Group B X 100 magnification.

Fig. 2. Micrographs of the epididymes of the animals in group B

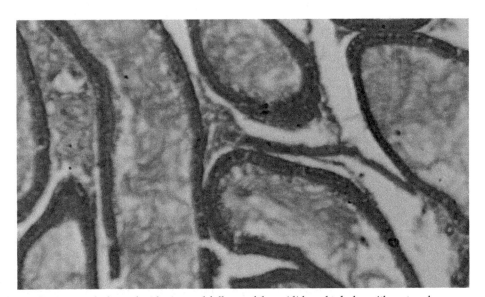

Group C micrograph showed widening and fullness of the epididymal tubules with matured spermatozoa. Group C X 100 magnification.

Fig. 3. Micrographs of the epididymes of the animals in group C

4. Discussion

There is increasing role and contribution of sesame lignans and other essential oils obtained from sesamum radiatum research to medicine in this present decade.

Moreover, sesamum radiatum leaves rich in trace minerals, vitamins, antioxidant lignans (phytoestrogens) and other essential oils as reflected in the GCMS findings, have the ability of improving fertility potential of the male reproductive tract with antimicrobial impact against the common infective agents of the reproductive tract.

Muller-Hinton Agar diffusion (MHA) method was extensively used to investigate the antibacterial activity of natural antimicrobial substance and plant extracts (Ahmed et al, 2010; Bankole et al, 2007; Shittu et al, 2006b). However, for solution/extracts with a low antimicrobial activity, one will need a large concentration or volume made possible with holes or cylinders using MHA rather than the disk method with limited applications (Bastner, 1994; Ahmed et al, 2010; Bankole et al, 2007; Shittu et al, 2006b). .

The GC-MS of the methanolic *Sesame radiatum* leaves extract did show the presence of mainly aromatic phenolic essential oils, which possess antimicrobial properties (Alma et al, 2003). For example, sesamol as one of the most potent antioxidants in the leaves was also reported in our previous study (Shittu et al, 2007c).

Moreover, the methanolic extracts showed antibacterial effect against *Staphylococcus aureus* only at a higher concentration. Unlike, the ethanolic extracts with no inhibitory activity against *Staphylococcus aureus* and was very effective against *Streptococcus pneumoniae* and *Candida albicans*, Hence, posses both antibacterial and antifungal activity (R´10s & Recio., 2005). This same natural antibacterial effect against common skin pathogens such as *Staphylococcus* and *Streptococcus* bacteria as well as common skin fungi including the athlete's foot fungus was reported in other similar study using the sesame oil (Sesame, 2000).

The pH of compounds in dilutions had also been found to modify the results outcome as usually observed in the case of phenolic or carboxylic compounds present in plants extracts, since studies have shown that the different effects of neutral essential oil are pH dependents. For example, anise oil has a higher antifungal activity at pH 4.8 than at 6.8, and *Cedrus deudora*was oil was most active at pH 9.0 (Janssen et al 1976).

In the present study, ethanolic extracts with lesser acidity was found to be more effective against *Candida albicans* at a lower pH than the methanolic extracts with no inhibitory activity against *Candida albican* as shown in table 1.

Moreover, the aqueous extract showed antifungal activity at a higher pH as seen in table 1. However, the antifungal activity of ethanolic extract was more potent than that of the aqueous extracts as reflected with lower MICs against *Candida albicans* with value of 28.2 µg/ml when compared to 31.9 µg/ml. obtained for the aqueous extract as shown in table 2.

This in a way reflect on the significance of the preservation of some of the active ingredient present in the leaves like sesame lignans such as sesaminol and its glucosides, which are water soluble in nature and extracted effectively during extraction processes of the Sesame leaves (R´10s & Recio., 2005). Hence, ethanol was more effective than methanol in extraction and preservation of the oily and water soluble active ingredients with proven anti-microbial properties especially against yeasts (Shittu et al, 2007c).

This preservation was further enhanced and improved using the modified Okogun` s method as supported by other previous report (Shittu et al, 2007c) and complementary to effective antimicrobial property of *sesamum radiatum* leaves (Shittu et al, 2006).

In addition, antimicrobial effectiveness of the different crude sesame leaves extracts were similar to that of standard antibiotics and antifungals used as reflected in the tables 4 and 5 respectively. More so, the zone of inhibition obtained especially against the *staphylococcus aureus* of the methanolic extract of sesame leaves (39.3 mm) was found to be higher than that of the primary standard antibiotic-cloxacillin (30.0mm) used in this study. This also implied a relative effectiveness of the *sesamum radiatum* leaves extract over the regular standard primary synthetic and expensive antibiotic available in the market.

It is actually the preservation of these rich nutritive constituents of aqueous *sesamum radiatum* leaves extracts that has contributed to the general state of well-being observed in all the treated animals during the whole experimental period with sesame-treated rats showing evidence of significant raw weight gained (P < 0.05). However, with ANOVA, no significant difference was observed in the raw animal weights compared to control.

Interestingly, other studies have reported the increasing application of stereological and morphometric techniques as new veritable approaches in modern medicine and biomedical sciences/researches in recent years (Mukerjee & Rajan, 2006, Shittu, 2006, 2010; Shittu et al, 2008b; Shittu et al, 2009).

In this present study, matured adult male rats were used based on the fact that morphometric study using light microscopy is best evaluated when the studied organ has attained a reasonably sizable dimension (Mukerjee & Rajan, 2006, Shittu, 2006, 2010; Shittu et al, 2008b; Shittu et al, 2009).

There was relative significant (P< 0.05) epididymal weight gain difference in the sesame-treated animal compared to the control as shown in table 6b. However, no significant changes in epididymal weights were observed in estradiol (high and low dose) treated golden hamsters (Jin *et al.,* 2005).

In the present study, it appeared that sesame-treated rats have more significant (P< 0.05) effects on the raw weights of the epididymis than testis as observed in other previous studies (Shittu, 2006, 2010; Shittu et al, 2008a; Shittu et al, 2009). In addition, this is actually a reflection of the more active site of action of sesame phytoestrogenic lignans as the epididymis is a known steroid responsive organ (Shittu, 2006, 2010). Hence, the activities of sesame is hormonally influenced as efferent ductile and epididymis of rats are also rich in estrogens receptors; a and b sub-types (Hess et al., 1997; Hess and Carnes, 2004; Shittu, 2006, 2010; Shittu et al, 2007a) and that any disruption of these receptors due to structural abnormalities in the efferent ductules or epididymis will lead to impairments of male fertility in mice (Hess, 1997; Hess & Carnes, 2004; Shittu, 2006, 2010).

Previous studies have also shown that the sectional tissues of studied organs are usually subjected to compression effect by 83% of their original dimension during their tissues processing stages, thereby necessitating the need of a correction factor. However, volume densities are not affected by this compression (Mouton, 2002; Shittu, 2006, 2010; Shittu et al, 2008b; Shittu et al, 2009) and hence, appeared to be more suitable for the present study.

In addition, the respective differential epididymal weights changes observed in the present study as seen in table 6 were well correlated with the tubular profiles of the epididymis especially, the tubular diameter for each group of animals as reflected in table 5, which further goes to support the above stated findings.

Moreover, the efferent ductile or epididymis is also rich in androgen receptors, the site of action for the testosterone (TT) and dihydrotestosterone (DHT) (Deslypere et al., 1992; Grino et al., 1990; Oliveira et al., 2003; Van-dekerckhove et al., 2000).

Contrary to speculation that phytoestrogen can disrupt and cause deleterious effects on the male reproductive developmental organs (Degen and Metzler, 1987). Our previous studies on *sesamum radiatum* leaves phytoestrogens have shown that sesame can indeed stimulate and enhance the release of quality matured spermatozoa from the testis into the epididymes as observed in the photomicrographs with evidence of matured spermatozoa fullness in the dilated epididymal lumens compared to the control group as shown in figure 1-3 (Shittu, 2006; 2010; Shittu et al, 2007a; Shittu et al, 2008a, Shittu et al, 2009) and this was also corroborated with significant (P< 0.05) higher epididymal tubular diameters observed in the sesame- treated groups compared to the control group as reflected in table 5b..

Moreover, various other reports are found confirming the epididymal presence of aromatase in human efferent ductules and proximal epididymis (Carpino et al., 2004) and cultured rat cells, (Wiszniewska, 2002). Thus, sesame phytoestrogenic lignans tend to   promote aromatization of testosterone to estradiol, such that, the low dose sesame will make available less endogenous estradiol and compete less, although there is synergism at this level between the testosterone and estradiol to favour spermatogenesis. However, the high dose, which will cause more estradiol production and compete more with dihydrotestosterone for aromatization to occur in its favour (Shittu, 2006, 2010; Shittu et al, 2007a; Shittu et al, 2008a; Shittu et al, 2009).

In addition, from the present study, it is postulated that sesame acts through mechanisms, which are dependent on the estrogens receptors (ER1 and ER2) binding and also cause estradiol (E2)-induced transactivation of the androgen receptor (AR), thereby ultimately influencing the hypothalamic-pituitary-testicular pathway as the case may be as evidenced in this present study and others (Shittu, 2006, 2010; Shittu et al, 2007a; Shittu et al, 2008a; Shittu et al, 2009).

Hence, we also hypothesized that the agonistic action of sesame radiatum leaves extract on the α-estrogens receptors is more pronounced than the β-estrogens receptors and with its rich antioxidative property, all contributed to enhancing spermatogenesis with improve male fertility as evident in present study.

5. Conclusion

The result confirmed the folkloric claims of the antimicrobial effectiveness of locally consumed Sesame leaves extracts against common skin infection and bacterial including yeast that are associated with infertility cases in this part of the world. In addition, Sesame leaves extract consumption enhances the quality of the spermatozoa produced with improvement in the storage capacity of the epididymes for these spermatozoa in a dose related manner.

6. Acknowledgements

The authors wish to appreciate the technical assistance of the staff of the Drug Quality Control Laboratory of LASUTH especially the duo of Martin A and Idowu B towards this study. We also appreciated the secretariat assistance of the trio of Solomon Shittu, Omolara Shittu and Moses Shittu towards this study. Jireh International Foundation provided the financial support for this study.

7. References

Adlercreutz, H.; Fotsis, T.; Bannwart, C.; Wähälä, K.;Mäkelä, T.; Brunow, G. & Hase, T.. (1986). Determination of urinary lignans and phytoestrogen metabolites, potential antiestrogens and anticarcinogens, in urine of women on various habitual diets. *J. Steroid Biochem.25(5b)*, 791-7

Ahmed, T.; Shittu, L. A. J.; Bankole, M. A.; Adesanya, O.A.; Bankole, M. N.; Shittu, R. K. & Ashiru, O. A. (2009.). Comparative Antimicrobial Studies Of Selected Antibiotics / Antifungal With Crude Extracts Of Sesame Radiatum Against Some Common Pathogenic Microorganisms. *Scientific Research & Essays.* 4 (6), 584-589

Aitken, J. & Fisher, H. (1994). Reactive oxygen species generation and human spermatozoa; the balance of benefits and risk. *Bioessays.* 16, 259-267.

Akpan-Iwo G; Idowu AA & Misari SM. (2006). Collection and evaluation of sesame (*Sesamum* spp.) germplasm in Nigeria. *IGPR/FAO.* 142, 59-62.

American Physiological Society. (2002). Guiding principles for research involving animals and human beings. *Am. J. Physiol. Regul. Integr. Comp.Physiol.*, 283(2), R281-3

Bankole, M A; Shittu, LAJ; Ahmed, T A; Bankole, M N, Shittu, R K, & Ashiru, O A. (2007). Synergistic Antimicrobial Activities of Phytoestrogens In Crude Extracts Of Two Sesame Species Against Some Common Pathogenic Microorganism. *Afr. J. Traditional, Complimentary Alternative Med.* 4(4), 427-433.

Bastner, A,; Pfeiffer, KP. & Bastner, H. (1994). Applicability of diffusion method required by the pharmacopoeias for testing antibacterial activity of natural compounds. *Pharmazie.* 49, 512-516.

Blouin, A,; Boender, RP. & Weibel, E. (1977).Distribution of organelles and membranes between hepatocytes and non hepatocytesin the rat liver parenchyma. *J Cell Bio.* 72, 441-455.

Carpino, A.; Romeo, F. & Rago, V. (2004). Aromatase immunolocalization in human ductuli efferentes and proximal ductus epididymis. *J. Anat, 204,* :217-20.

Clulow, J; Jones, RC; Hansen, LA, & Man, SY (1998). Fluid and electrolyte reabsorption in the ductuli efferentes testis. *J. Reprod. Fertil.* Suppl.53,:1-14.

Collins BM; Mclachlan JA & Arnold S (1997). The estrogenic and antiestrogenic activities of phytochemicals with the human receptor expressed in yeast. *Steroids* 62: 365–372.

Degen, G. H.. & Metzler, M. (1987). Sex hormones and neoplasia: genotoxic effects in short term assays. *Arch. Toxicol. 10*,264-78

De Kretser, DM. & Baker, HW. (1999). Infertility in men: recent advances and continuing controversies. *Journal of Clinical Endocrinology and Metabolism.* 84, 3443–3450.

Deslypere, JP; Young, M; Wilson, JD. & McPhaul, MJ. (1992). Testosterone and 5 -dihydro-testosterone interact differently with the androgen receptor to enhance transcription of the MMTV-CAT reporter gene. *Mol. Cell Endocrinol.* 88, 15-22.

Duty, SM; Silva, MJ; Barr, DB; Brock, JW; Ryan, L; Chen, Z; Herrick, RF; Christiani, DC. & Hauser, R. (2003). Phthalate exposure and human semen parameters. *Epidemiology.* 14, 269–277.

Eloff JNP. (1998). A sensitive and quick microplate method to determine the minimum inhibitory concentration of plants extract for bacteria, *Plant Med.* 64, 711-713.

Gill, LS (1992). *Ethnomedical uses of plants in Nigeria*, Uniben Press, Edo State, Nigeria, p. 212.

George, FW; Johnson, L. & Wilson, JD.(1989). The effect of a 5 alphareductase inhibitor on androgen physiology in the immature male rat. *Endocrinology.* 125, 2434-2438.

Grino, PB; Griffin, JE. &Wilson, JD (1990). Testosterone at high concentrations interacts with the human androgen receptor similarly to dihydrotestosterone. *Endocrinol.* 126, 1165-1172.

Hanilyn, PF. (1998). British Mycological Society Newsletter 3, 25-27.

Hess, R. A. & Carnes, K. The role of estrogen in testis and the male reproductive tract: a review and species comparison. *Anim. Reprod.,* 1:5-30, 2004..

Hess, RA; Gist, DH;, Bunick, D;, Lubahn, DB,;; Farrell, A;, Bahr, J,; Cooke PS. & Greene, GL (1997). Estrogen receptor (a & b) expression in the excurrent ducts of the adult male rat reproductive tract. J. Androl. 18: 602-611.

Hirose, N.;; Do(i, F.; Ueki, T.; Akazawa, K.; Chijiiwa, K.; Sugano, M.; Akimoto, K.; Shimizu, S. & Yamada, H. Suppressive effect of sesamin against 7,12- dimethylbenz[a]-anthracene induced rat mammary carcinogenesis. *Anticancer Res.,* 12:1259-65, 1992.

Izegbu, M. C.; Ojo, M. O. & Shittu,, L. A. J. (2005.). Clinicopathological patterns of testicular malignancies in Ilorin, Nigeria-a report of 8 cases. *J. Cancer Res. Ther.,*1(4):229-31,

Janssen, A.M. & Scheffer, J.J.C. (1975). Baerheim Svendsen, A. Antimicrobial activity of essential oils: a 1976–1986 literature review. Aspect of the test methods. *Planta Medica* 53, 395–398.

Jeng, KCG. &, Hou, RCW. (2005). Sesamin and Sesamolin: Nature`s therapeutic lignans. *Curr. Enzym. Inhi..* 1, 11-20.

Jin W, Arai KY; Watanabe G; Suzuki AK; Takahashi S, & Taya K. (2005). The Stimulatory Role of Estrogen on Sperm Motility in the Male Golden Hamster (Mesocricetus auratus). *Journal of Andrology,* 26 (4) 478-484

Johnson, L.A., T.M. Suleiman and E.M. Lucas. (1979). Sesame protein: A review and prospectus. *J. Am. Oil Chem. Soc.,* 56: 463-468

Kang, M.H, Kawai, Y, Naito M, Osawa, T. J. (1999). Nutr. 129:1885. In: Jeng KCG, Hou RCW. Sesamin and Sesamolin: Nature`s therapeutic lignans. Current Enzymes Inhibition, 1: 11-20, 2005.

Konan, AR; Datte, JY. & Yapo, PA. (2008). Nitric oxide pathway mediated relaxant effects of aqueous sesame leaves extract (*Sesamum radiatum* Schum & Thonn) in the guinea pig isolated aorta smooth muscle. *BMC Complimentary Altern. Med.,* www.iomedcentral.com/1472 6882 /8/:23.

Kuiper, G. G. J. M., Carlsson, B., Grandien, K., Enmark, E., Haggblad, J, Nilsson, S. & Gustafsson, J. (1997). Comparison of the ligand binding specificity and transcript tissue distribution of estrogen receptors a and b. *Endocrinology, 138*:863-70.

Leke, RJ; Oduma, JA; Bassol,-M S; Bacha, AM & Grigor, KM (1993). Regional and geographical variations in infertility: effects of environmental, cultural, and socioeconomic factors. *Environmental Health Perspectives.* (Supplement) 101(2)), 73-80.

Leridon,, H (1977).. *Human fertility. The basic components.* The University of Chicago Press, Chicago.

Martin, P. M.; Horwitz, K. B.; Ruyan, D. S. & McGuire, W.L. (1978). Phytoestrogen interaction with estrogen receptors in human breast cancer cells. *Endocrinology, 103*:1860-7,

Mitra, J & Chowdhury, M. (1994). Association of glycerylphosphoryl choline with human sperm and effect of capacitation on their metabolism. *Reprod Fertil Dev.* 6:679–685.

Mosher WD & Aral SO..(1985). Factors related to infertility in the United States, 1965-1976. *Sexual Transm Dis*; 12, 117-123.

Mouton PR. (2002). *Principles and Practices of Unbiased Stereology-Introduction for Bioscientists.* Baltimore Maryland: The John Hopkins University Press. 1-214

Mukerjee B, Rajan T. (2006). Morphometric Study of Seminal Vesicles of Rat in Normal Health and Stress Conditions. *JAnat Soc.* 55 (1), 31-36.

Murkies, A . (1998). Phytoestrogens–what is the current knowledge? *Aust. Fam. Physician, 27(1)*:S47-51.

Nascimento Gislene, G. F., Juliana Locatelli, Paulo C Freitas, and Giuliana L. Silva. (2000). .Antibacterial activity of plant extracts and phytochemicals on antibiotic resistant bacteria. *Brazilian J.Microbiol.* 31, 247-256

Nishimune Y & Tanaka H (2006). Infertility caused by polymorphisms or mutations in spermatogenesis-specific genes. *Journal of Andrology* 27 326–334.

Norris S. (2001). Reproductive infertility: Prevalence, causes, trends and treatments. *Parliamentary Research Branch (PRB 00-32E) Newsletter In brief,* Jamuary 2, 2001.

Obiajunwa EIFM, Adebiyi L, Omode PE (2005). Determination of Essential Minerals and Trace Elements in Nigerian Sesame Seeds, Using TXRF Technique. Pak. J. Nutri. 4(6): 393-395.

Okogun JI. 2000. *Methods of Medicinal Plants Extracts Preparation.* National institute of Pharmaceutical Research and Developments (NIPRD), Idu-Abuja, Nigeria,

Orgebin-Crist, MC (1967). Sperm maturation in rabbit epididymis. *Nature.* 216: 816-818.

Oliveira, C; Nie, R; Carnes, K; Franca, LR; Prins, GS; Saunders, PTK. &, Hess, RA. (2003). The antiestrogen ICI 182, 780 decreases the expression of estrogen receptor-alpha but has no effect on estrogen receptorbeta and androgen receptor in rat efferent ductules. *Reprod. Biol. Endocrinol..* 1, 75.

Penalvo, JL; Heinonen, SM; Aura, AM. & Adlercruetz, H. (2005). Dietary Sesamin is converted to enterolactone in humans. *J. Nutr.* 1056-1062.

R´ios ,JL. & Recio, MC. (2005). Medicinal plants and antimicrobial activity. *Journal of Ethnopharmacology.* 100:80–84.

Schwaab, V, Lareyre, JJ, Vernet , P; Pons, E; Faure, J; Dufaure, JP. & Drevet, JR. (1998)..
Characterization, regulation of the expression and putative roles of two glutathione
peroxidase proteins found in the mouse epididymis. *Journal of Reproduction and
Fertility.* (Suppl) 53, 157–162.

Schwartz, D. (1980).. La notion de f&condabilitt darts l'approche etiologique, diagnostique
et therapeutique de l'infeconditt. *J Gynecol Obstet Biol Reprod.* 9, :607-612.

Scott, TW; Wales, RG; Wallace, KC,. & White, IG.   (1963). Composition of ram epididymal
and testicular fluid and the biosynthesis of glycerylphosphorylcholine by the rabbit
epididymis. J. Reprod. Fertil. 6, 49–59.

Sesame. (2000). Sesame. *Aquaculture Research* August, 32: 623.

Sharpe, R. M. (2003). The 'oestrogen hypothesis'- where do we stand now? *Int. J. Androl.,*
26:2-15

Sharpe, RM & Irvine, DS (2004). How strong is the evidence of a link between
environmental chemicals and adverse effects on human reproductive health?
British Medical Journa.l 328, 447–451

Sharpe, R. M. & Shakkebeak, N. E. (1993). Are oestrogens involved in falling sperm counts
and disorders of the male reproductive tract? *Lancet. 341(8857),*:1392-5

Skakkebaek, NE (2003). Testicular dysgenesis syndrome. *Hormone Research.* 60 (Supplement
3), 49.

Shittu, L. A. J. (2006). *The effect of the aqueous crude leaves extract of Sesamum radiatum compared
to Mesterolone (proviron) on the adult male SpragueDawley rats testis and epididymis.*
MSc Dissertation. Lagos State University, College of Medicine, Ikeja, Nigeria,

Shittu, L. A. J. (2010). *Reproductive Impact Of Sesame Leaves Lignans In Adult Male SD Rats.*
LAP LAMBERT Academic AG & Co KG, ISBN: 978-3-8383-8206-7, USA,

Shittu, L.A.J,; Izegbu MC, Babalola OS, Adesanya OA, Ashiru OA (2005). Doctors`
knowlegde, attitude, and practise towards sperm- banking before cancer therapy in
Lagos Nigeria. *Nigerian Med. Practitioner.* 47(5), 96-98.

Shittu, L A. J; Babalola,, O. S; Adesanya, O. A; Jewo, I; Oyewopo, O.O. & Ashiru, O. A..
(2006a). Pregnancy outcome following swim up preparation of both fresh and
Cryopreserved spermatozoa. *Scientific Research &Essay.* 1 (3), 103-107,

Shittu, L. A. J.; Bankole, M. A.; Ahmed, T.; Aile, K.; Akinsanya, M. A.; Bankole, M. N.; Shittu,
R. K. and Ashiru, O. A. 2006b Differential antimicrobial activity of the various
crude leaves extracts of Sesame radiatum against some common pathogenic microorganisms. *Sci. Res. Essay.* 1(3), 108-11.

Shittu, L. A. J.; Bankole, M. A.; Oguntola, J. A.; Ajala, O.; Shittu, R. K.; Ogundipe, O. A.;
Bankole, M. N.; Ahmed, T. & Ashiru, O. A. 2007a.. Sesame Leaves Intake Improve
And Increase Epididymal Spermatocytes Reserve In Adult Male Sprague Dawley
Rat. *Scientific Research & Essay.,* 2(8,):319-24,

Shitu LAJ, Bankole MA, Ahmed T, Bankole MN, Shittu RK, Saalu CL, Ashiru OA (2007b).
Antibacterial and Antifungal Activities of Essential Oils of Crude Extracts of *Sesame
Radiatum* against Some Common Pathogenic Micro-organisms. *IJPT.* 6. 165-170.

Shittu LAJ, Bankole MA, Ogundipe OA, Fakade AK, Shittu RK, Bankole Marian N, Ahmed
T, Tayo AO, Ashiru OA (2007c). Weight reduction with improvement of serum

lipid profile and ratios of Sesame radiatum leaves diet in a non obses Sprague Dawley Rat. *Afr. J. Biotechnol.* 6(21): 2428-2433.

Shittu, L. A. J, Shittu, R. K, Adesite, S. O, Ajala, M. O, Bankole, M. A, Benebo, A. S, Tayo, A. O, Ogundipe, O. A, & Ashiru, O. A. (2008a). *Sesame radiatum* phytoestrogens stimulate spermatogenic activity and improve sperm quality in adult male Sprague Dawley rat testis. *Int. J. Morphol. , 26(3),*643-652

Shittu, L.A. J, Shittu, R K, Ogundipe, O, Tayo, A.O.& Osunubi, A.A.A. (2009). Hypoglycaemia and improved testicular parameters in *Sesamum radiatum* treated normo-glycaemic adult male Sprague Dawley rats. *African Journal of Biotechnology* Vol. 8 (12), 2878-2886, 17

Shittu, LA. J; Shittu, R K; Osinubi, A.A.A; & Ashiru, O A. (2008b). Stereological Evidences Of Epithelial Hypoplasia of Seminiferous Tubules Induced By Mesterolone In Adult Sprague-Dawley Rats. *African Journal of Metabolism & Endocrinology,* 7 (1),: 16 – 20

Shittu, L A J; Shittu, RK. &, Igbigbi P. (2010). Sesame Lignans Derivatives as Possible Selective Modulators for Both Estrogen Receptors A & B and Endothelial Nitric Oxide Synthetase (Enos) In Sprague Dawley Rat Penis (Postal Abstarct No- 33. *Proceeding of 6th Intelliegent System For Molecular Biology Students` Council Symposium,* Boston USA, July,

Thompson, L. U.; Robb, P.; Serraino, M. & Cheung, F. (1991). Mammalian lignan production from various foods. *Nutr. Cancer. 16,* :43-52

Thonneau, P.& Spira, A. (1990) . Prevalence of infertility: international of measurement data and problems. *European Journal of Obstetrics & Gynecology and Reproductive Biology.* 38, 43-52 43

Van-dekerckhove, P,; Lilford, R,; Vail, A,& Huges E. (2000). Androgen versus placebo or no treatment for idiopathic Oligo/asthenospermia, *Cochrane database System, Rev.* (2), CD000150.

Vos, JP; Dybing, E; Greim, HA; Ladefoged, O; Lambre, C; Tarazona, JV; Brandt, I, & Vethaak, AD. (2000). Health effects of endocrine –disrupting chemicals on wildlife, with special reference to the European situation. *Crit Rev. Toxicol.* 30, 71-133.

Wales RG; Wallace JC. & White, IG .(1966). Composition of bull epididymal and testicular fluid. *J. Reprod. Fertil.* 12, 139–152.

Weibel ER, Gomez DM. A principle for counting tissue structures on random sections. *J Appl Physiol,* 1962; 17: 343-348.

Whitten, P. L. & Naftolin, F. (1991). Effects of a phytoestrogen diet on estrogen-dependent *J. Natl. Cancer Ins.,* 83(8,:541-6

Wiszniewska, B.(2002). Primary culture of the rat epididymal epithelial cells as a source of oestrogen. *Andrologia,34,* 180-7

World Health Organization. (1987). Towards more objectivity in diagnosis and management of male infertility of a world health organization multicentres study. *Int. J. Androl.* Suppl. 7(10), 1-35

World Health Organization. (1991). *Infertility: a tabulation of available data on the prevalence of primary and secondary infertility.* Geneva, WHO, Programme on Maternal and Child Health and Family Planning, Division of Family Health.

Zini, A & Schlegel, PN. (1997). Identification and characterization of antioxidant enzyme mRNAs in the rat epididymis. *InternationalJournal of Andrology*. 20, 86–91.

Zuping, H.; Wai-Yee. C & Dym, M. (2006). Microarray technology offers a novel tool for the diagnosis and identification of therapeutic targets for male infertility. *Reproduction*. 132, 11–19

4

Antimicrobial and Antioxidant Activities of Some Plant Extracts

Elita Scio et al.*

Federal University of Juiz de Fora, Laboratory of Bioactive Natural Products,
Brazil

1. Introduction

Infectious diseases are the world's leading cause of premature deaths, killing almost 50,000 people every day. In recent years, drug resistance to human pathogenic bacteria has been commonly reported from all over the world (N'guessan et al., 2007). The abusive and indiscriminate use of antimicrobial compounds over many years is the main factor responsible for the appearance of the phenomenon of bacterial resistance to such compounds (Andremont, 2001). With increased incidence of resistance to antibiotics, natural products from plants could be interesting alternatives (Lu et al., 2007; Mbwambo et al., 2007). Some plant extracts and phytochemicals are known to have antimicrobial properties, and can be of great significance in therapeutic treatments. In the last few years, a number of studies have been conducted in different countries to demonstrate such efficacy (Benoit-Vical et al., 2006; Senatore et al., 2007; Singh et al., 2007). On the other hand, free radicals are known to be the major cause of various chronic and degenerative diseases. Oxidative stress is associated with pathogenic mechanisms of many diseases including atherosclerosis, neurodegenerative diseases, cancer, diabetes and inflammatory diseases, as well as aging processes. It is defined as an imbalance between production of free radicals and reactive metabolites, so-called oxidants, and it also includes their elimination by protective mechanisms, referred to as antioxidative systems. This imbalance leads to damage of important biomolecules and organs with potential impact on the whole organism. Antioxidants can delay, inhibit or prevent the oxidation of oxidizable materials by scavenging free radicals and diminishing oxidative stress (Duracková, 2010; Reuter et al., 2010). Natural antioxidants have been studied extensively for decades in order to find compounds protecting against a number of diseases related to oxidative stress and free radical-induced damage. To date, many plants have been claimed to pose beneficial health effects such as antioxidant properties (Kaur & Arora, 2009; Newman & Cragg 2007). According to World Health Organization (WHO), 65 - 80% of the world populations rely on traditional medicine to treat various diseases (Kaur & Arora, 2009). The WHO recommends

* Renata F. Mendes, Erick V.S. Motta, Paula M.Q. Bellozi, Danielle M.O. Aragão, Josiane Mello, Rodrigo L. Fabri, Jussara R. Moreira, Isabel V.L. de Assis and Maria Lúcia M. Bouzada

research into the use of the local flora for therapeutic purposes, with the intention of reducing the number of people excluded from effective therapy in the government health systems, which could constitute an economically viable alternative treatment of several diseases, especially in developing countries (Gonçalves et al., 2005; WHO, 2002). The potential of higher plants as source for new drugs is still largely unexplored. Among the estimated 250,000 - 500,000 plant species, only a small percentage has been investigated phytochemically and the fraction submitted to biological or pharmacological screening is even smaller (Mahesh & Satish, 2008). In this scenario, the screening of plant extracts has been of great interest to scientists for the discovery of new drugs effective in the treatment of several diseases, and about 20% of the plants or their extracts in the world have been submitted to biological or pharmacological tests (Rayne & Mazza, 2007; Suffredini et al., 2004). The phytochemical research based on ethnopharmacological information is considered an effective approach in the discovery of new agents from higher plants (Chen et al., 2008; Duraipiyan, 2006). Thus, in this study, methanol extracts of different parts of 70 species, most of them commonly used in Brazil for treating conditions likely to be associated with microorganisms, were evaluated for their antimicrobial and antioxidant activity. Furthermore, a phytochemical screening of the bioactive extracts was performed.

2. Materials and methods

2.1 Plant material

Specimens of 70 species (Table 1) were collected in Juiz de Fora, Minas Gerais, Brazil. A voucher specimen was deposited at the Herbarium Leopoldo Krieger (CESJ) of Federal University of Juiz de Fora.

2.2 Preparation of plant extracts

The dried parts of the plant (50 g each) were powdered and macerated with methanol (3 x 200 mL) for five days at room temperature. After evaporation of the solvent under reduced pressure, the respective methanol extracts were obtained. All the extracts were kept in tightly stoppered bottles under refrigeration (4 °C) until used for the biological testing and phytochemical analysis.

2.3 Antioxidant activity

2.3.1 DPPH assay

The free radical scavenging activity of samples and standard α-tocopherol solutions in methanol was determined based on their ability to react with stable 1,1-diphenyl-2-picrylhydrazyl (DPPH) free radical (Govidarajan et al., 2003). The plant samples at various concentrations (7.8 to 250 µg/mL) were added to a 152 µM solution of DPPH in methanol. After incubation at 37 °C for 30 min, the absorbance of each solution was determined at 517 nm. The antioxidant activity of the samples was expressed as IC_{50} (inhibitory concentration), which was defined as the concentration (in µg/mL) of sample required to inhibit the formation of DPPH radicals by 50%. Ascorbic acid, α-tocopherol, BHT, rutin and quercetin were used as positive control.

Family	Botanical name [Voucher number]	Common name	Plant parts used[a]	Ethnomedical uses (Albuquerque, 1989; Alice, 1995; Corrêa, 1984; Camargo, 1988; Corrêa et al., 1998; Lorenzi, 2000; Lorenzi & Matos, 2002; Matos, 2000; Moreira & Guarim-Neto, 2009; Morim, 2010; Panizza, 1998)
Amaranthaceae	*Alternanthera brasiliana* (L.) Kuntze [CESJ 48585]	Acônito-do-mato, caaponga, cabeça-branca	F, L	Diuretic, digestive, depurative, liver and bladder diseases, astringent, laxative, cough
Apocynaceae	*Allamanda cathartica* L. [CESJ 47443]	Alamanda, buiussu, carolina, cipó-de-leite	B, F, L, La	Scabies and lice elimination, purgative, parasitosis, fever, treatment of jaundice, complications of malaria, enlarged spleen, laxative
	Aspidosperma olivaceum Müll. Arg. [CESJ 49229]	Guatambu, guatambu-branco, guatambu-amarelo, tambu		No use reported
Asteraceae	*Acanthospermum australe* (Loefl.) Kuntze [CESJ 47438]	Picão-da prata, carrapicho-rasteiro, mata-pasto	AP	Liver diseases, diaphoretic, gonorrhea, malaria
	Achillea millefolium L. [CESJ 46087]	Novalgina, erva-de-carpinteiro, aquiléia, milefólio	L	Fever, head and general aches, colds indigestion
	Anthemis cotula L. [CESJ 48584]	Camomila-do-campo	F, L	Fever, gastrointestinal disorders, dysenteria, gouty arthritis
	Baccharis trimera (Less.) DC. [CESJ 46074]	Carqueja	L	Gastrointestinal and liver diseases, diabetes, inflammation
	Bidens segetum Mart. ex Colla [CESJ 47437]	Picão-do-mato		No use reported
	Carduus marianus L. [CESJ 48581]	Cardo-mariano, cardo-santo, cardo-de-nossa-senhora, cardo-branco	S, SB	Appetite stimulant, diuretic, tonic, liver cell regenerator, gastrointestinal disorders, bile flow stimulant, cirrhosis, hepatitis
	Matricaria chamomilla L. [CESJ 47435]	Camomila, camomila-romana, camomila-comum	F	Digestive, sedative, colic treatment, appetite stimulant, carminative
	Piptocarpha macropoda (DC.) Baker [CESJ 49448]			No use reported
	Solidago chilensis Meyen [CESJ 678]	Arnica, erva-de-lagarto, erva-lanceta, espiga-de-ouro	L	Stomachic, astringent

	Vernonanthura divaricata (Spreng.) H. Rob. [CESJ 49450]	Cambará-açu		No use reported
	Vernonia condensata Baker [CESJ 46086]	Boldo, alumã, alcachofra, figatil, cidreira-da-mata	L	Carminative, liver insufficiency, inflammation of the gallbladder, analgesic, syphilitic, appetite stimulant, liver and stomach disorders
Bignoniaceae	*Stenolobium stans* (L.) Seem [CESJ 46071]	Ipê-de-jardim, ipê-amarelo-de-jardim, ipêzinho-de-jardim	B, L	Diabetes, diuretic, tonic, antisyphilitic, vermifuge pains in the stomach
Bixaceae	*Bixa orellana* L. [CESJ 46077]	Urucum	S	Expectorant, laxative, stomachic, anti-bleeding, healing, dyspepsia liver and heart disorders, tuberculosis, skin problems, fever, inflammation
Commelinaceae	*Commelina robusta* Kunth [CESJ 50021]	Batata-ovo, manobi-açu, trapoeraba-açu	AP, L, R	Back pain, urinary tract infections with fever, trauma, wounds illnesses prevention
Euphorbiaceae	*Alchornea triplinervia* (Spreng.) Müll. Arg. [CESJ 49442]	Tapiá-vermelho, tapiá-guaçu-branco, pau-óleo	L	Gastric disturbances
	Acalypha brasiliensis Müll. Arg. [CESJ 50011]	Tapa-buraco		No use reported
Fabaceae	*Chamaecrista desvauxii* (Collad.) Killip [CESJ 23372]	Sene, acácia, carqueja-do-tabuleiro, flor-de-lilás, capim reis	L, R	Wounds in the uterus, worms, bowel, arthritis
	Samanea tubulosa (Benth.) Barneby & J.W. Grimes [CESJ 49743]	Amendoim-de-veado, árvore-da-chuva e pau-de-cangalha	L, SB	Colds and high blood pression
	Senna macranthera (DC. ex Collad.) H.S. Irwin & Barneby [CESJ 46159]	Manduirana, pau-fava, aleluia, mamangá, fedegoso		No use reported
	Senna multijuga (Rich.) H.S. Irwin & Barneby [CESJ 49783]	Pau-cigarra, canafístula, aleluia	S	Ophthalmic and skin infections
	Stylosanthes scabra Vogel [CESJ 47436]	Alfafa do nordeste, alfafa do campo		No use reported

Flacourtiaceae	*Casearia sylvestris* Sw. [CESJ 49218]	Guaçatonga, bugre-branco, café-bravo, café-de-frade	L, SB	Burns, cutaneous injuries, herpes, tonic, depurative, rheumatism, inflammation, analgesic, hemostatic, gastritis
Hypericaceae	*Vismia magnoliifolia* Schltdl. & Cham. [CESJ 49759]			No use reported
Lacistemataceae	*Lacistema pubescens* Mart. [CESJ 49751]	Espeto-vermelho, canela- vermelha, sabonete, cafezinho		No use reported
Lamiaceae	*Hyptis suaveolens* (L.) Poit [CESJ 46089]	Bamburral, erva-canudo, arbusto-selvagem	AP	Cramps, skin infections, respiratory tract infections, nasal congestion, fever, flu
	Ocimum basilicum L. [CESJ 46161]	Manjericão, alfavaca	L	Gastrointestinal disorders, fever, digestive, bacterial infections, parasitosis
	Peltodon radicans Pohl [CESJ 46158]	Paracari, hortelã-do-mato, rabugem-de-cachorro	AP	Expectorant, pertussis, cough, asthma, sneezing, carminative, dermatites, scorpion and snake bites, antispasmodic, syphilitic, parasitosis, diuretic
	Plectranthus neochilus Schltr. [CESJ 46580]	Boldo	L	Treatment of respiratory infections or related symptoms
	Salvia officinalis L. [CESJ 46579]	Sálvia, salva	AP	Infections diseases, astringent
Lauraceae	*Nectandra rigida* (Kunth) Nees [CESJ 49221]	Canela-amarela	B	Rheumatism
Lythraceae	*Cuphea ingrata* Cham. & Schltdl. [CESJ 47432]	Sete-sangrias-do-campo	WP	Fever, venereal diseases, rheumatism
Malpighiaceae	*Byrsonima variabilis* A. Juss. [CESJ 49240]	Murici		No use reported
Malvaceae	*Sida glaziovii* K. Schum. [CESJ 47439]	Guanxuma-branca		No use reported
Melastomataceae	*Miconia latecrenata* (DC.) Naudin [CESJ 49990]	Pixirica-preta		No use reported
	Tibouchina grandifolia Cogn. [CESJ 40445]	Orelha-de-onça		No use reported

	Tibouchina granulosa (Desr.) Cogn. [CESJ 49761]	Quaresmeira		No use reported
	Tibouchina mutabilis (Vell.) Cogn. [CESJ 46175]	Manacá		No use reported
	Trembleya parviflora (D. Don) Cogn. [CESJ 49219]	Manacá		No use reported
Monimiaceae	*Mollinedia schottiana* (Spreng.) Perkins [CESJ 48921]			No use reported
	Siparuna guianensis Aubl. [CESJ 49778]	Capitiú, caá-pitiú, erva-santa, fedorenta, negramina, negra-mena	SB	Carminative, stimulant, fever, antidispeptic, diuretic, muscle spasms prevention, headache, inflammation
Myrtaceae	*Eugenia cumini* (L.) Druce [CESJ 46601]	Jambolão, cereja, jamelão, jalão	B, Fr	Diabetes
	Myrcia splendens (Sw.) DC. [CESJ 49230]	Guamirim, folha-miúda		No use reported
Piperaceae	*Piper corcovadensis* (Miq.) C. DC. [CESJ 49993]	João-brandinho	L	Mucous membranes anesthesia (mouth), rheumathism, cough
Poaceae	*Cymbopogon citratus* (DC) Stapf. [CESJ 46582]	Capim-cheiroso, erva-cidreira, capim-cidreira, capim-limão	L	Calmant, gastrointestinal disorders, infections diseases, colic treatment, anxiety
Rosaceae	*Eriobotrya japonica* (Thunb.) Lindl. [CESJ 47434]	Nespereira, ameixeira	FR, L	Cough, asthma, chronic bronchitis, phlegm, high fever and gastroenteric disorders
	Rubus rosifolius Sm. [CESJ 48580]	Morango-silvestre, amora-do-mato	AP	Infectious and dolorous diseases
	Rubus urticifolius Poir. [CESJ 46583]	Nhambuí, árvore-preta, amora-do-silva	Fr	Throat diseases, diuretic
Rubiaceae	*Amaioua intermedia* Mart. [CESJ 49994]	Canela-de-veado, vachila, carvoeiro, pimentão-bravo, marmelada-brava		No use reported
Rutaceae	*Zanthoxylum rhoifolium* Lam. [CESJ 49782]	Mamica-de-cadela	L, SB	Toothache, earache, malaria

Sapindaceae	*Allophylus semidentatus* (Miq.) Radlk [CESJ 49774]	Fruta-de-faraó		No use reported
	Cupania oblongifolia Mart. [CESJ 49447]	Pau-magro, caboatã	B, L	Weight loss
	Sapindus saponaria L. [CESJ 46172]	Sabão-de-soldado	Fr, R, SB	Antitussive, adstringent, , calmant, diuretic, expectorant
Solanaceae	*Solanum sellowianum* Dunal [CESJ 49225]			No use reported
	Solanum swartzianum Roem. & Schult. [CESJ 49226]	Barbaso, fruta-de-pombo		No use reported
Tropaeolaceae	*Tropaeolum majus* L. [CESJ 46586]	Capuchinha, chaguinha, alcaparra-de-pobre, chagas, mastruço-do-peru	L	Scurvy, sepse, expectorant, urinary, gastrointestinal and dermatological disinfectant
Turneraceae	*Turnera subulata* Sm. [CESJ 47442]	Chanana, flor-do-Guarujá	R	Amenorrhea
Typhaceae	*Typha dominguensis* Pers. [CESJ 49773]	Taboa	F, R	Treatment of burns, wounds and inflammation, kidney stones and diarrhea
Urticaceae	*Cecropia pachystachya* Trécul [CESJ 46591]	Embaúba, umbaúba, torém	B, L	Cough, expectorant, asthma and diabetes
Verbenaceae	*Lippia pseudo-thea* Schauer [CESJ 46171]	Capitão-do-matto, câmara, chá-de-frade, chá-de-pedestre, cidrilha	L	Gastrointestinal disorders, expectorant, stimulant, rheumatism
	Lippia hermannioides Cham. [CESJ 46088]			No use reported
	Lippia alba (Mill.) N.E. Br. ex Britton & P. Wilson [CESJ 46177]	Erva-cidreira, erva-cidreira-do-campo, alecrim-do campo, salsa	L, R	Hypertension, stomach cramps, nausea, coughs, colds
	Lippia rubella (Moldenke) T.R.S. Silva & Salimena [CESJ 46178]			No use reported

	Lippia sidoides Cham. [CESJ 46180]	Alecrim-pimenta, alecrim-do-nordeste, estrepa-cavalo, alecrim-bravo	F, L	Allergic rhinitis, throat and mouth infections, antiseptic, skin and scalp disorders
	Lantana camara L. [CESJ 47441]	Camará, cambará, chumbinho, camará - de-chumbo	L	Treatment of respiratory diseases such as cough, bronchitis, pertussis, colds, flu, asthma, hoarseness, expectorant, antispasmodic, rheumatism, digestive, diuretic
	Aloysia floribunda M. Martens & Galeotti [CESJ 46584]			No use reported
Vitaceae	*Cissus verticillata* (L.) Nicolson & C.E. Jarvis [CESJ 46587]	Anil-trepador, cipó-pucá, cipó-puci, puçá, insulina, insulina-vegetal	AP, L	Tachycardia, hypertension, dropsy, anemia, leakage, tremors, activator of blood circulation, diabetes, anticonvulsant
Zingiberaceae	*Hedychium coronarium* J. König [CESJ 50022]	Gengibre-branco, lírio-do-brejo, lágrima-de-moça, lírio-branco, borboleta, lágrima-de-vênus	Fr, Rh	Arthritis, diabetes, headache and hypertension

ªAP, Aerial Parts; B, Bark; F, Flowers; Fr, Fruits; L, Leaves; La, Latex; R, Root; Rh, Rhizome; S, Seeds; SB, Stem Bark; WP, Whole Plant

Table 1. Ethnomedical data on medicinal plants.

2.3.2 Reducing power assay

The reducing power was determined by the method of Oyazu (1986), based on the chemical reaction of Fe(III) to Fe(II). Ten mg of each sample were mixed with potassium phosphate buffer (0.2 M, pH 6.6) (2.5 mL) and potassium ferricyanide (10 g/L) (2.5 mL). The mixture was incubated at 50 °C for 20 min. A 2.5 mL aliquot of 10% trichloroacetic acid was added to the mixture, which was then centrifuged at 3.000 g for 10 min. The upper layer of the solution (2.5 mL) was mixed with distilled water (2.5 mL) and 0.1 % $FeCl_3$ (0.5 mL), and the absorbance was measured at 700 nm. Ascorbic acid was used as reference material. All tests were performed in triplicate. Increase in absorbance of the reaction indicated the reducing power of the samples. A higher absorbance indicated a higher reducing power. EC_{50} (effective concentration) values ($\mu g/mL$) were calculated and indicate the effective concentration at which the absorbance was 0.5 for reducing power.

2.3.3 β-carotene - linoliec acid assay

In this assay, antioxidant capacity is determined by measuring the inhibition of the volatile organic compounds and the conjugated diene hydroperoxides arising from linoleic acid oxidation (Dapkevicius et al., 1998). A stock solution of β-carotene/linoleic acid mixture was prepared as follows: 50 μL of β-carotene (10 mg/mL) in chloroform (HPLC grade), 20 μL linoleic acid, 200 μL Tween 40 and 1 mL of chloroform was added. Chloroform was completely evaporated using a vacuum evaporator. Then, 30 mL of distilled water saturated with oxygen (30 min 100 mL/min) were added with vigorous shaking, and 250 μL of the reactive mixture and 10 μL of the extracts (40 μg/mL) were added in a microplate and incubated at 45 °C to accelerate oxidation reactions and start the bleaching of β-carotene. The absorbance readings were taken immediately at intervals of 15 min for 120 min in spectrophotometer at 470 nm (Duarte-Almeida et al., 2006). The same procedure was repeated with the antioxidant flavonoid quercetin as positive control, and a blank. After this incubation period, absorbances of the mixtures were measured at 490 nm. Antioxidative capacities of the extracts were expressed as percentage inhibition (1).

$$\text{Inhibition } (\%) = \frac{\text{control absorbance } - \text{ sample absorbance}}{\text{control absorbance}} \times 100 \qquad (1)$$

2.4 Antimicrobial assay

2.4.1 Microbial strains

The samples were evaluated against a panel of microorganisms, including the bacterial strains *Staphylococcus aureus* (ATCC 6538), *Pseudomonas aeruginosa* (ATCC 15442), *Salmonella enterica* serovar Typhimurium (ATCC 13311), *Shigella sonnei* (ATCC 11060), *Klebsiella pneumoniae* (ATCC 13866), *Escherichia coli* (ATCC 10536), *Bacillus cereus* (ATCC 11778), and the yeasts *Candida albicans* (ATCC 18804) and *Cryptococcus neoformans* (ATCC 32608).

2.4.2 Serial dilution assay for determination of the minimal inhibitory concentration (MIC)

The MIC of each extract was determined by using the broth microdilution techniques for bacteria and yeasts, respectively (Bouzada et al., 2009; NCCLS, 2002). MIC values were determined in RPMI 1640 buffered to pH 7.0 with MOPS for yeasts and Mueller Hinton broth (MHB) for bacteria. Bacterial strains were cultured overnight at 37 °C in Mueller Hinton agar (MHA). Yeasts were cultured for 48 h at 30 °C in Sabouraud dextrose agar (SDA). Sample stock solutions were two-fold diluted from 500 to 2.0 μg/mL (final volume = 80 μL) and a final DMSO concentration ≤ 1%. Then, RPMI or MHB (100 μL) was added onto microplates. Finally, 20 μL of 10^6 CFU/mL (values of 0.08 - 0.10 at 625 nm, according to McFarland turbidity standards) of standardized yeasts and bacterial suspensions were inoculated onto microplates and the test was performed in a volume of 200 μL. Plates were incubated at 30 °C for 48 h for yeasts and at 37 °C for 24 h for bacteria. The same tests were performed simultaneously for growth control (RPMI + yeast and MHB + bacteria) and sterility control (RPMI or MHB + extract). The MIC values were calculated as the highest dilution showing complete inhibition of the tested strain. Chloramphenicol and Amphotericin B were used as reference drugs for bacteria and yeasts, respectively.

2.5 Phytochemical studies

A portion of each extract that was subjected for the biological screening was used for the identification of the major secondary metabolites employing the protocols described by Matos (1997). Briefly, the extract (1 mg/mL) was submitted to the following identification reactions: The characterization for tannins was performed by gelatin, iron salt and lead acetate reactions. Triterpenoids and sterols were investigated by Liebermann-Burchard reagent and the alkaloids analysis was done by precipitation reactions with the reagents of Dragendorff, Bouchardat, Mayer and Bertrand. For the research of flavonoids, the reactions of Shinoda and aluminum chloride were employed and the presence of saponins was determined by the formation of foam.

2.6 Statistical analysis

DPPH, reducing power and β-carotene/linoleic acid assays were carried out in triplicates. The results were expressed as mean ± standard deviation (SD). All statistical analysis were conducted using Graph Pad Prism software.

3. Results and discussion

The paper describes the antimicrobial and antioxidant activities and the phytochemical profile of some methanol extracts belonging to Brazilian traditional medicinal plants, most of them commonly used for treating conditions likely to be associated with microorganisms.

The major classes of phytocompounds of the bioactive extracts are presented in Table 2.

Plant species	Part tested[a]	Phytocompounds[b]					
		Al	Tr	St	Ta	Sa	Fl
Alternanthera brasiliana	AP	-	-	+	-	-	+
Allamanda cathartica	L	+	-	+	+	-	+
Acanthospermum australe	AP	+	-	+	+	+	+
Achillea millefolium	L	+	-	+	-	-	+
Anthemis cotula	L	-	+	-	-	-	+
Anthemis cotula	F	-	-	+	-	-	-
Baccharis trimera	AP	-	-	+	+	-	-
Bidens segetum	L	-	-	+	+	-	+
Carduus marianus	L	-	-	+	+	-	+
Matricaria chamomilla	L	+	+	-	+	-	+
Piptocarpha macropoda	L	+	+	-	+	-	+
Solidago chilensis	L	+	+	-	+	+	+
Vernonanthura divaricata	L	+	-	+	+	-	+
Stenolobium stans	L	+	-	+	+	-	+
Bixa orellana	L	+	-	+	+	+	+
Alchornea triplinervia	L	+	+	-	-	-	-
Acalypha brasiliensis	L	+	+	-	+	-	+
Chamaecrista desvauxii	L	+	+	-	+	-	+
Samanea tubulosa	L	+	+	-	+	-	+
Senna macranthera	L	+	-	+	+	-	+
Senna multijuga	F	+	+	-	+	-	+
Stylosanthes scabra	A	-	-	+	+	-	+
Casearia sylvestris	L	+	-	+	+	+	+
Vismia magnoliifolia	L	-	+	-	+	-	+

Plant species	Part tested[a]	Phytocompounds[b]					
		Al	Tr	St	Ta	Sa	Fl
Lacistema pubescens	L	-	+	-	+	-	+
Hyptis suaveolens	L	+	-	+	-	-	+
Ocimum basilicum	L	+	-	+	+	-	+
Peltodon radicans	L	-	+	-	-	-	+
Salvia officinalis	L	+	-	+	-	+	+
Nectandra rigida	L	-	+	-	+	-	+
Cuphea ingrata	AP	+	-	+	+	+	+
Byrsonima variabilis	L	+	+	-	+	+	+
Sida glaziovii	AP	-	-	+	-	+	+
Miconia latecrenata	L	+	-	+	-	+	+
Tibouchina grandifolia	L	+	+	-	+	-	+
Tibouchina granulosa	L	-	-	+	+	-	-
Tibouchina mutabilis	L	+	-	+	+	+	-
Eugenia cumini	L	+	+	-	-	-	+
Myrcia splendens	L	+	-	+	+	-	-
Piper corcovadensis	L	-	-	+	-	+	-
Eriobotrya japonica	L	+	-	+	-	-	+
Rubus rosifolius	L	+	-	+	+	+	+
Amaioua intermedia	L	-	+	-	-	-	+
Cupania oblongifolia	L	-	+	-	+	-	+
Sapindus saponaria	Fr	+	+	-	+	+	-
Solanum swartzianum	L	+	-	+	+	-	+
Tropaeolum majus	F	+	+	-	-	-	+
Turnera subulata	L	+	-	+	+	-	+
Cecropia pachystachya	L	+	+	-	+	-	+
Lippia pseudo-thea	L	+	+	-	+	+	+
Lippia hermannioides	L	+	+	-	+	-	+
Lippia alba	AP	+	-	+	+	+	+
Lippia rubella	AP	+	+	-	+	+	+
Lippia sidoides	AP	+	+	-	+	-	+
Lantana camara	L	-	-	+	+	-	+
Lantana camara	F	-	+	-	+	-	+
Aloysia floribunda	L	-	+	-	-	-	+
Cissus verticillata	L	+	-	+	-	-	+

[a]AP, Aerial Parts; F, Flowers; Fr, Fruits; L, Leaves. [b]Al, Alkaloids; Tr, Triterpenes; St, Sterols; Ta, Tannins; Sa, Saponins; Fl, Flavonoids

Table 2. Phytocompounds of methanol extracts of the active medicinal plants.

| Plant species | Part tested[a] | MIC (µg/mL)[b,c] | | | | | | | | |
		Sa	Pa	Bc	Ss	St	Ec	Kp	Ca	Cn
Alternanthera brasiliana	AP	-	-	-	-	-	-	-	39	-
Allamanda cathartica	L	-	-	-	-	-	-	-	39	-
Achantospermum australe	AP	-	-	-	-	-	-	-	39	-
Anthemis cotula	L	-	-	-	-	-	-	-	39	-
Anthemis cotula	F	-	-	-	-	156	-	-	39	-
Baccharis trimera	AP	-	-	-	-	-	-	-	-	39
Bidens segetum	L	-	156	156	5	156	-	-	-	-
Carduus marianus	L	-	-	-	-	-	-	-	39	-
Matricaria chamomilla	L	300	78	-	-	-	-	-	-	-
Piptocarpha macropoda	L	-	-	78	-	-	-	-	78	300
Solidago chilensis	L	-	-	-	-	-	-	-	39	-
Vernonanthura divaricata	L	-	-	-	-	-	-	-	-	156
Bixa orellana	L	-	-	-	-	-	-	-	156	-
Alchornea triplinervia	L	-	-	-	-	-	-	-	-	78
Acalypha brasiliensis	L	-	-	-	-	-	-	-	-	78
Chamaecrista desvauxii	L	5	5	-	5	78	-	300	-	-
Samanea tubulosa	L	39	39	39	-	-	-	-	300	156
Senna macranthera	L	-	-	156	300	156	-	-	-	-
Senna multijuga	F	300	78	39	156	78	300	39	-	20
Stylosanthes scabra	AP	-	2	39	5	-	-	-	-	-
Casearia sylvestris	L	-	-	-	-	-	-	-	-	-
Vismia magnoliifolia	L	-	-	-	39	-	-	-	300	156
Lacistema pubescens	L	-	-	-	39	-	-	-	-	-
Nectandra rigida	L	-	-	300	-	-	-	-	-	-
Cuphea ingrata	AP	-	-	39	-	-	-	-	39	-
Sida glaziovii	AP	-	-	-	-	-	-	-	39	-
Miconia latecrenata	L	-	-	-	-	-	-	-	-	300
Tibouchina grandifolia	L	5	-	-	-	300	-	-	-	-
Tibouchina granulosa	L	-	39	39	39	-	-	-	-	-
Eugenia cumini	L	-	-	-	-	-	-	-	-	39
Myrcia splendens	L	-	-	300	-	-	-	-	-	-
Piper corcovadensis	L	-	-	-	-	-	-	-	-	78
Rubus rasaefolius	L	-	-	-	-	-	-	-	39	-
Amaioua intermedia	L	-	-	-	-	-	-	-	-	78
Cupania oblongifolia	L	-	39	39	39	-	39	-	-	-
Sapindus saponaria	Fr	-	-	-	-	-	-	-	156	300
Solanum swartzianum	L	-	-	-	-	-	-	-	-	78
Tropaeolum majus	F	-	-	-	-	-	-	-	-	39
Turnera subulata	L	-	-	-	-	-	-	-	78	-
Cecropia pachystachya	L	-	-	-	-	-	-	-	-	39
Lippia pseudothea	L	-	-	156	-	-	-	-	-	-
Lippia hermannioides	L	-	-	78	-	-	-	-	-	-
Lippia sidoides	AP	-	-	78	-	-	-	-	-	-
Lantana camara	L	-	-	-	-	-	-	-	39	-
Lantana camara	F	-	-	-	-	-	-	-	39	-

Plant species	Part tested[a]	MIC (μg/mL)[b,c]								
		Sa	Pa	Bc	Ss	St	Ec	Kp	Ca	Cn
Aloysia floribunda	L	5	-	-	-	-	-	-	39	-
Cissus verticillata	L	-	-	-	-	-	-	-	-	156
Positive Controls										
Chloramphenicol		63	16	1.0	1.0	1.0	16	4.0		
Amphotericin B									0.08	0.04

[a]AP, Aerial Parts; F, Flowers; Fr, Fruits; L, Leaves

[b]Sa, *Staphylococcus aureus*; Pa, *Pseudomonas aeruginosa*; St, *Salmonella enterica* serovar Typhimurium; Ss, *Shigella sonnei*; Kp, *Klebsiella pneumoniae*; Ec, *Escherichia coli*; Bc, *Bacillis cereus*. [c]means MIC ≥ 300 μg/mL

Table 3. Antimicrobial activity of methanol extracts of the medicinal plants.

The results of the antimicrobial screening of the most active extracts are summarized in Table 3. The MIC values presented in this study for the extracts tested ranged from 300 to 5 μg/mL. All the extracts exhibited activity against at least one organism tested. According to Cos et al. (2006), plant extracts with MIC values below 100 μg/mL are very promising. So, *Bidens segetum*, *Chamaecrista desvauxii* and *Stylosanthes scabra* presented a very strong activity against *Shigella sonnei* with MIC of 5 μg/mL. *Chamaecrista desvauxii* and *Stylosanthes scabra* were also very active against *Pseudomonas aeruginosa* with MIC of 5 and 20 μg/mL, respectively. Against *Staphylococcus aureus*, the extracts of *Tibouchina grandifolia*, *Chamaecrista desvauxii* and *Aloysia floribunda* presented an outstanding activity with MIC of 5 μg/mL. On the other hand, *Senna multijuga* displayed a broader spectrum of antibacterial activity, showing activity against all bacteria tested with MIC values varying from 300 to 39 μg/mL (Table 3). Infections still cause about one-third of all deaths worldwide and are the leading cause of death, mainly because of disease in developing countries.

S. sonnei, a gram-negative bacterium, is a significant cause of gastroenteritis in both developing and industrialized countries (Boumghar-Bourtchai et al., 2008). People infected with *Shigella* develop diarrhoea, fever and stomach cramps starting a day or two after they are exposed to the bacterium. It is typically associated with mild self-limiting infection (DeLappe et al., 2003). Recently, there has been a rise in strains resistant to multiple antibiotics. *P. aeruginosa*, an increasingly prevalent opportunistic human pathogen, is the most common gram-negative bacterium found in nosocomial infections. Three of the more informative human diseases caused by *P. aeruginosa* are bacteremia in severe burn victims, chronic lung infection in cystic fibrosis patients, and acute ulcerative keratitis in users of extended-wear soft contact lenses (Lyczak et al., 2000). *S. aureus* is a gram-positive bacterium that commonly colonises human skin and mucosa (e.g. inside the nose) without causing any problems. However, if either of these is breached due to trauma or surgery, *S. aureus* can enter the underlying tissue, creating its characteristic local abscess lesion, and if it reaches the lymphatic channels or blood can cause septicaemia (Harris et al., 2002). Antifungal properties were presented by 35 extracts. Among them, *Acanthospermum australe*, *Sida glaziovii*, *Cuphea ingrata*, *Lantana camara*, *Allamanda cathartica*, *Anthemis cotula*, *Carduus marianus*, *Alternanthera brasiliana*, *Rubus rosifolius*, *Solidago chilensis*, and *Aloysia floribunda* demonstrated a strong anti-candida activity with MIC of 39 μg/mL. By the other side, extracts from *Cecropia pachystachya*, *Eugenia cumini*, *Baccharis trimera*, and *Tropaeolum majus* were active against *C. neoformans* with MIC values of 39 μg/mL, being *Senna multijuga* the most active with MIC of 20 μg/mL. Candidiasis is a common infection of the skin, oral cavity, esophagus, gastrointestinal tract, vagina and vascular system of humans. Although most infections occur in patients who are immunocompromised or debilitated in some other way, the organism most often responsible for disease, *Candida albicans*, expresses several virulence factors that contribute to pathogenesis (Calderone & Fonzi, 2001).*Cryptococcus neoformans* is an encapsulated basidiomycete yeast responsible for disseminated infections in immunosuppressed patients. Meningoencephalitis and pneumonia are the most frequent visceral presentations of the disease, but other rare presentations have been reported (Braga et al., 2007; Charlier-Woerther et al., 2011). Some of the most active species had already been studied for their antimicrobial effects elsewhere. The essential oil of different parts of *B. segetum* presented antifungal activity (Nascimento et al., 2008). Flavonoids isolated from the leaves of *T. grandifolia* demonstrated antifungal activity against the phytopathogenic fungus *Cladosporium cucumerinum* (Kuster et al., 2009). Dichlorometane extract of *A. australe* showed positive results against *Bacillus subtilis, Micrococcus luteus, Listeria monocytogenes* and *S. aureus* (Vivot et al., 2007). Antimicrobial efficacy of flavonoids and crude alkaloids of *L. camara* was found against *C. Albicans, Proteus mirabilis, S. aureus, E. coli,* and *Trichophyton mentagrophytes* (Sharma & Kumar, 2009). The iridoid isolated from *A. cathartica* presented fungitoxicity against some dermatophytes that causes dermatomycosis (Tiwari et al., 2002). The wound healing activity of this specie has also been tested, and it presented significant results in tests *in vivo* (Nayak et al., 2006). Flavonoids from *A. cotula* flowers showed interesting antimicrobial activity against both gram-negative and gram-positive microorganisms (Quarenghi et al., 2000). Quercetin isolated from the ethyl acetate extract of *A. brasiliana* presented antibacterial action against *S. aureus* (Silva et al., 2011). Antimicrobial activity of aqueous and hydroalchoolic fractions from *R. rosifolius* leaves showed activity against *E. coli, S. aureus, P. aeruginosa* and *C. albicans* (Mauro et al., 2002) and *B. trimera* was active against *S. aureus* and *E. coli* (Avancini et al., 2000). The antifungal activity of the leaf oil of *S. chilensis* was assayed by paper disk agar diffusion test and showed that human pathogenic dermatophytes were very sensitive (Vila et al., 2002). The crude hydroalcoholic extract of *S. cumini* was active against *Candida krusei* and against multi–resistant strains of *P. aeruginosa, K. pneumoniae* and *S. aureus* (de Oliveira et al., 2007). However, antimicrobial activity for *C. desvauxii, S. scabra, A. floribunda, S. multijuga, S. glaziovii, C. ingrata, C. marianus, C. pachystachya* and *T. majus* were reported here for the first time. Preliminary phytochemical analysis revealed that almost all the antimicrobial extracts showed flavonoids and tannins in their chemical composition (Table 2). Flavonoids are a broad class of plant phenolics that are known to possess antimicrobial activity, essentially by enzyme inhibition of DNA gyrase (Cushnie & Lamb, 2005). The mode of tannins antimicrobial action may be related to their ability to inactivate microbial adhesions, enzymes, cell envelope transport protein, etc. They also complex with polysaccharides (Ya et al., 1988). Condensed tannins have been determined to bind cell walls of ruminal bacteria, preventing growth and protease activity (Jones et al., 1994). However, the extracts tested also contain triterpenoids, sterols, saponins and alkaloids. Saponins are known to interact with cell membranes, increasing permeability and producing cell damage (Francis et al., 2002). In this sense, saponins may be involved in antimicrobial properties. The mechanism of action of some alkaloids is attributed to their ability to intercalate with DNA (Phillipson & O'Neill, 1989). The antimicrobial activity of triterpenes and sterols may be related to lipophilic components of plant extracts. This components increase permeability and loss of cellular components, and a change variety of enzyme systems, including those involved in the production of cellular energy and synthesis of structural components, inactivating or destroying genetic material (Bagamboula et al., 2004; Kim et al., 1995). The antioxidant hability of the extracts was also measured.

Natural antioxidants have been studied extensively for decades in order to find compounds protecting against a number of diseases related to oxidative stress and free radical-induced damage. Antioxidants are believed to play a very important role in the body defense system against reactive oxygen species (ROS), which are the harmful byproducts generated during normal cell aerobic respiration (Gutteridge & Halliwell, 2000). There is a number of assays designed to measure overall antioxidant activity/reducing potential, as an indication of host total capacity to withstand free radical stress. DPPH assay is very convenient for the screening of large numbers of samples of different polarity because of its high throughput. It evaluates the ability of antioxidants to scavenge free radicals. These antioxidants donate hydrogen to free radicals, leading to non-toxic species and therefore to inhibition of the propagation of lipid oxidation. Hydrogen-donating ability is an index of primary antioxidants (Lugasi et al., 1998). Among all extracts, 24 showed an outstanding antioxidant activity with $IC_{50} \leq 10$ µg/mL. *Cecropia pachystachya, Tibouchina mutabilis, Cupania oblongifolia,* and *Myrcia splendens* were the most active $(IC_{50} \leq 3$ µg/mL) (Table 4).

Plant species	Part tested[a]	DPPH (IC_{50} µg/mL ± SD)	Reducing power (EC_{50} µg/mL ± SD)	β-carotene/linoleic acid (% I ± SD)
Achillea millefolium	L	12.30 ± 1.16	14.86 ± 0.33	37.82 ± 8.70
Bidens segetum	L	6.52 ± 2.61	24.43 ± 0.06	67.67 ± 4.60
Stenolobium stans	L	7.45 ± 0.67	16.35 ± 0.30	41.98 ± 3.27
Bixa orellana	L	8.07 ± 0.71	23.42 ± 0.03	78.75 ± 3.30
Alchornea triplinervia	L	11.20 ± 1.09	> 53.64	60.69 ± 1.16
Hyptis suaveolens	L	11.70 ± 1.43	30.48 ± 0.34	51.42 ± 9.82
Ocimum basilicum	L	8.17 ± 1.46	14.66 ± 0.01	32.76 ± 11.20
Peltodon radicans	L	4.46 ± 1.32	23.23 ± 0.07	50.33 ± 14.30
Salvia officinalis	L	9.59 ± 0.50	19.44 ± 0.06	61.66 ± 2.80
Nectandra rigida	L	6.63 ± 0.63	13.19 ± 0.08	52.10 ± 12.10
Byrsonima variabilis	L	10.7 ± 2.47	33.71 ± 0.08	31.67 ± 1.80
Tibouchina granulosa	L	7.50 ± 0.42	10.05 ± 0.61	62.37 ± 3.17
Tibouchina mutabilis	L	1.56 ± 0.24	5.54 ± 0.10	69.05 ± 8.60
Myrcia splendens	L	2.90 ± 0.20	12.31 ± 0.38	49.34.±.2.31
Eriobotrya japonica	L	11.90 ± 0.87	13.98 ± 0.34	65.50 ± 2.00
Cupania oblongifolia	L	2.22 ± 0.10	6.29 ± 0.08	47.48 ± 4.8
Cecropia pachystachya	L	2.11 ± 0.40	7.70 ± 0.22	79.28 ± 2.80
Lippia hermannioides	L	3.99 ± 0.30	13.68 ± 0.42	54.90 ± 5.22
Lippia alba	AP	5.43 ± 0.34	14.40 ± 0.02	47.62 ± 27.50
Lippia rubella	AP	3.79 ± 0.27	10.27 ± 0.10	10.60 ± 5.60
Lantana camara	L	4.54 ± 0.26	14.04 ± 0.,02	55.03 ± 8.80
Lantana camara	F	9.82 ± 1.79	27.99 ± 0.07	61.84 ± 9.20
Amaioua intermedia	L	8.41 ± 1.22	12.22 ± 0.08	58.13 ± 0.70
Positive controls				
Ascorbic acid		1.80 ± 0.12	4.27 ± 0.06	
α-tocopherol		2.26 ± 0.14		
BHT		10.5 ± 1.06		
Quercetin		0.98 ± 0.20		91.52 ± 1.50
Rutin		2.52 ± 0.60		

[a]AP, Aerial Parts; F, Flowers; L, Leaves

Table 4. Antioxidant activity of methanol extracts of the selected medicinal plants.

The total antioxidant activity of the extracts is constituted by individual activities of each of the antioxidant compounds. Moreover, these compounds render their effects via different mechanisms such as radical scavenging, metal chelating activity, inhibition of lipid peroxidation, quenching of singlet oxygen, and so on to act as antioxidants. Even if a sample exhibits high activity with one method, it does not always show similar good results with all other methods. Therefore, it is essential to evaluate samples accurately by several methods. Hence, the antioxidant activity for those extracts was also evaluated by reducing power and β-carotene/linoleic acid assays. The reducing ability of a compound generally depends on the presence of reductants, which exhibited antioxidative potential by breaking the free radical chain, by donating a hydrogen atom. Antioxidant action of the reductones is based on the breaking of free radicals chain by the donation of a hydrogen atom. Reductones are believed not only to react directly with peroxides, but also prevent peroxide formation by reacting with certain precursors (Jamuna et al. 2010). The results found using this assay showed an outstanding antioxidant property of *C. pachystachya, T. mutabilis, C. oblongifolia,* and *M. splendens* and suggested that compounds present in those extracts were good electron and hydrogen donors, and could terminate the radical chain reaction by converting free radicals into more stable products. When employing β-carotene/linoleic acid assay, the more active inhibitors of β-carotene bleaching were *C. pachystachya, T. mutabilis* and *B. orellana* which showed values greater than 75% of inhibition. Interestingly, *C. oblongifolia* and *M. splendens* were not so effective in quenching β-carotene. It is well known that the value of this method appears to be limited to less polar compounds. They exhibit stronger antioxidative properties in emulsions because they concentrate at the lipid:air surface, thus ensuring high protection of the emulsion itself. On the other hand, polar antioxidants remaining in the aqueous phase are more diluted and are thus less effective in protecting the lipid (Koleva et al., 2002). It is well known that plants which possess antioxidative and pharmacological properties are related to the presence of phenolic compounds, specially phenolic acids and flavonoids (Fabri et al., 2009). Antioxidant activity had also been detected for *C. pachystachya* (Aragão et al., 2010) and *B. orellana* (Chisté et al., 2011). For *T. mutabilis, C. oblongifolia and M. splendens,* the antioxidant capacities were reported here for the first time. Polyphenolic compounds such as flavonoids and tannins found in the extracts (Table 2) are considered to be the major contributors to the antioxidant activity of medicinal plants. The antioxidant activities of polyphenols were attributed to their redox properties, which allow them to act as reducing agents, hydrogen donators and singlet oxygen quenchers, as well as their metal chelating abilities (Vladimir-Knezevic et al., 2011). It would seem that a great part of the extracts tested in this study for antimicrobial activity does not possess antioxidant effects (Table 3 and 4).

3. Conclusion

The results obtained represent a worthwhile expressive contribution to the characterization of antimicrobial and antioxidant activity of plant extracts of traditional medicinal plants from Brazilian flora and justify, in part, the popular uses of some of these species.

4. Acknowledgment

The authors are grateful to Fundação de Amparo a Pesquisa do Estado de Minas Gerais (FAPEMIG) and the Universidade Federal de Juiz de Fora (UFJF)/Brazil for financial support, to Dr. Fatima Regina Salimena for the botanical identification of the species, and to Delfino Antônio Campos for his technical assistance.

5. References

Albuquerque, J.M. (1989). Plantas medicinais de uso popular. Ministério da Educação, ABEAS, ISBN 85-85234-05-9, Brasília, Brazil

Alice, C.B.; Siqueira, N.C.S.; Mentz, L.A.; Silva, G.A.A.B. & José, K.F.D. (1995). Plantas Medicinais de Uso Popular. Atlas Farmacognóstico, Ulbra, ISBN: 85-8569212X, Canoas, Brazil

Andremont, A. (2001). The Future Control of Bacterial Resistance to Antimicrobial Agents. American Journal Infect Control, Vol.29, No. 4, (August 2001), pp. 256-258, ISSN 0196-6553

Aragão, D.M.O; Guarize, L.; Lanini, J.; Garcia, R.M.G. & Scio, E. (2010). Hypoglycemic Effects of *Cecropia pachystachya* in Normal and Alloxan-induced Diabetic Rats. Journal of Ethnopharmacology, Vol.128, No.3, (April 2010), pp. 629-633, ISSN 0378-8741

Avancini, C. A. M.; Wiest, J. M. & Mundstock, E. (2000). Atividade Bacteriostática e Bactericida do Decocto de Baccharis trimera (Less.) D.C., Compositae, Carqueja, como Desinfetante ou Anti-Séptico. Arquivo Brasileiro de Medicina Veterinária e Zootecnia, Vol.52, No.3, (June 2000), pp. 230-234, ISSN 1678-4162

Bagamboula, C. F.; Uyttendaele, M. & Debevere, J. (2004). Antimicrobial and Antioxidative Activities of the Essencial oils and Methanol Extracts of Salvia cryptanha (Montbret et Aucher ex Benth.) and Salvia multicaulis (Vahl.). Food Chemistry, Vol.84, No.4, (March 2004), pp. 519-525, ISSN 0308-8146

Benoit-Vical, F.; Grellier, P.; Abdoulaye, A.; Moussa, I.; Ousmane, A. & Berry, A. (2006). In vitro and in vivo Antiplasmodial Activity of Momordica balsamina Alone or in a Traditional Mixture. Chemotherapy, Vol.52, No.6, (September 2006), pp. 288-292, ISSN 1421-9794

Boumghar-Bourtchai, L.B.; Kurkdjian, P.M.; Bingen, E.; Filliol, I.; Dhalluin, A.; Ifrane,S.A.; Weill, F-X. & Leclercq, R. (2008). Macrolide-Resistant Shigella sonnei. Emerging Infectious Diseases, Vol.14, No.8, (August 2008), pp. 1297-1299, ISSN 1080-6040

Bouzada, M.L.M; Fabri, R.L.; Nogueira, M.; Konno, T.U.P.; Duarte, G.G. & Scio, E. (2009). Antibacterial, Cytotoxic and Phytochemical Screening of Some Traditional Medicinal Plants in Brazil. Pharmaceutical Biology, Vol.47, No.1, (January 2009), pp. 44-52, ISSN 1388-0209

Braga, F.C.; Bouzada, M.L.M.; Fabri, R.L.;. Matos, M.O.; Moreira, F.O.; Scio, E. & Coimbra, E.S. (2007). Antileishmanial and Antifungal Activity of Plants Used in Traditional Medicine in Brazil. *Journal of Ethnopharmacology*, Vol.111, No.2, (May 2007), pp. 396-402, ISSN 0378-8741

Calderone, R.A. & Fonzi, W.A. (2001). Virulence Factors of Candida albicans. Trends in Microbiology, Vol.9, No.7, (July 2001), pp. 327-335, ISSN 0966-842X

Chen, I.N.; Chen-Chin, C.; Chang-Chai, N.G.; Chung-Yi, W.; Yuan-Tay, S. & Tsu-Liang, C. (2008). Antioxidant and Antimicrobial Activity of Zingiberaceae Plants in Taiwan. Plant Foods for Human Nutrition, Vol.63, No.1, (December 2007), pp. 15-20, ISSN 0921-9668

Chisté, R.C.; Mercadante, A.Z.; Gomes, A.; Fernandes, E.; Lima, J.L.F.C. & Bragagnolo, N. (2011). In vitro Scavenging Capacity of Annatto Seed Extracts Against Reactive

Oxygen and Nitrogen Species. *Food Chemistry*, Vol.127, No.2, (July 2011), pp. 419-426, ISSN 0308-8146

Camargo, M.T.L.A. (1988). Plantas medicinais e de rituais afro-brasileiros, Almed, ISBN 85-274-0545-8, São Paulo, Brazil

Charlier-Woerther, C.C.; Fenoll, C.; Michel, C.B.; Valeyre, D.; Lortholary, O. & Masquelet, A.C. (2011). Cryptococcal myositis and Sarcoidosis. Lettres à la rédaction / Médicine et maladies infectieuses, Vol.41, No.5, (May 2011), pp. 267-272, ISSN 0399-077X

Corrêa, A.D; Siqueira-Batista, R. & Quintas, L.E.M. (1998). Plantas Medicinais: do Cultivo à Terapêutica, Vozes, ISBN 85-3261995-9, Petrópolis, Brazil

Corrêa, M.P. (1984). Dicionário de Plantas Úteis do Brasil e das Exóticas Cultivadas, Ministério da Agricultura, ISBN 9788573594218, Rio de Janeiro, Brazil

Cos, P.; Vlietinck, A.J.; Berghe, D.V. & Maes, L. (2006). Anti-infective Potential of Natural Products: How to Develop a Stronger in vitro 'Proof-of-Concept'. Journal of Ethnopharmacology, Vol.106, No.3, (July 2006), pp. 290-302, ISSN 0378-8741

Cushnie, T.P.T. & Lamb, A.J. (2005). Antimicrobial Activity of Flavonoids. *International Journal of Antimicrobial Agents*, Vol.26, No.5, (November 2005), pp. 343-356, ISSN 0924-8579

Dapkevicius, A.; Venskutonis, R.; Beek, T. A. & Linssen, P. H. (1998). Antioxidant Activity of Extracts Obtained by Different Isolation Procedures from Some Aromatic Herbs Grown in Lithuania. Journal of the Science of Food and Agriculture, Vol.77, No.1, (March 1999), pp. 140-146, ISSN 0022-5142

DeLappe, N.; O'Halloran, F.; Fanning, S.; Corbett-Feeney, G.; Cheasty, T. & Cormican, M. (2003). Antimicrobial Resistance and Genetic Diversity of Shigella sonnei Isolates from Western Ireland, an Area of Low Incidence of Infection. Journal of Clinical Microbiology, Vol.41, No.5, (May 2003), pp. 1919-1924, ISSN 0095-1137

Duarte-Almeida, J.M.; Santos, R.J Dos; Genovese, M.I. & Lajolo, F.M. (2006). Avaliação da Atividade Antioxidante Utilizando Sistema β -caroteno/Acido linoléico e Método de Seqüestro de Radicais DPPH•. Ciência e Tecnologia de Alimentos, Vol.26, No.2, (June 2006), pp. 446-452, ISSN 0101-2061

Duracková, Z. (2010). Some Current Insights into Oxidative Stress. Physiological Research, Vol.59, No.4, (November 2009), pp. 459-469, ISSN 0862-8408

Duraipiyan, V.; Ayyanar, M. & Ignacimuthu, S. (2006). Antimicrobial Activity of Some Ethnomedical Plants Used by Paliyar Tribe from Tamil Nadu, India. BMC Complementary and Alternative Medicine, Vol.6, No.35, (October 2006), pp. 1-7, ISSN 1472-6882

Fabri, R.L.; Nogueira, M.S.; Braga, F.G.; Coimbra, E.S. & E. Scio (2009). Mitracarpus frigidus Aerial Parts Exhibited potent Antimicrobial, Antileismanial and Antioxidant Effects. Bioresource Technology, Vol.100, No.1, (January 2009), pp. 428-433, ISSN 09608524

Francis, G.; Kerem, Z.; Makkar, H.P.S. & Becker, K. (2002). The Biological Action of Saponins in Animal Systems: a Review. British Journal of Nutrition, Vol.88, No.6, (December 2002), pp. 587-605, ISSN 0007-1145

Gonçalves, A.L.; Alves Filho, A. & Menezes, H. (2005). Estudo Comparativo da Atividade Antimicrobiana de Extratos de Algumas Árvores Nativas. Arquivos do Instituto Biológico, Vol.72, No.3, (September 2005), pp. 353-358, ISSN 0020-3653

Govidarajan, R.; Rastogi, S.; Vijayakumar, M.; Shirwaikar, A.; Rawat, A.K.S.; Mehrotra, S. & Pushpangadan, P. (2003). Studies on the Antioxidant Activities of Desmodium gangeticum. Biological & Pharmaceutical Bulletin, Vol.26, No.10, (October 2003), pp. 1424-1427, ISSN 1347-5217

Gutteridge, J. M. C. & Halliwell, B. (2000). Free Radicals and Antioxidants in the Year 2000 - A Historical Look to the Future. Annals of the New York Academy of Sciences, Vol.899, No.1, (January 2000), pp. 136-147, ISSN 0077-8923

Harris, L.G.; Foster, S.J. & Richards, R.G. (2002). An Introduction to Staphylococcus aureus and Techniques for Identifying and Quantifying S. aureus Adhesins in Relation to Adhesion to Biomaterials: Review. European Cells & Materials Journal, Vol.4, No.1, (December 2002), pp. 39-60, ISSN 1473-2262

Jamuna, K.S.; Ramesh, C.K.; Srinivasa, T.R. & Raghu, K.L. (2010). Comparative Studies on DPPH and Reducing Power Antioxidant Properties in Aqueous Extracts of some Common Fruits. Journal of Pharmacy Research, Vol.3, No.10, (September 2010), pp. 2378-2380, ISSN 0974-6943

Jones, G.A.; Mcallister, T.A.; Muir, A.D. & Cheng, K.J. (1994). Effects of Sainfoin (Onobrychis viciifolia Scop.) Condensed Tannins on Grotwn and Proteolysis by Four Strains of Ruminal Bacteria. Applied and Environmental Microbiology, Vol.60, No.4, (April 1994), pp. 1374-1378, ISSN 1098-5336

Kaur, G.J. & Arora, D.S. (2009). Antibacterial and Phytochemical Screening of Anethum graveolens, Foeniculum vulgare and Trachyspermum ammi. BMC Complementary and Alternative Medicine, Vol.9, No.30, (August 2009), pp. 1-10, ISSN 1472-6882

Kim, J.M.; Marshall, M.R.; Cornell, J.A.; Preston, J.F. & Wei, C.I. (1995). Antibacterial Activity of Carvacrol, Citral and Geraniol against Salmonella typhymurium in Culture Medium and on Frish Cubers. Journal of Food Science, Vol.60, No.6, (November 1995), pp. 1364-1368, ISSN 0022-1147

Koleva, I.I.; Beek Van, T.; Linssen, J.P.H.; Groot, A. & Evstatieva, L.N. (2002). Screening of Plant Extract for Antioxidant Activity: a Comparative Study on Three Testing Methods. Phytochemical Analysis, Vol.13, No.1, (January/February 2002), pp. 8-17, ISSN 1099-1565

Kuster, R.M.; Arnold, N. & Wessjohann, L. (2009). Anti-fungal flavonoids from Tibouchina grandifolia. Biochemical Systematics and Ecology, Vol.37, No.1, (February 2009), pp. 63-65, ISSN 0305-1978

Lorenzi, H. (2000). Plantas Daninhas do Brasil - Terrestres, Aquáticas, Parasitas e Tóxicas, Plantarum, ISBN 85-86714-27-6, São Paulo, Brazil

Lorenzi, H. & Matos, F.J.A. (2002). Plantas Medicinais no Brasil: Nativas e Exóticas Cultivadas, Plantarum, ISBN 85-86714-18-6, São Paulo, Brazil

Lu, Y.; Zhao, Y.P.; Wang, Z.C.; Chen, S.Y. & Fu, C.X. (2007). Composition and Antimicrobial Activity of the Essential Oil of Actinidia Macrosperma from China. Natural Product Research, Vol.21, No.3, (March 2007), pp. 227-233, ISSN 1478-6419

Lugasi, A.; Horvahovich, P. & Dworschák, E. (1999). Additional Information to the in vitro Antioxidant Activity of Ginkgo biloba L. Phytotherapy Research, Vol.13, No.2, (March 1999), pp. 160-162, ISSN 1099-1573

Lyczak, J.B.; Cannon, C.L. & Pier, G.B. (2000). Establishment of Pseudomonas aeruginosa Infection: Lessons from a Versatile Opportunist. Microbes and Infection, Vol.2, No.9, (July 2000), pp. 1051–1060, ISSN 1286-4579

Mahesh, B. & Satish, S. (2008). Antimicrobial Activity of Some Important Medicinal Plant against Plant and Human Pathogens. World Journal of Agricultural Sciences, Vol.4, No.4(S), pp. 839-843, ISSN 1817-3047

Matos, F.J.A. (1997). Introdução à Fitoquímica Experimental, EUFC, ISBN 85-7282-026-4, Fortaleza, Brazil

Matos, F.J.A. (2000). Plantas Medicinais - Guia de Seleção e Emprego de Plantas Usadas em Fitoterapia no Nordeste do Brasil, UFC, ISBN 85-7485008-X, Fortaleza, Brazil

Mauro, C.; Cardoso, C.M.Z.; Schultze, C.; Yamamichi, E.; Lopes, P.S.; Marcondes, E.M.C.; Miranda, J.P.; Arruda, D.A.O.; Frota, M. & Pacheco, A.L. (2002). Estudo Botânico, Fitoquímico e Avaliação da Atividade Antimicrobiana de Rubus rosaefolius Sm. - Rosaceae. Revista Brasileira de Farmacognosia, Vol.12, Suppl.1, pp. 23-25, ISSN 0102-695X

Mbwambo, Z.H.; Moshi, M.J.; Masimba, P.J.; Kapingu, M.C, & Nondo R,S. (2007). Antimicrobial Activity and Brine Shrimp Toxicity of Extracts of Terminalia brownii Roots and Stem. BMC Complementary and Alternative Medicine, Vol.7, No.9, (March 2007), pp. 1-5, ISSN 1472-6882

Moreira, D. L. & Guarim-Neto, G. (2009). Usos Múltiplos de Plantas do Cerrado: Um Estudo Etnobotânico na Comunidade Sítio Pindura, Rosário Oeste, Mato Grosso, Brasil. Polibotánica, No.27, (April, 2009), pp. 159-190, ISSN 1405-2768

Morim, M.P. (2010). Samanea, In: Lista de Espécies da Flora do Brasil, 05.27.2011. Available from: <http://floradobrasil.jbrj.gov.br/2010/FB023141>

N'guessan, J.D; Dinzedi, M.R.; Guessennd, N.; Coulibaly, A.; Dosso, M.; Djaman, A.J. & Guede-Guina, F. (2007). Antibacterial Activity of the Aqueous Extract of Thonningia sanguinea Against Extended-Spectrum-β- Lactamases (ESBL) Producing Escherichia coli and Klebsiella pneumoniae Strains. Tropical Journal of Pharmaceutical Research, Vol.6, No.3, (September 2007), pp. 779-783, ISSN 1596-5996

Nascimento, A.; Moreno, P.R.H; Souza. A. & Young, M.C.M. (2008). Chemical Composition and Antimicrobial Activity of the Essential oil from Bidens segetum Mart. Ex Colla Leaves, Flowers and Fruits. Planta Medica, Vol.74, No.9, (July 2008), pp. 1199-1199, ISSN 0032-0943

NCCLS (National Committee for Clinical Laboratory Standards) (2002). Reference Method for Broth Dilution Antifungal Susceptibility Testing of Yeasts. Approved Standard M27-A2 - P. National Committee for Clinical Laboratory Standards. Wayne, P.A.

Nayak, S.; Nalabothu, P.; Sandiford, S. & Bhogadi, V. (2006). Evaluation of Wound Healing Activity of Allamanda cathartica L. and Laurus nobilis. L. Extracts on Rats. BMC Complementary and Alternative Medicine, Vol.6, No.12, (April 2006), pp.1-6, ISSN 1472-6882

Newman, D.J. & Cragg, G.M. (2007). Natural Products as Sources of New Drugs Over the Last 25 Years. Journal of Natural Products, Vol.70, No.3, (March 2007), pp. 461-477, ISSN 0163-3864

de Oliveira, G.F.; Furtado, N.A.C.; Silva, A.A.; Martins, C.H.G.; Bastos, J.K.; Cunha, W.R. & Silva, M.L.D.E. (2007). Antimicrobial Activity of Syzygium cumini (Myrtaceae) Leaves Extract. Brazilian Journal of Microbiology, Vol.38, No.2, (June 2007), pp. 381-384, ISSN 1517-8382

Oyazu, M. (1986). Studies on Product of Browning Reaction Prepared from Glucose Amine. Japanese Journal of Nutrition, Vol.44, No.9, pp. 307-315, ISSN 0021-5147

Panizza, S. (1998). Plantas que Curam - Cheiro de Mato, Ibrasa, ISBN 85-3480067-7, São Paulo, Brazil

Phillipson, J.D. & O'Neil, M.J. (1989). New Leads to the Treatment of Protozoal Infections Based on Natural Product Molecules. Acta Pharmaceutica Nordica, Vol.1, No.1, pp. 131-144, ISSN 1100-1801

Quarenghi, M.V.; Tereschuk, M.L.; Baigori, M.D. & Abdala, L.R. (2000). Antimicrobial Activity of Flowers from Anthemis cotula. Fitoterapia, Vol.71, No.6, (December 2000), pp. 710-712, ISSN 0367-326X

Rayne, S. & Mazza, G. (2007). Biological Activities of Extracts from Sumac (Rhus spp.): A Review. Plant Foods for Human Nutrition, Vol.62, No.4, (August 2007), pp. 165-175 ISSN 0921-9668

Reuter, S.; Gupta, S.C.; Chaturvedi, M.M. & Aggarwal, B.B. (2010). Oxidative Stress, Inflammation, and Cancer: How are They Linked? Free Radical Biology & Medicine, Vol.49, No.11, (December 2010), pp. 1603-1616, ISSN 0891- 5849

Senatore, F.; Rigano, D.; Formisano, C.; Grassia, A.; Basile, A. & Sorbo, S. (2007). Phytogrowth-Inhibitory and Antibacterial Activity of Verbascum sinuatum. Fitoterapia, Vol.78, No.3, (April 2007), pp. 244-247, ISSN 0367-326X

Sharma, B. & Kumar, P. (2009). Bioefficacy of Lantana camara L. Against some Human Pathogens. Indian Journal of Pharmaceutical Sciences, Vol.71, No.5, (September - October 2009), pp. 589-593, ISSN 0250-474X

Silva, L.C.; Pegoraro, K.A.; Pereira, A.V.; Esmerino, L.A.; Cass, Q.B.; Barison, A. & Beltrame, F.L. (2011). Antimicrobial Activity of Alternanthera brasiliana Kuntze (Amaranthaceae): a Biomonitored Study. Latin American Journal of Pharmacy, Vol.30, No.1, (April 2010), pp. 147-153, ISSN 0326-2383

Singh, G.; Maurya, S.; de Lampasona, M.P. & Catalan, C.A. (2007). A Comparison of Chemical, Antioxidant and Antimicrobial Studies of Cinnamon Leaf and Bark Volatile Oils, Oleoresins and Their Constituents. Food and Chemical Toxicology, Vol.45, No.9, (September 2007), pp. 1650-1661, ISSN 0278-6915

Suffredini, I.B.; Sader, H.S.; Gonçalves, A.G.; Reis, A.O.; Gales, A.C.; Varellal, A.D. & Younes, R.N. (2004). Screening of Antibacterial Extracts from Plants Native to the Brazilian Amazon Rain Forest and Atlantic Forest. Brazilian Journal of Medical and Biological Research, Vol.37, No.3, (March 2004), pp. 379-384, ISSN 0100-879X

Tiwari, T. N.; Pandey, V. B. & Dubey, N. K. (2002). Plumieride from Allamanda cathartica as an Antidermatophytic Agent. Phytotherapy Research, Vol.16, No.4, (June 2002), pp. 393-394, ISSN 0951-418X

Vila, R.; Mundina, M.; Tomi, F.; Furlan, R.; Zacchino, S.; Casanova, J. & Caniguera, S. (2002). Composition and Antifungal Activity of the Essential Oil of Solidago chilensis. Planta Medica, Vol.68, No.2, (February 2002), pp. 164-167, ISSN 0032-0943

Vladimir-Knezević, S.; Blazeković, B.; Stefan, M.B.; Alegro, A.; Koszegi, T. & Petrik, J. (2011). Antioxidant Activities and Polyphenolic Contents of Three Selected Micromeria Species from Croatia. Molecules, Vol.16, No.2, (February 2011), pp. 1454-1470, ISSN 1420-3049

Vivot, E.; Massa, R; Cruanes, M.J.; Munoz, J,D.; Ferraro, G.; Gutkind, G. & Martino, V. (2007). In vitro Antimicrobial Activity of Six Native Species from Entre Rios Flora (Argentini). Latin American Journal of Pharmacy, Vol.26, No.4, (July - August 2007), pp. 563-566, ISSN 0326-2383

WHO (World Health Organization) (2002). Traditional Medicine - Growing Needs and
    Potential. World Health Organization Policy Perspectives on Medicines. Bulletin of
    the World Health Organization, Vol.80, No.2, (May 2002), pp.1-6, ISSN 0042-9686
Ya, C.; Gaffney, T.H. & Haslam, E. (1988). Carbohydrate-polyphenol complexation. In
    Chemistry and Significance of Condensed Tannins, R.M. Hemingway & J.J.Karchesy
    (Eds.), 553, Plenum Press, ISBN 0306433265, New York, USA

5

Phytochemical and Antibacterial Studies of the Hexane Extract of *Alchornea cordifolia* Leaf

G.O. Adeshina[1,*], O.F. Kunle[2], J.A. Onaolapo[1],
J.O. Ehinmidu[1] and L.E. Odama[3]
*[1]Department of Pharmaceutics and Pharmaceutical Microbiology,
Ahmadu Bello University, Zaria,
[2]Department of Medicinal Plant Research,
National Institute for Pharmaceutical Research and Development, Idu – Abuja,
[3]Department of Biological Sciences, Kogi State University, Anyingba,
Nigeria*

1. Introduction

Alchornea cordifolia (Schum. & Thonn.) Muel. Arg. (Euphorbiaceae) is also known as Agyama in Ghana, Susu bolonta in Sierra Leone, Casamance bugong in Senegal, Tschiya in Togo, Bondji in Cameroon, Ewe ipa, Ubobo and Bambami in Nigeria. It is geographically distributed in secondary forest usually near water, moist or marshy places and it grows to a considerable height but is always of a shrubby or scrambling habit.

The plant leaf extracts have been reportedly used in various African countries such as Senegal in the treatment of venereal diseases, conjunctivitis, dermatoses, stomach ulcers, bronchitis, cough, toothache (Le Grand and Wondergem, 1987; Le Grand, 1989). In Zaire it was used in the treatment of urinary tract infections, infected wounds, diarrhoea, cough, dental caries, chest pain and anaemia (Kambu *et al.*, 1990; Muanza *et al.*, 1994). In Sierra Leone it was used for diarrhoea and piles (Dalziel, 1956; Macfoy and Sama, 1990) and in Nigeria for gonorrhoea, yaws, rheumatic pain and cough (Gbile and Adeshina, 1986; Ogungbamila and Samuelson, 1990).

A variety of plants or materials derived from plants are been used for the prevention and treatment of diseases virtually in all cultures. The potential of herbal medicines and medicinal plant research results in health care is no longer in doubt, having gained recognition in several nations of the world and the World Health Organisation (WHO).

Secondary metabolites which constitute important source of the pharmaceutical preparations have been reportedly isolated from different parts of plants. Some of these compounds have been reported to be present in *A. cordifolia* such as flavonoids (Ogungbamila and Samuelson, 1990), alkaloids and tannins (GHP, 1992), inulin and alchornine (Abdullahi *et al.*, 2003).

This work tends to investigate the phytochemical components and antibacterial activities of hexane extract.

2. Materials and methods

2.1 Collection, identification and preparation of plant leaf

Alchornea cordifolia leaves were collected in October from Abuja, Nigeria. They were authenticated in the herbarium of the National Institute for Pharmaceutical Research and Development (NIPRD), Abuja, Nigeria where a voucher with specimen number 4334 was kept for future reference. The leaves were air-dried at room temperature and then reduced to powder using mortar and pestle.

2.2 Preparation of the extract and its derived fractions

Using the Soxhlet extractor, 300 gm of the powdered leaves was extracted with 450 ml of hexane at room temperature until all the extractable components were exhausted. The extract was concentrated, dried, weighed and kept in a dessicator until needed.

Hexane extract was analysed for chemical composition using the bioassay-guided fractionation by employing the Accelerated Gradient Chromatography (AGC) technique. Silical gel G (E-Merck, Germany) was used as an absorbent. Gradient elution was effected using hexane and ethyl acetate sequentially with increasing polarity. A total of 77 fractions were collected. The thin layer chromatography (TLC) analyses of the fractions were carried out using Whatman TLC plates of size 10 × 20 cm precoated with K5 silical gel 150A (Whatman Limited Maidstone, England). The chromatograms were developed using solvent mixture specific for separating alkaloid compounds especially hexane and ethyl acetate, 3:1. After development, the chromatograms were dried and detection was made using ultra-violet light at both wavelength 254 nm and 365 nm. Similar fractions were pooled together giving 33 fractions.

2.3 Phytochemical screening of the hexane extract

The extract was subjected to phytochemical analysis to detect the presence of the chemical constituents using standard protocol (Trease and Evans 1996).

2.4 Extraction of the secondary metabolites

Extraction of the secondary metabolites present in the hexane extract was also carried out using standard methods of Marcek (1972).

3. Antimicrobial activity

3.1 Purification of organisms

The organisms: *Pseudomonas aeruginosa* ATCC 10145, *Staphylococcus aureus* ATCC 12600 and *Escherichia coli* ATCC 11775 were collected from the Department of Pharmaceutical Microbiology, University of Benin, Benin City, Nigeria. While the clinical isolalates *Pseudomonas aeruginosa*, *Staphylococcus aureus*, *Escherichia coli* and *Proteus sp.* were from the

Staff Clinic, National Institute for Pharmaceutical Research and Development, Abuja, Nigeria. The organisms were confirmed by sub-culturing into Nutrient broth and incubated at 37ºC for 18 hours.

They were further streaked on the Nutrient agar and incubated at 37ºC for 18 hours. Biochemical tests were used to confirm the organisms. The organisms were kept on agar slants at 4ºC until needed.

3.2 Preparation of inoculums

Eighteen-hour broth culture of the test organism was suspended into sterile nutrient broth. It was standardized according to National Committee for Clinical Laboratory Standards (NCCLS, 2002) by gradually adding normal saline to compare its turbidity to McFarland standard of 0.5 which is approximately 1.0×10^6 cfu/ml.

3.3 Susceptibility testing

The washed overnight broth cultures were diluted appropriately using sterile normal saline to 0.5 McFarland scales (0.5 McFarland is about 10^6 cfu/ml). The molten sterile nutrient agar (20 ml) was poured into sterile petri dish and allowed to set. The sterile nutrient agar plate was flooded with 1.0 ml of the standardized test organism and the excess was drained off and dried at 30ºC for 1 hr. A sterile cork borer (No. 4) was used to bore equidistant cups into the agar plate. One drop of the molten agar was used to seal the bottom of the bored hole, so that the extract will not sip beneath the agar. 0.1ml of the different concentrations (0.625 – 20.0 mg/ml) of the extract was added to fill the bored holes. Negative control was prepared by putting 0.1 ml of pure solvent in one of bored hole and aqueous solution of 2 µg of Gentamicin (for Gram positive bacteria) and 4 µg of Gentamicin (for Gram negative bacteria) (Sweetman, 2005) in another bored hole which served as positive control. One hour pre-diffusion time was allowed, after which the plates were incubated at 37°C for 18 h. The zones of inhibition were then measured in millimeter. The above method was carried out in triplicates and the mean of the triplicate results was taken.

3.4 Minimum Inhibitory Concentration (M.I.C.) and Minimum Bactericidal Concentration (M. B. C.)

The M.I.C. was determined by agar dilution method. Ten millilitre (10 ml) volume of double strength melted Mueller-Hinton agar at 45°C was diluted with equal volume of the test extract in graded concentrations of 0.625 – 20.0 mg/ml. These were poured aseptically into sterile Petri dishes and dried at 37°C for 1 h with the lid slightly raised. The solidified leaf extract-agar admixture plates were inoculated with 2.0 µl of standardized 18 h culture test organism. The inocula were allowed to diffuse into the test agar plates for 30 min. The test agar plates were then incubated at 37°C for 18 h. The M.I.C. value was taken as the least concentration of the extract showing no detectable growth.

The M. B. C. was carried out by inoculating the concentration of the extract in the test agar plates showing no visible growth into sterile nutrient broth test-tubes containing inactivating agents 3% v/v Tween 80. These test-tubes were then incubated at 37°C for 24 h after which they were examined for presence or absence of growth.

3.5 Preliminary antimicrobial activity test of the various fractions from the hexane extract

Exactly 5.0 ml of 20.0 mg/ml of the fraction was incorporated into 5.0 ml molten double strength sterile nutrient agar kept at 45°C and poured into sterile Petri dishes and allowed to set. The test organism was streaked on the poured plate and incubated at 37°C for 24 hours after which the activity/no activity was observed.

4. Results

The hexane extract (HE) of *Alchornea cordifolia* leaves was brown in colour. There was a yield of 40.22% of the extract.

The phytochemical screening of the hexane extract of *A. cordifolia* leaf revealed the presence of tannins, alkaloids, flavonoids and phenol with tannins having the highest percentage yield of 6.8 (Table 1).

Secondary Metabolites	Yield (%)
Tannins	6.8
Alkaloids	5.9
Flavonoids	4.2
Phenol	3.2

Table 1. Percentage yield of the secondary metabolites from the hexane extract of *A. cordifolia* leaf.

The susceptibility of the bacteria species to the secondary metabolites of the plant showed that test *Staphylococcus aureus* was more susceptible to the secondary metabolites than the other bacteria species (Table 2). The zones of inhibition observed from tannins and saponin were larger than those from the other metabolites (Table 2).

Test bacteria species	Zones of inhibition (mm)			
	Tannin	Saponin	Alkaloids	Phenols
Ps.aeruginosa	24± 0.1	20± 0.2	16± 0.0	14± 0.0
Ps.aeruginosa ATCC 10145	21± 0.1	19± 0.1	18± 0.1	15 ± 0.1
Staph. aureus	26± 0.3	21 ± 0.1	20± 0.0	17± 0.2
Staph. aureus ATCC 12600	22 ± 0.1	18± 0.2	21± 0.1	16± 0.0
E.coli	19± 0.2	16± 0.2	16± 0.0	13± 0.1
E.coli ATCC 11775	15± 0.0	14 ± 0.2	12± 0.1	11± 0.3
Proteus sp.	20± 0.0	22± 0.3	17 ± 0.2	12 ± 0.1

Table 2. Susceptibility of the bacterial species to the secondary metabolites of the hexane extract of *A. cordifolia* leaf.

The clinical isolate of *Staphylococcus aureus* was more susceptible to the hexane extract of the plant leaf than the other bacterial species (Table 3).

The lowest Minimum Inhibitory Concentration of the hexane extract was found to be 2.5mg/ml against *Staph. aureus* and *Staph. aureus* ATCC 12600 (Table 4).

Test bacteria	Zones of Inhibition (mm)					
	20mg/ml	10mg/ml	5mg/ml	2.5mg/ml	1.25mg/ml	GTM
Ps.aeruginosa	13± 0.2	11± 0.1	NI	NI	NI	31 ± 0.0
Ps.aeruginosa ATCC 10145	11± 0.0	NI	NI	NI	NI	32 ± 0.2
Staph. aureus	23± 0.0	19± 0.1	18± 0.2	14± 0.2	NI	23± 0.0
Staph. aureus ATCC 12600	22± 0.2	17± 0.0	15± 0.1	12± 0.2	NI	25 ±0.1
E.coli	11± 0.2	NI	NI	NI	NI	20±0.2
E.coli ATCC 11775	16± 0.1	14± 0.3	11± 0.1	NI	NI	22±0.0
Proteus sp.	15± 0.2	13± 0.0	11± 0.1	NI	NI	21±0.0

The results are expressed as mean ± standard deviation, GTM = Gentamicin, NI = No Inhibition.

Table 3. Susceptibility of the bacterial species to different concentrations of the hexane extract of *A. cordifolia leaf*.

Test Bacteria	MIC (mg/ml)	MBC (mg/ml)
Ps. aeruginosa	20	NA
Ps.aeruginosa ATCC 10145	NA	NA
Staph. aureus	2.5	5
Staph. aureus ATCC 12600	2.5	5
E .coli	20	NA
E. coli ATCC 11775	10	20
Proteus sp.	10	20

Key: NA – No Activity

Table 4. M. I. C. and M. B. C. of the hexane extract against the test bacteria species.

Fractions	Ps. aeruginosa	Ps. aeruginosa ATCC 10145	Staph. aureus	Staph. aureus ATCC 12600	E. coli	E. coli ATCC 11775	Proteus sp.
HEF$_{1-17}$	-	-	-	-	-	-	-
HEF$_{18}$	-	-	IN	-	-	IN	IN
HEF$_{19}$	-	-	IN	-	-	IN	IN
HEF$_{20}$	-	-	IN	IN	-	IN	IN
HEF$_{21}$	+	+	+	+	-	-	-
HEF$_{22}$	-	-	IN	-	-	-	-
HEF$_{23}$	-	-	IN	-	-	-	-
HEF$_{24}$	-	-	IN	-	-	-	-
HEF$_{25}$	-	-	IN	-	-	-	-
HEF$_{26}$	IN	IN	IN	IN	-	-	-
HEF$_{27}$	+	+	+	+	IN	IN	IN
HEF$_{28}$	+	+	+	+	+	+	+
HEF$_{29}$	IN	IN	IN	IN	IN	IN	IN
HEF$_{30}$	+	+	+	+	+	+	+
HEF$_{31}$	+	+	-	-	-	-	-
HEF$_{32}$	-	-	IN	IN	-	-	-
HEF$_{33}$	-	-	-	-	+	+	+

KEY: - = No Activity, IN = Inhibitory or bacteristatic, + = Activity or bactericidal

Table 5. Antibacterial activity of fractions of hexane extract of *Alchornea cordifolia*.

The hexane extract fractions (HEF) $_{1-17}$ showed no antibacterial activity against any of the bacteria species while HEF_{29} had bacteristatic effect and HEF $_{28, 30}$ had bactericidal effect against all the bacteria species (Table 5).

5. Discussion

The results from the phytochemical screening of the hexane extract revealed the presence of tannins, saponins, alkaloids and phenol. Several plants which are rich in tannins have been shown to possess antibacterial activities against a number of microorganisms (Doss et al., 2009). Saponnins though are haemolytic on red blood cells, are harmless when taken orally and they have beneficial properties of lowering cholesterol levels in the body (Amos-Tautua et al., 2011). Alkaloids have been shown to possess both antibacterial (Erdemoglu et al., 2009) and antidiabetic (Costantino et al., 2003) activities. Phenols and phenolic compounds have been extensively used in disinfections and remain the standard with which other bactericides are compared (Uwumarongie et al., 2007).

The antibacterial activities exhibited by the secondary metabolites: tannins, saponins, alkaloids, and phenols extracted from the hexane extract of A. cordifolia leaf can be responsible for the antibacterial activity of the extract. The presence of secondary metabolites in plants have been reported to be responsible for their antibacterial properties (Rojas et al., 2006; Nikitina et al., 2007; Udobi et al., 2008; Rafael et al., 2009; Adeshina et al., 2010). The broad spectrum of antibacterial activity showed by the hexane extract against Gram positive and Gram negative bacteria can be attributed to the presence of the secondary metabolites. All the secondary metabolites showed more antibacterial activity against the gram-positive bacteria than the gram-negative bacteria. This is similar to the results of Adeshina (2005) who discovered that tannins, saponin, alkaloid and phenol from the leaf methanol, water and ethyl acetate extracts of Alchornea cordifolia had antibacterial activities against gram-positive bacterial strains more than gram-negative bacteria. Banso and Adeyemo (2007) also detected that tannins and alkaloids from Dichrostachys cinerea possessed antibacterial activities against gram-positive bacterial strains more than gram-negative bacteria.

The hexane extract appeared to be more active against the gram positive bacteria, Staph. aureus, than the Gram negative bacteria species. Gram negative bacteria are known to be resistant to the action of most antibacterial agents including plant based extracts and these have been reported by many workers (Kambezi and Afolayan, 2008; El-Mahmood, 2009). Gram negative bacteria have an outer phospholipids membrane with the structural lipopolysaccharide components, which make their cell wall impermeable to antimicrobial agents.

The bactericidal action of HEF_{28} and HEF_{30} against all the tested bacteria species can be an indication that these fractions possess the active ingredients responsible for antibacterial activity of the hexane extract of Alchornea cordifolia leaf. HEF_{21} and HEF_{27} displayed notable antibacterial activities against Staph. aureus and Pseudomonas aeruginosa that is of great importance because the infections cause by these bacteria are known to be difficult to control. Staphylococcus aureus has been reported by many workers to have developed resistance to most antibiotics and Pseudomonas aeruginosa is an opportunistic organism which has been reported to readily receive resistance carrying plasmid from other bacteria species (Wiley et al., 2008). HEF_{33} also showed noteworthy bactericidal action against the tested enteric bacteria-*E. coli* and *Proteus sp.* Enteric bacteria are known to transmit resistance plasmid among themselves (Brooks *et al.*, 2008) therefore developing resistance to many antibiotics. In view of all these observations, these fractions: HEF_{28}, HEF_{30}, HEF_{21}, HEF_{27} and HEF_{33} can further be worked on to get their structures and other necessary properties needed for formulation into newer antibiotics.

In conclusion, the hexane extract and fractions of *Alchornea cordifolia* leaf possess broad spectrum of antibacterial activity against the test bacteria species. Five out of the thirty-three fractions displayed potential antibacterial activity that can be explored as remedy for human bacterial infections. The results obtained from this work gives high hope for the development of new antibacterial agents.

6. References

[1] Abdullahi M, Mohammad G, Abdukadir NU. (2003). Medicinal and Economic Plants of Nupe Land, 1st edition, Jube-Evans Books and Publications, Bida, Nigeria. pp. 106-107.

[2] Adeshina GO, Onaolapo JA, Ehinmidu JO, Odama LE. (2010). Phytochemical and Antimicrobial Studies of the Ethyl Acetate Extract of *Alchornea cordifolia* Leaf found in Abuja, Nigeria. J. Med. Plants Res. 4(8): 649-658.

[3] Adeshina GO. (2005). Phytochemical and Antimicrobial Studies of the Leaf of *Alchornea cordifolia* (Schum. & Thonn.) Muell. Arg. (Euphorbiaceae). A Ph.D thesis of the Ahmadu Bello University, Zaria, Nigeria.

[4] Amos-Tautua, B.M.W., Angaye, S.S., Jonathan, G. (2011). Phytochemical Screening and Antimicrobial Activity of the Methanol and Chloroform Extracts of *Alchornea cordifolia*. J. Emerging Trends Engineer. App. Sci. 2(3): 445-447.

[5] Banso A, Adeyemi SO. (2007). Evaluation of Antibacterial Properties of Tannins Isolated from *Dichrostarchys cinerea*. Afr. J. Biotechnol. 6(15): 1785-1787.

[6] Brooks GF, Butel JS, Morse SA. (2004). Jawetz, Melnick and Adelberg's Medical Microbiology. 24th ed. Lange Med. Brooks/McGraw-Hill. pp. 203 - 642.

[7] Costantino L, Raimondi L, Pirisimo R, Brunetti T, Pessoto P, Giannessi F, Lins AP, Barlocco D, Antolini L, El-Abady, SA. Isolation and Pharmacological Activities of the *Tecoma stans* Alkaloids. 11 Farmaco 58(9): 781-785.

[8] Dalziel JM. (1956). The Useful Plants of West Tropical Africa, 3rd edition, Crown Agents for Oversea Government and Administration, Millbank, London. pp. 455.

[9] Doss A, Mohammed Mubarak H, DHanabalan R. (2009). Antibacterial Activity of Tannins from the leaves of *Solanum trilobatum* Linn. Indian J. Sci. Technol. 2(2): 41-43.

[10] El-Mahmood AM. (2009). Antibacterial activity of crude extracts of *Euphorbia hirta* against some bacteria associated with enteric infections, J. Med. Plants Res. 3(7):498-505.

[11] Erdemoglu N, Ozkan S, Tosun F. (2007). Alkaloid Profile and Antimicrobial Activity of *Lupirius angustifolius* L. Alkaloid Extract . Phytochem. Reviews. 6(1): 197-201.

[12] Gbile ZO, Adeshina SK. (1986). Nigerian Flora and its Pharmaceutical Potentials, Mediconsult, 31:7-16.

[13] Ghana Herbal Pharmacopoiea. (1992). Alchornea, 1st edition, The advent Press, Accra, pp. 7-8.

[14] Kambezi L. Afolayan, AJ. (2008). Extracts from *Aloe ferox* and *Withania somnifera* inhibit *Candida. Albicans* and *Neisseria gonorrhea*. Afr. J. Biotechnol. 7 (1):012-015.

[15] Kambu K, Tona L, Kaba S, Cimanga K, Mukala N. (1990). Antispasmodic Activity of Extracts Proceeding of Plant, Antidiarrhoeic Traditional Preparations used in Kinshasa, Zaire, Ann Pharm FR. 48(4):200-208.

[16] Le Grand A, Wondergem PA. (1987). Antiinfective Phytotherapy of the Savannah Forests of Senegal (East Africa), An Inventory, J. Ethnopharmacol. 21(2):109-125.

[17] Le Grand A. (1989). Anti-infectious Phytotherapy of the Tree-Savannah, Senegal (West Africa) III; A Review of the Phytochemical Substances and Anti-microbial Activity of 43 Species, J. Ethnopharmacol. 25(3):315-338.

[18] Macfoy CA, Sama AM.(1990). Medicinal Plants in Pujehun District of Sierra Leone, J. Ethnopharmacol. 30(3):610-632.

[19] Marcek K. (1972). Pharmaceutical Application of Thin Layer and Paper Chromatography, 2nd edition, Elsevier Publishing Company, London, pp. 357-369.

[20] Muanza DN, Kim BW, Euter KL, Williams L. (1994). Antibacterial and Antifungal Activities of Nine Medicinal Plants from Zaire, Int. J. Pharmacog. 32(4):337-345.

[21] National Committee for Clinical Laboratory Standard (2002). Performance Standard for Antimicrobial Disc Susceptibility Testing. Twelfth International Supplement. Approved standard M100-S12. National Committee for Clinical Laboratory Standards, Wayne, Pa.

[22] Nikitina VS, Kuz`mina LYu, Melentíev AL, Shendel GV. (2007). Antibacterial activity of Polyphenolic Compounds Isolated from Plants of Geraniaceae and Rosaceae families. Appl. Biochem. Microbiol. 43(6): 629 - 634.

[23] Ogungbamila FO, Samuelsson G. (1990). Smooth Muscle Relaxing Flavonoids from *Alchornea cordifolia*. Acta. Pharm. Nordica. 2(6): 421- 422.

[24] Rafael L, Teresinha N, Moritz JC, Maria IG, Eduardo MD, Tania SF. (2009). Evaluation of Antimicrobial and Antiplatelet Aggregation Effect of *Solidago chilensis* eyen. Int. J. Green Pharm. 3: 35 – 39.

[25] Rojas JJ, Ochoa VJ, Ocampo SA, Muñoz J. (2006). Screening for Antimicrobial Activity of Ten Medicinal Plants Used in Colombian Folkloric Medicine: A Possible Alternative in the Treatment of Non-nosocomial Infections. BMC Complementary Altern. Med. 6: 2.

[26] Sweetman, S. (2005). Sweetman S (Ed), Martindale: The Complete Drug Reference. London: Pharmaceutical Press. Electronic version.

[27] Trease EG, Evans WC. (1993).Textbook of Pharmacognosy. 3 rd ed. London: Bailliere Tindal; 1993. p. 81-90, 268-98.

[28] Udobi CE, Onaolapo JA, Agunu A. (2008). Antibacterial Activities and Bioactive Components of the Aqueous Fraction of the Stem Bark of *Parkia bigblobosa* (JACQ) (Mimosaceae). Nig. J. Pharm. Sci. 7(1): 49-55.

[29] Uwumarongie, OH., Obasuyi,O and Uwumarongie, EG (2007). Phytochemical Analysis and Antimicrobial Screening of the Root of Jatropha tanjorensis. Chem. Tech. J. 3: 445-448.

[30] Wiley JM, Sherwood LM, Woolverton CJ. (2008). Presscott, Harley and Klein's Microbiology. 7th ed. McGraw-Hill Companies, Inc; pp. 859-882.

6

Antioxidant Activity of European Mistletoe (*Viscum album*)

Simona Ioana Vicas[1], Dumitrita Rugina[2] and Carmen Socaciu[2]
[1]University of Oradea, Faculty of Environmental Protection, Oradea
[2]University of Agricultural Sciences and Veterinary Medicine,
Department of Chemistry and Biochemistry, Cluj-Napoca,
Romania

1. Introduction

European mistletoe (*Viscum album L.*) is an evergreen, hemi-parasitic plant, normally found growing on a variety of trees, especially pine, poplar, apple trees, locus trees etc. Although there are many varieties of mistletoe, including the American (*Phorandendron serotinum* or *Phorandendron flavescens*), the European (*Viscum album L.*), and the Korean (*Viscum album L. coloratum*), most investigative work has been done on European mistletoe.

Traditionally, the genus *Viscum*, has been placed in its own family *Viscaceae*, but recent genetic research by APG II (The Angiosperm Phylogeny Group, 2003) system shows this family to be correctly placed within family Santalaceae (Fig. 1).

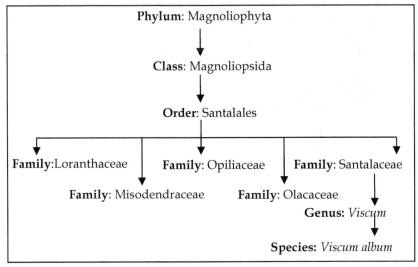

Fig. 1. Scientific classification of species *Viscum album* (according to APG II system).

Different species of *Viscum* are capable of parasitizing a large number of host species. From a review of literature, Barney et al., 1998, identified 452 host species of *Viscum album* (96 genera and 44 families). For *V. album* ssp. *album* 190 hosts have been identified, for *V. album* ssp. *abieties* 10 hosts, and for *V. album* ssp. *austriacum* 16 hosts are known (Zuber, 2004).

The genus *Viscum* are woody hemi-parasitic shrubs with branches 15–80 cm long, which grow on different host trees. Mistletoe tend to form a globular shape (Fig. 2, a) which may reach over 1 m in diameter. The foliage is dichotomously or verticillately branching, with opposite pairs of green leaves (Fig 2, c and d) which perform some photosynthesis (minimal in some species, notably *V. nudum*), but with the plant drawing its mineral and water needs from the host tree. The leaves are narrowly obovate (Fig. 2, b), approximatelly three or four times as long than broad. The color of leaves are dark green, and present three distinct veins and two less distinct veins running parallel to the leaf margin (Fig. 2, b). In young leaves, the veins are visible on both sides, while in older leaves they are mainly seen on the underside (Büssing, 2000). *V. album* is dioecious, i.e. part of the plants is female, the other part is male. Flowers are highly reduced and inconspicuous, greenish-yellow color, and 1–3 mm diameter (Fig. 2, c). The fruit is a berry, white, when mature, containing one seed embedded in very sticky juice (Fig. 2, e).

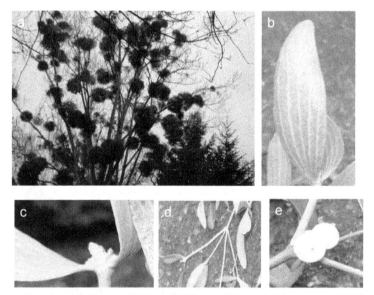

Fig. 2. *Viscum album* morphology. a. Image of *Viscum album* growing on poplar (*Populus nigra*); b. Aspect of leave; c. The flower of mistletoe; d. Stem branched; e. Adult berry containing one seed (Vicas et al., 2009a).

In recent years, antioxidants derived from natural resources, mainly from plants, have been intensively used to prevent oxidative damages. Natural antioxidants have also some advantages over synthetic ones, being obtained easily and economically and have slight or negligible side effects.

Aqueous extracts of the European mistletoe have been widely used for decades as alternative treatment and adjuvant cancer therapy, particularly in Germany, Austria and Switzerland. The European mistletoe extracts are used in an adjuvant cancer therapy because of their immunostimulatory and simultaneously cytotoxic properties. These effects are usually more evidence for the whole extracts than for purified mistletoe lectins and viscotoxins alone (Eggenschwiler et al., 2007).

Different mistletoe preparations are available for the treatment of cancer. Abnobaviscum®, Helixor, Iscador®, Iscucin® and Isorel® are produced according to anthroposophical methods; other mistletoe preparations include Cefalektin®, Eurixor® and Lektinol®. Iscador was first proposed for the treatment of cancer in 1920, by Rudolf Steiner, PhD, (1861-1925), founder of the Society for Cancer Research, in Arlesheim, Switzerland and introduced in the treatment of human cancer as early as 1921. The anthroposophical preparations are available from different host trees such as oak, apple, pine and others. Harvesting procedure is standardized, and the juices from summer and winter harvests are mixed together. The total extract of mistletoe extracts is considered essential for full effectiveness and concentration of its compounds is ensured through process standardization (http://wissenschaft.mistel-therapie.de/- Mistletoe in cancer treatment).

Mistletoe can biosynthesize their own compounds, but it can take some nutrients from the host trees. It has been suggested that pharmacologically active compounds may pass from the host trees to the parasitic plants (Büssing and Schietzel., 1999).

The main ingredients of the *Viscum album* extract are its three ribosome inactivating proteins or lectins (mistletoe lectins, ML) ML-1, ML-2, and ML-3 (Hajtó et al., 2005), the glycoprotein binding with D-galactose and N-acetyl-D-galactosamine, viscotoxins (VT) (Urech et al., 2006), as well as, oligo- and polysaccharides, alkaloids (Khwaja et al., 1980). The flavonoid patterns of *V. album* from various hosts were investigate by Becker and Exner (1980). They identified quercetin and a series of quercetin methyl ethers, which may be assumed to be accumulated on the plant surface. The epicuticular material of the *V. album* contains preferably the flavonol quercetin and its methyl derivatives, occasionally also the flavonol kaempferol and some of its methyl derivatives, and rarely the flavanone naringenin (Haas et al., 2003).

It has been suggested that pharmacologically active compounds may pass from the host trees to the parasitic plants (Büssing and Schietzel., 1999).

In recent years, the research studies were focused on the antioxidant activity of mistletoe (Onay-Ucar et al. 2006; Leu et al., 2006; Yao et al., 2006; Shi et. al., 2006; Vicas et al., 2009b; Choudhary et al., 2010).

Many plant extracts exhibit efficient antioxidant properties due their phytoconstituents, such as phenolics, especially phenolic acids and flavonoids (Aqil *et al.*, 2006; Miliauskas *et al.*, 2004) and carotenoids (Stahl and Sies, 2003).

To evaluate the antioxidant capacities of plant extracts, numerous *in vitro* methods have been developed. DPPH (2,2-diphenyl-1-picrylhydrazyl), ORAC (oxygen radical absorbance capacity), Trolox equivalent antioxidant capacity (TEAC), and ferric-reducing ability (FRAP) are among the more popular methods that have been used (Wu *et al.*, 2004). The advantages and disadvantages of these methods have been fully discussed in several reviews (Cao and Prior, 1998; Frankel and Meyer, 2000; Prior and Cao, 1999; Sánchez-Moreno, 2002).

The aim of our research studies are focused, the first, on screening of bioactive compounds (phenolic acid and flavonoids) from leaves and stems of *V. album* that are growing on different host trees, and the second we evaluated the antioxidant activity of *V. album'* leaves and stems.

2. HPLC fingerprint of bioactive compounds from *Viscum album*

To analyze the bioactive compounds, leaves and stems of *V.album* were harvested in July 2009, from five different host trees located in the Borod-Gheghie region, North-West of Romania country. The mean annual rainfall is 500-700 mm/an. The mean annual minimum and maximum temperatures were -22.3⁰C and 35⁰C, respectively (20-yr averages). The mean annual air temperature is 9.2 ⁰C. The area is opened to West, the frequent air mass is oriented to western circulation, transporting oceanic air, cold and humid. Multi-annual average wind speed is 4.1 m/sec. The mistletoe samples have been harvested at the approximate same height, the trees where from it has been harvested having the same soil (brown soil) and climate conditions. The host trees were located in semi-shaded to sunny area (Vicas et al., 2010). The plant materials were labeled according to the host trees, thus: *Acer campestre* (VAA), *Mallus domestica* (VAM), *Fraxinus excelsior* (VAF), *Populus nigra* (VAP) and *Robinia pseudoacacia* (VAR) for easy identification. A voucher specimen of the plants was deposited in the herbarium of the Environmental Protection Faculty from University of Oradea.

The leaves and stems of *V. album* from different host trees were dried rapidly, in an oven at 90⁰C, for 48 hours, in order to prevent enzymatic degradation (Markham, 1982). The dried plant material was stored in a sealed plastic bag for HPLC analysis. After weighing out a portion of the dried material (approximately 1 g), extraction was carried out with ethanol 70% (1:10, w/v). The mixture was stirred for 24 hours in the dark, and then it was centrifuged for 5 minutes, at 3000 rpm. The ethanol fraction of the supernatant was removed using a rotary evaporator. Further, the aqueous extract was subjected to acid hydrolysis (1N HCl) for 2 hours, at 80⁰C. The aglycones were extracted 3 times with ethyl acetate by continuous stirring and then centrifuged at 5000 rpm, for 5 minutes. The solvent was removed by flushing the samples with nitrogen. The residue resulting after evaporation was dissolved in ultrapure water (300 μl), filtered throught 0.45 μm filters (Millex-LG, Millipore), and subjected to HPLC analysis.

A Shimadzu HPLC system equipped with a LC20AT binary pump, a degaser, a SPD-M20A diode array detector (Shimadzu Corp., Kyoto, Japan) and a SUPELCOSIL ™ LC-18 column (Sigma-Aldrich Co), 5μm, 25 cm x 4.6 mm was used. Gradient elution was performed with mobile phase A, composed of methanol: acetic acid: double distilled water (10:2:88 v/v/v) and mobile phase B, comprising methanol: acetic acid: double distilled water (90:3:7 v/v/v), at a flow rate of 1.0 ml/min. All solvents were HPLC grade solvents, filtered through a 0.45-μM membrane (Millipore, U.S.A.) and degassed in an ultrasonic bath before use. The chromatograms were monitored at 280 and 360 nm. The following pure standards were used to quantify the bioactive compounds in the leaves and stems of mistletoe: betulinic acid, gallic acid, protocatechuic acid, gentisic acid, chlorogenic acid, p-OH benzoic acid, caffeic acid, syringic acid, salicilyc acid, p-coumaric acid, ferulic acid, sinapic acid, trans-cinamic acid, naringenin, quercetin, kaempherol and rosmarinic acid. The quantification was made by comparison to calibration curves with pure standards, in the range 0.48 to 500.0 μg/ml. The regression coeficients of calibration curves ranged between 0.9812 and 0.9999. Integration and data analysis were made using Origin 7.0 software.

Quantitative data regarding the phenolic compounds composition of mistletoe extracts are shown in Tab. 1.

We identified and quantified 17 compounds from mistletoe samples (Tab. 1), including a pentacyclic triterpene (betulinic acid), 12 phenolic acids (gallic acid, protocatechuic acid, gentisic acid, chlorogenic acid, p-OH benzoic acid, caffeic acid, syringic acid, salicilyc acid, p-coumaric acid, ferulic acid, sinapic acid, and trans-cinamic acid) and 4 polyphenols (naringenin, quercetin, kaempherol and rosmarinic acid). The Fig. 3 presents the chemical structure of bioactive compounds investigated.

These compounds were identified according to their retention time and the spectral characteristics of their peaks compared with standards, as well as by spiking the sample with individual standards. Phenolic compounds are found usually in nature as esters and rarely as glycosides or in free form. Thus, hydrolysis was needed for their identification and quantitative determination. Flavonoids are also present in plants in the form of glycosides. Each flavonoid may occur in a plant in several glycosidic combinations. For this reason, hydrolysis was used to release the aglycones which were further investigated by HPLC.

Quantitative HPLC analysis of *V. album* showed a higher content of bioactive compounds in the leaves compared with stems (Tab. 1). In the case of leaves from *V. album* hosted by *Acer campestre* (VAA), seven phenolic acids and three polyphenols were identified, while in the stem of mistletoe we found only one phenolic acid (trans-cinnamic acid). Caffeic acid was the dominant compound (13.61 μg/g dry matter) in the leaves of mistletoe. Kampherol and rosmarinic acid were presented in both, leaves and stems, while quercetin was identified only in leaves.

The mistletoe hosted by *Fraxinus excelsior* (VAF) contains nine phenolic acids, and two flavonoids. HPLC chromatograms of phenolic acids from leaves and stems of *Viscum album* hosted by *Fraxinus excelsior* are presented in Fig. 4. Concentration of para-coumaric acid in the VAF sample was 1.82 μg/g dry matter, but we have not identified it in other mistletoe extracts. Caffeic acid was found to have the higest values both in leaves (13.98 μg/g dry matter) and stems (15.86 μg/g dry matter). Kaempherol was also present both in leaves (7.30 μg/g dry matter) and stems (3.66 μg/g dry matter), while quercetin was present only in leaves (6.05 μg/g dry matter).

In case of *V. album* collected from *Populus nigra* (VAP), ferrulic acid was a dominant compound in the set of phenolic acids both in leaves (11.52 μg/g dry matter) and in stems (6.14 μg/g dry matter). Salycilic acid was also present in VAP leaves (8.4 μg/g dry matter) and stems (2.3 μg/g dry matter), while in the other mistletoe samples it was detected only in leaves.

The HPLC chromatogram of mistletoe hosted by *Mallus domestica* (VAM) showed seven phenolic acids in leaves. Betulinic acid was present only in this mistletoe, both in leaves (1.87 μg/g dry matter) and stems (2.05 μg/g dry matter). Also, like in mistletoe hosted by *P.*

COMP. NO.	BIOACTIVE COMPOUNDS	VAA *Acer campestre*		VAF *Fraxinus excelsior*		VAP *Populus nigra*		VAM *Mallus domestica*		VAR *Robinia pseudocacia*	
		leaves	stems	leaves	stems	leaves	stems	leaves	stems	leaves	stems
Pentacyclic triterpene											
1.	Betulinic acid	nd	nd	nd	2.35 ±0.03	nd	nd	1.87 ±0.20	2.05 ±0.05	nd	nd
Phenolic acids											
2.	Gallic acid	nd	nd	nd	nd	nd	nd	nd	nd	39.93 ±0.4	nd
3.	Protocatechuic acid	nd	nd	5.06 ±0.03	3.87 ±0.01	2.58 ±0.01	0.45 ±0.01	4.10 ±0.32	nd	nd	2.01 ±0.2
4.	Gentisic acid	nd	nd	nd	nd	nd	nd	nd	nd	nd	nd
5.	Chlorogenic acid	4.70 ±0.01	nd	2.74 ±0.02	1.27 ±0.2	nd	nd	nd	nd	nd	nd
6.	para-OH benzoic acid	10.16 ±0.1	nd	10.81 ±0.02	nd	1.25 ±0.02	nd	1.02 ±0.11	nd	nd	nd
7.	Cafeic Acid	13.61 ±0.04	nd	13.98 ±0.01	15.86 ±0.03	nd	5.34± 0.03	6.39 ±0.23	6.81 ±0.004	nd	nd
8.	Syringic acid	nd	nd	1.11 ±0.04	12.13 ±0.01	nd	nd	nd	1.32 ±0.02	nd	nd
9.	Salicilyc acid	6.70 ±0.03	nd	2.70 ±0.03	nd	8.4 ±0.01	2.3 ±0.05	1.80 ±0.01	nd	nd	nd
10.	para-coumaric acid	nd	nd	1.82 ±0.001	nd	nd	nd	nd	nd	nd	nd
11.	Ferulic acid	7.58 ±0.001	nd	8.99 ±0.02	8.06 ±0.02	11.52 ±0.1	6.14 ±0.11	7.81 ±0.01	6.88 ±0.01	9.93 ±0.01	nd
12.	Sinapic acid	5.41 ±0.3	nd	12.35 ±0.01	4.82 ±0.04	7.17 ±0.3	nd	2.11 ±0.02	1.13 ±0.01	19.32 ±0.01	nd
13.	Trans-cinnamic acid	5.41 ±0.04	1.23 ±0.03	nd	3.07 ±0.05	nd	nd	nd	nd	nd	nd
Flavonoids											
14.	Naringenin	nd	nd	nd	nd	nd	nd	nd	nd	nd	nd
15.	Quercetin	0.93 ±0.01	nd	6.05 ±0.02	nd	3.25 ±0.01	nd	0.36 ±0.02	nd	7.90 ±0.01	nd
16.	Kampherol	2.74 ±0.01	3.32±0. 001	7.30 ±0.01	3.66 ±0.01	nd	nd	nd	nd	7.58 ±0.01	6.38 ±0.01
Polyphenol											
17.	Rosmarinic acid	1.94 ±0.002	1.81	nd	1.27 ±0.01	0.8 ±0.2	2.0 ±0.001	1.12 ±0.01	1.08 ±0.02	nd	nd
	Total phenolic acids	53.57	1.23	59.56	49.08	30.92	14.23	23.23	16.14	69.18	2.01
	Ratio leaves/stems of phenolic acid	43.51:1		1.2:1		2.2 : 1		1.4:1		34.4:1	
	Total phenolic acid (leaves +stem)	54.80		108.64		45.15		39.37		71.19	
	Total flavonoids (leaves +stem)	6.99		17.01		3.25		0.36		21.86	

Table 1. Quantitative HPLC analysis of bioactive aglicones of phenolics (μg/g dry matter*) from leaves and stems of *V. album* harvested from different hosts, on July 2009 (Vicas et al.,2011a).

nigra, ferulic acid was the main compound in leaves and stems (7.81 µg/g dry matter, and 6.88 µg/g dry matter, respectively) of VAM samples.

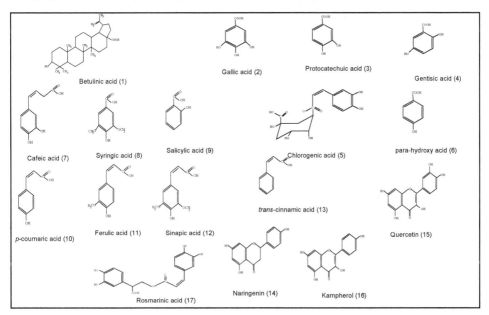

Fig. 3. Bioactive compounds investigated in the leaves and stem of *V.album*.

The main compound in *V. album* hosted by *Robinia pseudoacacia* (VAR) was gallic acid (39.93 µg/g dry matter), which has not been found in the other samples studied.

We did not detect gentisic acid in any sample, nor naringenin, while quercetin was identified only in stems.

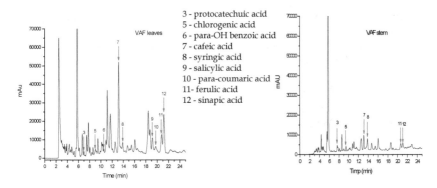

Fig. 4. HPLC chromatograms, used to fingerprint and evaluate quantitatively phenolic acids from leaves and stems of *V.album* harvested from *Fraxinus excelsior* (VAF) (Vicas et al., 2011a).

Phenolic acids represent the major fraction of bioactive compounds in all *V. album*. A high variability of phenolic acid rations between leaves and stems was observed. While, VAA and VAR had high ratios (43.51:1 and 34.41:1, respectively) the lowest ratios were observed in the case of VAF and VAM (1.21:1 and 1.44:1, respectively).

In our study, the mistletoe hosted by *Fraxinus excelsior* (VAF) proved to be the richest in phenolic acids (108.64 µg/g dry matter), followed by VAR (71.19 µg/g dry matter), VAA (54.80 µg/g dry matter), VAP (45.15 µg/g dry matter) and VAM (39.37 µg/g dry matter).

The total polyphenols from leaves and stems of *V. album* decreased in the following order: VAR > VAF > VAA > VAP > VAM.

Luczkiewicz *et al.* (2001), analyzed the phenolic acids present in mistletoe plants hosted by six different hosts. They found that in mistletoe hosted by *Mallus domestica*, the main compound was rosmarinic acid (17.48 mg %), while in mistletoe hosted by *Populus nigra*, the dominant component was chlorogenic acid (12.34 mg %).

Condrat *et al.*, (2009) investigated also nine phanerogam plants (including the European mistletoe) for their flavonoid content and antioxidant activity. Quercetin and kaempferol concentrations were found to be very low in mistletoe extracts (0.20 µmol/g dry matter, and 0.16 µmol/g dry matter, respectively).

Our study revealed that the flavanone naringenin was not present in all the varieties of *Viscum album* investigated. This result is in agreement with the study of Haas *et al.*, (2003) that did not find naringenin in all subspecies of *V. album* analysed, but they found it, rarely, in epicuticular waxes, in *V. cruciatum*. They also found flavonols (quercetin and occasionally kaempherol, along with some of their methyl derivatives) in epicuticular material of *V. album*.

3. Antioxidant activity of *Viscum album*

Phenolic compounds have attracted the interest of many researchers because they are powerful antioxidants and can protect the human body from oxidative stress. The antioxidant activity of phenolics is mainly due their redox properties.

The present study inquired a variety of *in vitro* tests, based on the capacity to scavenge free radicals. On the basis of the chemical reactions involved, major antioxidant capacity can be divided into two categories: i) hydrogen atom transfer (HAT) and ii) single-electron transfer (SET) reaction – based assay. HAT-based procedures measure the classical ability of an antioxidant to quench free radicals by hydrogen donation (ORAC method):

$$X^{.} + AH \rightarrow XH + A^{.}, \text{ where } AH = \text{any H donor}$$

SET-based method detects the ability of a potential antioxidant to transfer one electron to reduce a species, including metals, carbonyls, and radicals (TEAC method):

$$X^{.} + AH \rightarrow X^{-} + AH^{+}$$

$$AH^{+} + H_2O \leftrightarrow A^{.} + H_3O^{+}$$

$$X^{-} + H_3O^{+} \rightarrow XH + H_2O$$

$$M(III) + AH \rightarrow AH^{+} + M(II)$$

For the determination of antioxidant activity of mistletoe extract through different methods, we used fresh leaves and stems (2 g) that were homogenized with 10 ml distilled water, or with 10 ml 98% ethanol using an Ultra Turax homogenizator, for 1 minute. This mixture was centrifuged (10 000 rpm, at 4^0C, for 10 minutes) and the supernatants were filtered through a filter paper. The filtrate was used for the antioxidant activity measurements and total phenolics content.

3.1 DPPH inhibition by mistletoe extracts

A rapid, simple and inexpensive method to measure antioxidant capacity of plant extracts involves the use of the free radical, 2,2-Diphenyl-1-picrylhydrazyl (DPPH). DPPH is widely used to test the ability of compounds to act as free radical scavengers or hydrogen donors, and to evaluate antioxidant activity of extracts. The reaction involves a colour change from violet to yellow (Fig.5) that can be easily monitored using a spectrophotometer at 515 nm.

The DPPH radical-scavenging activity was determined using the method proposed by Brand-Williams et al., (1995). The reaction was performed in 12 well-plate. A volume of 200 µl sample and 1.4 ml DPPH solution (80 µM) were added to each microplate well. The decrease in the absorbance of the resulting solution was monitored at 515 nm for 30 min. The percentage of scavenging effect of different extracts against DPPH radicals, was calculated using the following equation:

$$\text{DPPH scavenging effect (\%)} = [(A_0 - A_s) \times 100] / A_0 \tag{1}$$

Where, A_0 is absorbance of the blank, and A_S is absorbance of the samples at 515 nm

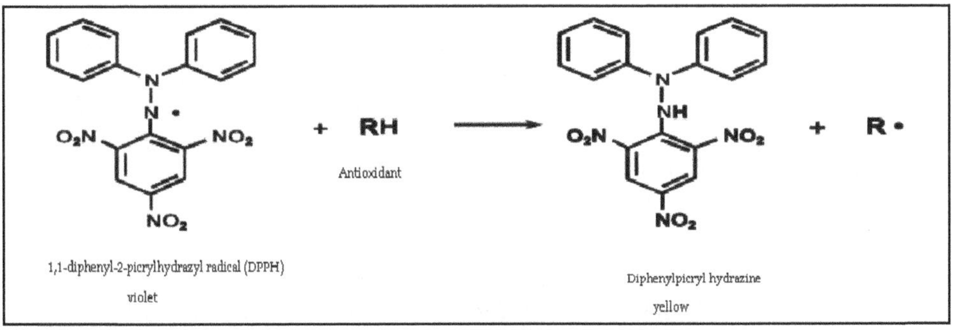

Fig. 5. The structure of DPPH radical and its reduction by an antioxidant.

The comparative antioxidant activity of *V.album* leaves hosted by different host trees, evaluated by the DPPH method shown significantly differences ($p < 0.001$) regarding to DPPH scavenging effect (%) of aqueous and ethanol extracts in leaves and stems (Vicas et al., 2011a).

The results showed that DPPH scavenging effect of aqueous extracts from mistletoe leaves varied between 11.49 %, in the case of mistletoe growing on *Robinia pseudoacacia* (VAR), to 2.22 % in the case of VAM (mistletoe growing on *Mallus domestica*). Higher DPPH scavenging effect was observed in the ethanol extracts, with values ranging from 77.19% (VAF) to 50.47 % (VAA).

The DPPH scavenging effect of extracts of mistletoe stems was lower than that of leaf extracts. No antioxidant activity was detected in aqueous extracts of VAF and VAM stems.

In all samples, stem extracts have lower antioxidant activity than the corresponding leaf extracts, also in the case of ethanol extracts.

Similar results were obtained by Önay-Uçar et al.,(2006), who investigated the antioxidant activity of methanol extracts of V.album grown on different host trees. Their results showed that mistletoe hosted by Robinia pseudocacia (VAR) exhibited 73.44% inhibition of DPPH, and mistletoe hosted by Acer campestre (VAA) presented 59.52% inhibition of DPPH. The slight differences between our results and theirs can be assigned to the solvent used for extraction and/or to environmental factors.

Sharma and Bhat (2010), showed that the absorbance profiles of DPPH were highest in a buffered methanol solution, followed by methanol and ethanol solutions. Higher absorbance in methanol solutions implies better sensitivity vis-à-vis ethanol solutions of DPPH.

Roman et al., (2009) investigated the efficiency of ultrafiltration process on the antioxidant activity of aqueous extract of V. album. The values obtained by the DPPH assay ranged between 66.2% and 88.2% DPPH inhibition for mistletoe concentrated extracts. The correlation coefficient between data of DPPH inhibition and total protein content was 0.94, suggesting that, besides the phenolic compounds of Viscum extracts, viscolectins have a great contribution to the radical scavenging activity.

Other research paper (Oluwaseun and Ganiyu, 2008) investigated the antioxidant properties of methanol extracts of V. album isolated from cocoa and cashew trees in the South Western part of Nigeria. The scavenging ability of each methanol extract against DPPH followed a dose-dependent pattern (0-10 mg/ml). The free radical scavenging ability of the V. album extract from cocoa tree performs better than that from cashew tree, a fact that is in agreement with the total phenol content of the two extracts (182 mg /100 g, and 160 mg /100 g, respectively).

Papuc et al., 2010, investigate the free radicals scavenging activity of ethanol extract from mistletoe. The scavenging activity calculated for V. album in % inhibition was 7.2%.

When the activities of the same type of mistletoe extracts, collected from the same host tree, but in different seasons, were compared using the DPPH assay, it was found that the antioxidant activity was, in general, higher in spring (Vicaş et al., 2008). The values obtained in May 2008 by the DPPH assay varied from 42.2 % DPPH inhibition for V. album growing on Robinia pseudocacia (VAR) to 17.4 % DPPH inhibition for V. album growing on Populus nigra (VAP). In July, the VAR extracts exhibited the highest capacity to scavenge free radicals (46.91%), but the VAA and VAP extracts lost their antioxidant activity. The differences may be explained by the different environmental factors (temperature, water, irradiation, etc.).

The antioxidant activity of the *V. album* extract from *Robinia pseudoacacia* has the highest, especially in the case of DPPH method (11.49 ±0.04 % for VAR leaves aqueous extracts harvesting in July; 76.60± 0.02% for VAR leaves ethanol extracts harvesting December) and this is also in agreement with total phenolic content (Vicas *et al.,* 2011b).

3.2 ORAC method

The ORAC method measures antioxidant inhibition of peroxyl radical-induced oxidations, and thus reflects classical radical chain breaking antioxidant activity by hydrogen atom transfer. The ORAC assay was performed essentially as described by Huang *et al.,*(2002). A volume of 150 μl of working solution of sodium fluorescein (4 x 10^{-3} mM) was added to 25 μl samples, in a 12 well-microplate. The plate was allowed to equilibrate by incubating it for a minimum of 30 minutes in the Synergy™ HT Multi-Detection Microplate Reader (BioTek Instruments, Winooski, VT) at 37°C. Reaction was initiated by the addition of 25 μl of 2,2′-azobis(2-amidino-propane) dihydrochloride (AAPH) solution (153 mM) and the fluorescence was then monitored kinetically with data taken every minute, at 485 nm, 20 nm bandpass excitation filter, and a 528 nm, 20 nm bandpass emission filter. ORAC values were calculated as described by Cao and Prior (1999). The area under the curve (AUC) and the Net AUC of the standards and samples were determined using equations 2 and 3 respectively.

$$AUC = 0.5 + (R2 / R1) + (R3 / R1) + (R4 / R1) + 0.5(Rn / R1) \qquad (2)$$

$$Net\ AUC = AUC_{sample} - AUC_{blank} \qquad (3)$$

Where R1- fluorescence value at the initiation of reaction and Rn - fluorescence value after 30 min.

The standard curve was obtained by plotting the Net AUC of different Trolox concentrations against their concentration (6.25 – 100 μM). ORAC values of samples were then calculated automatically using Microsoft Excel to interpolate the sample's Net AUC values against the Trolox standard curve.

The values obtained by ORAC assays varied from 10.73 ± 1.90 mM Trolox equivalents/g fresh matter for the VAP ethanol leaf extract, to 1.52 ± 1.25 mM Trolox equivalents/g fresh matter for the VAM aqueous stem extract. According to the results obtained in the ORAC assay, there was no significant differences between the antioxidant capacity of leaves and stems for all variants of mistletoe investigated, except for the aqueous leaf extracts of VAA *vs* VAM (p < 0.01), and for the aqueous stem extracts of VAA *vs* VAM (p < 0.05). The highest values were recorded in the case of VAA aqueous leaf extract (5.49 mM Trolox equivalents/g fresh matter) and VAP ethanol leaf extract (10.73 mM Trolox equivalents/g fresh matter) (Vicas et al. 2011a).

3.3 TEAC method

The TEAC is a spectrophotometric method, widely used for the assessment of antioxidant activity of various substances. This method measures the ability of compounds to scavenge the 2,2'-azino-bis(3-ethylbenzthiazoline-6-sulphonic acid) (ABTS) radical cation in relation to Trolox. The blue/green ABTS+ chromophore radical is produced through the reaction between ABTS and potassium persulfate. In the presence of an antioxidant the ABTS+ radical changes from blue/green to colorless depending on antioxidant capacity of compound, its concentration and the duration of the reaction. ABTS was dissolved in distilled water to a 7 mM concentration. ABTS+ was produced by reacting ABTS stock solution with 2.45 mM potassium persulfate and allowing the mixture to stand, in the dark, at room temperature for 12-16 h before use. ABTS stock solution was diluted with ethanol in order to obtain an absorbance of 0.70 ± 0.02 at 734 nm. After addition of 17 µl of extract to 170 µl of diluted ABTS+, the interaction between the antioxidants and the ABTS+ was monitored spectrophotometrically at 734 nm (Arnao et al. 2001). The results were expressed in mM Trolox equivalent/g fresh matter.

Based upon the conducted research, it has been found that all mistletoe extracts (aqueous or ethanol, leaf or stem) have the ability of scavenging cation-radicals ABTS+. According to the results obtained with TEAC assays, there were significant differences (p < 0.001) between all the extracts investigated (Vicas et al. 2011a). The highest level of scavenging radicals was detected in water extracts, and ethanol extracts had the lowest deactivation level. Aqueous leaf and stem extracts of mistletoe growing on *Acer campestre* (VAA) recorded the highest TEAC values (678.72 ± 0.00 mM equivalent Trolox/g fresh matter, and 577.94 ±0.01 mM equivalent Trolox/g fresh matter, respectively), while for the ethanol extracts the highest level of scavenging cation-radicals ABTS+ was recorded for leaves from VAF (461.09 ±0.11 mM equivalent Trolox/g fresh matter) and for stems from VAP (306.68 ± 0.01 mM equivalent Trolox/g fresh matter). We may suppose that water extracts had the highest antioxidant activity because they contain more bioactive compounds with the ability of scavenging cation-radicals ABTS+, as compared to ethanol extracts (Vicas et al. 2011a).

3.4 Folin-Ciocalteu method

Total phenolic content was determined by the Folin-Ciocalteu method (Singleton et al., 1999). Mistletoe extract (23 µl) was mixed with 1817 µl distillated water, 115 µl Folin-Ciocalteu reagent (dilution 1:10, v/v) and 345 µl of 15% Na_2CO_3 solution, and the mixture incubated at room temperature, in the dark, for 2 hours. The absorbance was measured at 765 nm using a spectrophotometer (BioTek Synergy). The calibration curve was linear for the range of concentrations between 0.1-0.5 mg/ml gallic acid. The results were expressed in mg gallic acid equivalents (GAE)/g fresh matter). In aqueous leaf extracts, the highest polyphenolic content was found in VAR (200.51 ± 0.00 mg GAE/g fresh matter, while the lowest value was 176.87 ± 0.003 mg GAE/g fresh matter for VAM. The values obtained for total phenolics in both, aqueous and ethanol extracts, decreased in the order: VAR > VAF > VAP > VAA > VAM. The mistletoe stem extracts contained lower levels of phenolics than the leaf extracts, in both solvents. The lowest level of total phenolics was recorded for VAF and VAA aqueous stem extracts (58% and 54,97% less that leaves, respectively). In the other extracts (VAM or VAR), the differences between leaves and stems were not significant.

In a recent research paper Vicas et al., (2011 b) presented comparatively the total phenolic content from leaves of mistletoe, in three different periods (May, July and December). Generally, the content of total phenolic was higher in aqueous extract comparative with ethanol extract. In aqueous leaves extract, the highest phenolic content was found in VAR

(209.51 ± 0.01 mg GAE/ g fresh matter), harvesting in May, while the lowest value was 83.93 ± 0.001 mg GAE/ g fresh matter for VAF, harvesting in July. The mistletoe stem extracts contained lower levels of phenolics, comparing with leaves, in both solvents. In the ethanol extract, the highest phenolic content was found in VAM (58.97 ± 0.009 mg GAE/ g fresh matter), harvesting in December, followed by VAA extract (51.96 ± 0.006 mg GAE/ g fresh matter). These results can be explained by the influence of harvesting time on the chemical composition and antioxidant activity.

There are many research studies that have established a correlation between the total phenol content of plants and their antioxidant properties (Kılıçgün and Altıner, 2010; Song et al., 2010; Tosun et al., 2009; Alali et al., 2007).

3.5 FRAP method

Considering the antioxidant potential of European mistletoe components (leaves and stems) due to their content in phenolic derivatives (phenolic acids and flavonoids) and carotenoids, and their specific hydrophilic and lipophilic character, respectively, we measured comparatively the „lipophilic" and hydrophilic" antioxidant capacity, based on the reducing power of such antioxidants against the ferric tripyridyltriazine (Fe(III)-TPTZ) complex (Fig.6). Statistical correlations between their phenolic or carotenoid concentrations and hydrophilic / lipophilic antioxidant activities, in relation to their location (leaves *versus* stems) are also reported.

Mistletoe extracts for total phenolic content and hydrophilic and lipophilic antioxidant activity were prepared as presented in Fig. 7. Shortly, 10 g leaves or stems were mixed with 25 ml methanol (MeOH), and then the slurries were kept at 4^0C for 12 hours. After centrifugation for 20 minutes, the supernatant was recovered and stored at – 20^0 C until the hydrophilic antioxidant activity (HAA) was assayed. The pellet was dissolved in acetone, homogenized and sonicated to extract the lipophilic components submitted to lipophilic antioxidant activity (LAA) analysis. The homogenates were centrifuged for 20 minutes, and the supernatant was recovered and stored at – 20^0 C until assayed

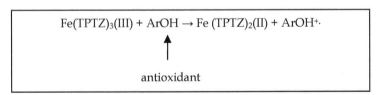

$$Fe(TPTZ)_3(III) + ArOH \rightarrow Fe(TPTZ)_2(II) + ArOH^{+\cdot}$$

antioxidant

Fig. 6. Reducing power of an antioxidants against the ferric tripyridyltriazine (Fe(III)-TPTZ) complex.

The ferric reducing antioxidant power (FRAP) assay was used to determine both hydrophilic and lipophilic antioxidant activities. The assay was determined according to the method of Benzie and Strain (1996) with some modifications. The FRAP assay consists in the ferric tripyridyltriazine (Fe(III)-TPTZ) complex reduction to the ferrous tripyridyltriazine (Fe(II)-TPTZ) by an antioxidant at low pH. The stock solutions included: 300 mM acetate buffer; 250 mg $Fe_2(SO_4)_3 \cdot H_2O$ dissolved in 50 ml distillated water; 150 mg TPTZ and 150 μl HCl, dissolved in 50 ml distillated water. The working FRAP solution was freshly prepared by mixing 50 ml acetate buffer, 5 ml $Fe_2(SO_4)_3 \cdot H_2O$ solution and 5 ml TPTZ solution. Mistletoe extracts (100 µl) were allow to react with 500 µl FRAP solution and 2 ml distilled water, for 1 h, in dark. The final colored product (ferrous tripyridyltriazine complex) was quantified by VIS absorption at 595 nm. As positive antioxidant control we used ascorbic acid (AA) and obtained a standard linear curve, between 5 and 100 mg/l vitamin C. The antioxidant activity (HAA and LAA) was expressed in mg/l AA equivalents/ g fresh weight.

We noticed no semnificative differences between the HAA values from leaves and stems hydrophilic fractions, but mistletoe leaves extract originating from *Mallus domestica* (VAM) and *Fraxinus excelsior* (VAF) and all stem extracts have shown the highest antioxidant activity, (0.14 ± 0.12 and 0.13 ± 0.11mg/l vitamin C equivalent / g of fresh leaves).

Meanwhile, LAA is significantly lower (around 100 times) comparing to HAA, in both leaves and stems. No significant differences were noticed between stem and leaves of mistletoe extract. Overall, we observed better antioxidant capacity for VAF and VAM.

A reason for low LAA values (which can be due to low carotenoid concentrations found in acetone extract) can be also the overlapping of carotenoids absorption (450 nm) and the color developed during FRAP method (UV-Vis absorbtion at 595 nm), observed also by other authors who studied vegetable extracts (Ou *et al.*, 2002).

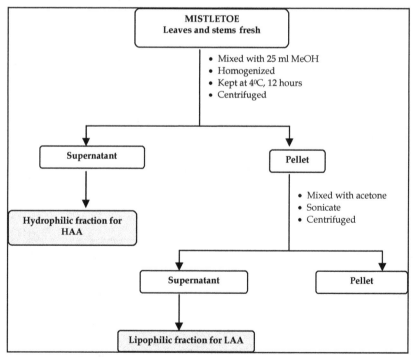

Fig. 7. Flow sheet of extraction of mistletoe extract for the determination of antioxidant activity of hydrophilic and lipophilic fractions (HAA and LAA, respectively). (Vicas et al., 2009b).

Total phenolics concentration was determined by the Folin-Ciocalteu method, and total carotenoids content from the lipophilic and hydrophilic fraction was determined by the VIS absorption at 470 nm, using a β-carotene (0.001-0.004 mg/ml) standard curve. The total carotenoids content was expressed based on β-carotene equivalents (β-carotene; mg/g fresh weight).

The total phenolics and carotenoids content were measured in methanol and acetone extracts. Methanol extract showed relatively high phenolics content (between 0.65 and 0.40 mg GAE/g fresh weight), which are known as the major natural hydrophilic antioxidants.

The phenolics content did not differ significantly between leaves and stems in the methanol extract. But, in the acetone extract the content in the phenolic compounds are 100 time lower comparing to the methanol extract (from 0.015 to 0.002 mg GAE/g FW). Generally, the acetone extracts gave lower values of phenolics and carotenoids than methanol extract. The leaves had, in both solvents, higher concentrations of phenolics and carotenoids, comparing with stems. The stem acetone extract did not contain any carotenoids. Mistletoe leaves originating *Acer campestre* (VAJ), followed by VAM and VAF showed higher concentrations of phenolics, and also carotenoids especially in methanol.

The HAA values, as determined by FRAP method, were significantly correlated with the values of phenolics content, as determined by Folin-Ciocalteu assay (R^2 = 0.9363) in the case of leaves, and R^2 = 0.761 in the case of stems, as shown in Fig. 8. The LAA values, as determined by FRAP method, were slightly correlated with the carotenoids content (R^2 = 0.6327) (Fig. 8A), and meanwhile HAA were no correlated with carotenoids (R^2 = 0.168) (Fig. 8 B) (Vicas et al., 2009b).

The methanol extracts of *V. album* demonstrated to be rich in phenolic compounds, potential antioxidants with ferric reducing ability. Mistletoe leaves originating from *Acer campestre* (VAJ), followed by VAM and VAF showed higher concentrations of phenolics, and also carotenoids, superior to acetone extracts. Meanwhile, VAF and VAM showed higher HAA and LAA activities. These data suggest that the antioxidant capacity slightly differs depending on the host trees.

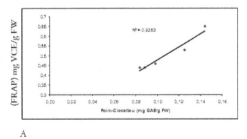   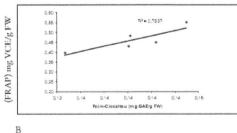

A   B

Fig. 8. Correlations found between the HAA, as determined by FRAP method, and total phenolics concentration values (GAE units) of mistletoe leaves (A) and stems (B) (Vicas et al., 2009b).

Other authors (Onay-Ucar et al., 2006) also reported that antioxidant capacity of *V. album* extract differ depending on the time of harvest and nature of the host trees. Similar results were obtained by Oluwaseun and Ganiyu (2007), who evaluated the antioxidant activity of methanol extract of *V. album* leaves from two hosts (cocoa and cashew trees), showing that mistletoe from cocoa tree had higher total phenol content (182 mg/100g) than that from cashew tree (160 mg/100g), the main reason of their antioxidant capacity. Therefore, that the total phenolic content, more than carotenoids content can serve as a useful indicator for the antioxidant activities of mistletoe extracts. Carotenoids are less available also for extraction, being linked to proteins in the photosynthetic apparatus in leaves, a possible.

4. Conclusion

The influence of the host tree may have a key role in the phenolic composition of mistletoe leaves or stems. The mistletoe hosted by *Fraxinus excelsior* (VAF) proved to be the richest in phenolic acids (108.64 µg/g dry matter), followed by VAR (71.19 µg/g dry matter), VAA (54.79 µg/g dry matter), VAP (45.15 µg/g dry matter) and VAM (39.37 µg/g dry matter), as determined by HPLC. The total polyphenols from leaves and stems of *V. album* decreased in the following order: VAR > VAF > VAA > VAP > VAM.

In aqueous leaf extracts, the highest polyphenol content was found in VAR (200.51 ± 0.00 mg GAE/ g fresh matter, while the lowest value was 176.87 ± 0.003 mg GAE/ g fresh matter for VAM. The values obtained for total phenols in both, aqueous and ethanol extracts, decreased in the order: VAR > VAF > VAP > VAA > VAM. The mistletoe stem extracts contained lower levels of phenols, as compared to leaves, in both solvents.

The bioactive compounds and the antioxidant activity are present in leaves and also in stems, in all the mistletoe samples examined (aqueous and ethanol). Of the samples examined, the best results were obtained with ethanol extract of VAF, followed by VAR.

As it has been observed by other authors (Cao and Prior, 1998), the values obtained for the antioxidant capacity of an extract depend greatly on the methodology used. The antioxidant potential is reflected by a more complex synergy of active molecules, not only phenols.

The differences in antioxidant activity between leaves and stems of mistletoes harvested from different trees can be attributed to environmental factors such as season, climate and temperature which can significantly affect the accumulation of the antioxidant components in the plant tissue.

5. Acknowledgment

This work was supported by CNCSIS-UEFISCSU, project number 1120, PN II – IDEI 696/2008, Romania.

6. References

Alali, F.Q.; Tawaha, K.; El-Elimat, T.; Syouf, M.; El-Fayad, M.; Abulaila, K.; Nielsen, S.J.; Wheaton, W.D.; Falkinham, J.O. 3rd; & Oberlies, N.H. (2007). Antioxidant activity and total phenolic content of aqueous and methanolic extracts of Jordanian plants: an ICBG project. *Natural Product Resarch*, Vol. 21, No.12, pp. 1121-1231, ISSN 1478-6427

Aqil, F.; Ahmad, I.; Mehmood, Z. (2006). Antioxidant and free radical scavenging properties of twelve traditionally used Indian medicinal plants. *Turkish Journal of Biol*ogy, Vol. 30, pp. 177-183, ISSN 1300 0152

Arnao, M.B.; Cano, A.; Alcolea, J.F.; Acosta M. (2001). Estimation of free radical quenching activity of leaf pigment extracts. *Phytochemical Analysis*, Vol. 12, pp. 138-143, ISSN: 1099-1565

Barney, C.W.; Hawksworth, F.G.; Geils, B.W. (1998). Hosts of *Viscum album*. European Journal of Forest Pathology, Vol. 28, pp. 187-208, ISSN 1439-0329

Becker, K. & Exner, J.(1980). Vergleichende Untersuchungen von Misteln verschiedener Wirtsbäume and Hand der Flavonoide und Phenolcarbonsäuren, Z. *Pflanzenphysiol*, Vol.97 pp.417-428

Benzie, I.F. & Strain J. J. (1996). The ferric reducing ability of plasma (FRAP) as a measure of "antioxidant power": The FRAP assay. *Analytical Biochemistry*, Vol. 239, pp. 70-76, ISSN 0003-2697

Büssing A. & Schietzel M. (1999). Apoptosis-inducing properties of *Viscum album* L. extracts from different host trees, correlate with their content of toxic mistletoe lectins. *Anticancer Research*, Vol. 19, pp. 23-28, ISSN 0250-7005

Büssing, A. (2000). Mistletoe. The genus Viscum. 2nd ed. Harwood Academic Publishers, pp. 31-41, ISBN 90-5823-092-9, Amsterdam, The Netherlands

Cao, G. & Prior, R.L. (1998). Comparison of different analytical methods for assessing total antioxidant capacity of human serum. Clinical Chemistry, Vol. 44, pp. 1309-1315, ISSN 0009-9147

Choudhary, M.I.; Maher, S.; Begum, A.; Abbaskhan, A.; Ali, S.; Khan, A.; Rehman, S.; Rahman A. (2010). Characterization and Antiglycation Activity of Phenolic Constituents from *Viscum album* (European Mistletoe). *Chemical and Pharmaceutical Bulletin*. Vol. 58, No. 7, pp. 980-982, ISSN 0009-2363

Condrat, D.; Szabo, M.R.; Crisan, F.; Lupea A-X. (2009). Antioxidant activity of some phanerogam plant extracts. *Food Science and Technology Research* Vol.15, No.1, pp. 95-98, ISSN 1344-6606

Eggenschwiler, J.; Balthazar, L.; Stritt, B.; Pruntsch, D.; Ramos, M.; Urech, K.; Rist, L.; Simões-Wüst, Viviani, A. 2007. Mistletoe lectins is not the only cytotoxic component in fermented preparations of *Viscum album* from white fir (*Abies pectinata*), BMC Complementary and Alternative Medicine, Vol. 7 No.14, pp. 1-7, ISSN 1472-6882

Haas, K.; Bauer, M., Wollenweber, E. (2003). Cuticular waxes and flavonol aglycones of mistletoes. *Zeitschrift für Naturforschung*, Vol.58c, pp. 464-470, ISSN 0932-0784

Hajtó, T.; Hostanska, K.; Gabius, H.J. (1989). Modulatory potency of the β-galactoside-specific lectin from mistletoe extract (Iscador) on the host defense system in vivo in rabbits and patients. *Cancer Research*. Vol. 49, pp. 4803-4808, ISSN 0008-5472

Huang, D.; Ou, B.; Hampsch-Woodill, M.; Flanagan, J.A.; Prior, R.L. (2002). High-throughput assay of oxygen radical absorbance capacity (ORAC) using a multichannel liquid handling system coupled with a microplate fluorescence reader in 96-well format. *Journal of Agricultural and Food Chemistry.* Vol.50, No. 16, pp. 4437-4444, ISSN 0021-8561

Khwaja, T.; Varven, J.; Pentecost, S.; Pande, H. (1980). Isolation of biologically active alkaloids from Korean mistletoe*Viscum album, coloratum , Cellular and Molecular Life Sciences*, Vol. 36, No.5, 599-600, ISSN 1420-682X

Kiliçgün, H. & Altiner, D. (2010). Correlation between antioxidant effect mechanisms and polyphenol content of *Rosa canina. Pharmacognosy Magazine*, Vol. 6, No. 23, pp. 238-241, ISSN 0973-1296

Leu, Y-L.; Hwang, T-L.; Chung, Y-M.; Hong P-Y. (2006). The inhibition of superoxide anion generation in human neutrophils by Viscum coloratum. *Chemical and Pharmaceutical Bulletin*, Vol. 54, pp. 1063-1066, ISSN 0009-2363

Luczkiewicz, M.; Cisowski, W.; Kaiser, P.; Ochocka, R.; Piotrowski A. (2001). Comparative analysis of phenolic acids in mistletoe plants from various hosts. *Acta Poloniae Pharmaceutica-Drug Research*, Vol. 58 No. 5, pp. 373-379, ISSN 0001-6837

Markham, K.R. (1982). Techniques of Flavonoid Identification. Academic Press. Ed., New York, pp.15-16

Miliauskas, G.; Venskutonis, P.R.; vanBeek T.A. (2004). Screening of radical scavenging activity of some medicinal and aromatic plant extracts. *Food Chemistry*, Vol. 85, pp. 231-237, ISSN 0308-8146

Mistletoe preparations in cancer treatment, (September 2009) Available from http://wissenschaft.mistel-therapie.de/- Mistletoe in cancer treatment

Oluwaseun, A.A. & Ganiyu O. (2007). Antioxidant properties of methanolic extracts of mistletoes (*Viscum album*) from cocoa and cashew trees in Nigeria. African Journal of Biotechnology, Vol. 7 No. 17, pp. 3138-3142 ISSN 1684-5315

Onay-Ucar, E.; Karagoz, A.; Arda, N. (2006). Antioxidant activity of *Viscum album* ssp. *album*. *Fitoterapia* Vol. 77, pp. 556-560, ISSN 0367-326X

Ou, B.; Huang, D.; Hampsch-Woodill, M.; Flanagan, J.A.; Deemer E. K. (2002). Analysis of antioxidant activities of common vegetables employing oxygen radical absorbance capacity (ORAC) and ferric reducing antioxidant power (FRAP) assays: a comparative study. *Journal of Agricultural and Food Chemistry*, Vol. 50, pp. 3122-3128, ISSN 0021-8561

Papuc, C.; Crivineanu, M.; Goran G.; Nicorescu V.; Durdun N. (2010). Free Radicals Scavenging and Antioxidant Activity of European Mistletoe (*Viscum album*) and European Birthwort (*Aristolochia clematitis*), *Revista de Chimie. (Bucharest)*, Vol. 61, No. 7, pp. 619-622, ISSN 0034-7752

Roman, G.P.; Neagu, E.; Radu G.L. (2009). Antiradical activities of *Salvia officinalis* and *Viscum album* L. Extracts concentrated by ultrafiltration process. *Acta Sci. Pol. Technol. Aliment* Vol. 8 No. 3, pp. 47-58, ISSN 1644-0730

Sharma, O.P. & Bhat T.K. (2010). DPPH antioxidant assay revisited. *Food Chemistry* Vol.113, pp 1202-1205, ISSN 0308-8146

Shi, Z-M.; Feng, P.; Jiang, D-Q.; Wang X-J. (2006). Mistletoe alkali inhibits peroxidation in rat liver and kidney. *World Journal Gastroenterology* Vol.12, pp. 4052-4055.

Singleton, V.L.; Orthofer, R.; Lamuela-Raventos R.M. (1999). Analysis of total phenols and other oxidation substrates and antioxidants by means of Folin-Ciocalteu reagent. *Methods Enzymology*, Vol. 299, pp. 152-178, ISSN 0076-6879

Song, F.L.; Gan, R.Y.; Zhang, Y.; Xiao, Q.; Kuang, L.; Li, H.B. (2010). Total phenolic contents and antioxidant capacities of selected chinese medicinal plants. *International Journal of Molecular Sciences* Vol.11, No.6, pp. 2362-2372, ISSN 1422-0067

Stahl, W. & Sies, H. (2003), Antioxidant activity of carotenoids, *Molecular Aspects of Medicine*, Vol. 24, No. 6, pp. 345-351, ISSN 0098-2997

The Angiosperm Phylogeny Group (2003). An update of the Angiosperm Phylogeny Group classification for the orders and families of flowering plants: APG II. Botanical Journal of the Linnean Society, Vol. 141, No. 4, pp. 399-436, ISSN 0024-4074

Tosun, M.; Ercisli, S.; Sengul, M.; Ozer, H.; Polat, T.; Ozturk, E. (2009). Antioxidant properties and total phenolic content of eight Salvia species from Turkey. *Biological Research*, Vol. 42, No. 2, pp. 175-181, ISSN 0716-9760

Urech, K.; Schaller, G.; Jäggy, C. (2006). Viscotoxins, mistletoe lectins and their isoforms in mistletoe (*Viscum album* L.) extracts Iscador, Arzneimittelforschung, Vol. 56, No. 6A, pp. 428-434, ISSN: 0004-4172

Vicas, S., Laslo, V.; Pantea, S.; Bandici, G., (2010). Chlorophyll and Carotenoids Pigments from Mistletoe (*Viscum Album*) Leaves using Different Solvents. *Analele Universitatii din Oradea, Fascicula Biologie*, TOM XVII, No. 2, pp. 213-218, ISSN 1224-5119

Vicas, S.; Rugină, D.; Leopold, L.; Pintea, A.; Socaciu, C. (2011a). HPLC Fingerprint of Bioactive Compounds and Antioxidant Activities of *Viscum album* from Different Host Trees, *Notulae Botanicae Cluj-Napoca*, Vol. 39, No. 1, pp. 48-57, ISSN 0255-965X

Vicas, S.; Rugina, D.; Socaciu, C. (2011b). Comparative Study about Antioxidant Activities of *Viscum Album* from Different Host Trees, Harvested in Different Seasons, *Journal of Medicinal Plant Research* , Vol. 5 No. 11, pp. 2237-2244, ISSN 1996-0875

Vicas, S.; Rugina, D.; Pantea, S.; Socaciu, C. (2009a). The Morphological Features and UV-VIS Analysis of Some Taxonomic Markers of Genus *Viscum, Bulletin UASVM, Agriculture Cluj-Napoca*, Vol. 66 No. 1, ISSN 1843 - 5246

Vicas, S.; Prokisch, J.; Rugina, D.; Socaciu C. (2009b). Hydrophilic and Lipophilic Antioxidant Activities of Mistletoe (*Viscum album*) as determined by FRAP method. *Notulae Botanicae Cluj-Napoca* Vol. 37 No.2, pp. 112-116, ISSN 0255-965X

Vicas, S.; Rugina, D.; Socaciu C. (2008). Antioxidant activities of Viscum album's leaves from various host trees. *Bulletin UASVM, Agriculture Cluj-Napoca*, Vol. 65, No. 1, pp. 327-332, ISSN 1843 - 5246

Wu, X.; Beecher, G.R.; Holden, J.M.; Haytowitz, D.B.; Gebhardt, S.E.; Proir R.L. (2004). Lipophilic and hydrophilic antioxidant capacities of common foods in the United State. *Journal of Agricultural and Food Chemistry*, Vol. 52, pp. 4026-4037, ISSN 0021-8561

Yao, H.; Liao, Z-X.; Wu, Q.; Lei, G-Q.; Liu, Z-J.; Chen, D-F.; Chen, J-K.; Zhou, T-S. (2006). Antioxidative flavanone glycosides from the branches and leaves of *Viscum coloratum*. *Chemical and Pharmaceutical Bulletin,* Vol. 54, pp. 133-135, ISSN 0009-2363

7

Antioxidant and Anti-Inflammatory Activities of *Sasa quelpaertensis* Leaf Extracts

Se-Jae Kim, Joon-Ho Hwang, Hye-Sun Shin,
Mi-Gyeong Jang, Hee-Chul Ko and Seong-Il Kang
Department of Biology and Sasa Industry Development Agency,
Jeju National University, Jeju,
Republic of Korea

1. Introduction

Oxidative stress plays a critical role in the pathogenesis of inflammation (Winrow et al., 1993), which is a physiological response that protects the body from stimuli including infections and tissue injury. The magnitude of the inflammatory response is crucial, and insufficient responses result in immunodeficiency, which can lead to infection and cancer. Excessive responses cause morbidity and mortality from diseases such as rheumatoid arthritis, Crohn's disease, atherosclerosis, diabetes, Alzheimer's disease, multiple sclerosis, and cerebral and myocardial ischemia (Tracey, 2002). Inflammation is associated with a wide range of inflammatory mediators that initiate inflammatory responses, recruit and activate other cells to the site of inflammation, and subsequently resolve the inflammation (Gallin & Snyderman, 1999). The expression of pro-inflammatory mediators such as cytokines, chemokines, adhesion molecules, iNOS, and COX-2 involves nuclear factor-κB (NF-κB) (Baeuerle & Baltimore, 1996; Hayden & Ghosh, 2004). Mitogen-activated protein kinases (MAPKs) pathways are also reportedly stimulated by inflammatory mediators (Guha & Mackman, 2001).

The genus *Sasa* (Poaceae) is composed of perennial plants commonly known as bamboo grasses, and various *Sasa* species are widely distributed in Asian countries including China, Japan, Korea, and Russia (Okabe et al., 1975). *Sasa* leaves have been used in traditional medicine for their anti-inflammatory, antipyretic, and diuretic properties (Bae, 2000). Bamboo leaves have also been used in clinical settings to treat hypertension, cardiovascular disease, and cancer (Shibata et al., 1975).

Many recent studies have described the beneficial health effects of *Sasa* species leaves, which have been used as alternative medicines. *S. albomarginata* extract reportedly has anticancer properties (Shibata et al., 1979). Both lignin and polysaccharide preparation from *Sasa* species reportedly have antitumor properties (Suzuki et al., 1968; Yamafuji & Murakami, 1968). Two polysaccharide preparations (GK1 and GK2) from *S. kurilensis* was found to negatively affect the growth of Sarcoma-180 implanted in mice (Raidaru et al., 1997). Also, Sasa Health, an alkaline extract derived from *S. senanensis* leaves containing polysaccharides, chlorophyllin, lignin, and flavonoids, reportedly has a protective effect on spontaneous mammary tumorigenesis (Tsunoda et al., 1998) and Her2/NeuN mammary tumorigenesis (Ren et al., 2004). Researchers have also recently reported that *S. senanensis* leaf extracts have antioxidant and immunostimulation-mediated antitumor properties (Kurokawa et al., 2006; Seki et al., 2008). Hagasewa et al. (2008) reported antioxidant C-glycosyl flavones in the leaves of *S. kurilensis* var. *gigantea*. Extract from *S. borealis* leaves reportedly improves chronic high glucose-induced endothelial apoptosis (Choi et al., 2008), as well as insulin resistance by modulating inflammatory cytokine secretion in high fat diet-induced obese C57/BL6J mice (Yang et al., 2010). Park et al. (2007) reported four antioxidant flavone glycosides (tricine-7-O-β-D-glucopyranoside, isoorientin, apigenin 6-C-β-D-xylopyranosyl-8-C-β-D-glucopyranoside, isoorientin 2-O-α-L-rhamnoside) from *S. borealis*. Two phenolic compounds, (–)-syringaresinol and tricin, isolated from *S. borealis*, exhibited P-glycoprotein inhibitory properties in adrimiamycin-resistant human breast cancer, MCF-7/ARD (Jeong et al., 2007).

S. quelpaertensis Nakai is another bamboo grass. It is a native Korean plant that grows only on Mt. Halla on Jeju Island, South Korea. This small bamboo grass has recently been the focus of much attention due to its potential biomass as well as its role as an invasive plant that inhibits the growth of other plants in the habitat on Jeju Island. Young leaves of *S. quelpaertensis* are used for a popular bamboo tea, but their beneficial health effects and the bioactive compounds contained in the plant have not yet been identified. Thus, systematic research about using its leaves as an industrial bio-resource is increasingly required. As a first step to evaluating the potential of *S. quelpaertensis* leaves as nutraceuticals, in this study, we investigated the anti-oxidative and anti-inflammatory activities of *S.quelpaertensis* leaf extract.

2. Materials and methods

2.1 Reagents

Dulbecco's modified Eagle's medium (DMEM), fetal bovine serum (FBS), and penicillin-streptomycin (PS) were obtained from Gibco-BRL (Grand Island, NY, USA). Antibody against inducible NOS (iNOS) was purchased from Calbiochem (San Diego, CA, USA), and antibody against cyclooxygenase-2 (COX-2) was obtained from Becton Dickinson (Mountain View, CA, USA). Anti-phospho-extracellular signal-regulated kinase (ERK1/2) was acquired from Santa Cruz Biotechnology (Santa Cruz, CA, USA). Antibodies against ERK1/2, JNK1/2, phospho-JNK1/2, p38, and phospho-p38 were obtained from Cell Signaling Technology (Beverly, MA, USA). The lactate dehydrogenase (LDH) Cytotoxicity Detection Kit was purchased from Takara Shuzo Co. (Otsu, Shiga, Japan). Protein assay reagent was purchased from Bio-Rad Laboratories Inc. (Hercules, CA, USA). Trizol reagent was purchased from Molecular Research Center Inc. (Cincinnati, OH, USA), lipopolysaccharide (LPS) (*Escherichia coli* 026:B6) and 3-(4,5-dimethylthiazol-2-yl)-2,5-diphenyl tetrazolium bromide (MTT) were purchased from Sigma (St. Louis, MO, USA). All other reagents were acquired from Sigma.

2.2 Preparation of extracts

S. quelpaertensis leaves were collected in October 2010, from Mt. Halla on Jeju Island, South Korea. A dried powder of the *S. quelpaertensis* leaves was extracted using 80% methanol

(MeOH) at room temperature for 48 h. This procedure was repeated twice. The combined extract was concentrated on a rotary evaporator under reduced pressure and freeze-dried to a powder. The dried extract was dissolved in water and then fractionated using the organic solvents n-hexane (hexane), ethyl acetate (EtOAc), and n-butanol (BuOH) at room temperature. Each fraction was concentrated on a rotary evaporator under reduced pressure and freeze-dried to a powder.

2.3 Measurement of antioxidant activities

2.3.1 DPPH radical scavenging assay

2,2-Diphenyl-1-picrylhydrazyl (DPPH) radical scavenging activity was examined according to the method reported by Tateyama et al. (1997) with slight modifications. Briefly, the extracts were mixed with methanol and then added to 0.4 mM DPPH in methanol. After 20 min of incubation in the dark at room temperature, the reduction in the DPPH free radical was measured by absorbance, which was read using a microplate reader (Bio-Tek Instruments, Winooski, VT, USA) at 517 nm. Trolox and BHA, a stable antioxidant, were used as a reference control and pure methanol was used as a control sample. Three replicates were made for each test sample. The radical scavenging activity of samples, expressed as percent inhibition, was calculated according to the follow formula: % inhibition $= (A0/AX)/A0 \times 100$, where $A0$ and AX are the absorbance values of the blank sample and the tested samples, respectively. The results were indicated as IC_{50}, which is the 50% inhibitory concentration of DPPH radical scavenging activity.

2.3.2 NO scavenging activity

Nitric oxide (NO) scavenging activity was measured using the method described by Feelisch and Stamler (1996) with slight modifications. Sodium nitroprusside (SNP) in an aqueous solution at physiological pH spontaneously generates nitric oxide, which can be measured using the Griess reagent system. The reaction solution containing 1 mM SNP in phosphate-buffered saline (PBS) (pH 7.4) was mixed with the extract, followed by incubation at room temperature for 3 h. Then, the reaction solution was mixed with an equal volume of Griess reagent (1% sulfanilamide and 0.1% naphthylethylenediamine in 5% phosphoric acid). The absorbance at 540 nm was recorded using a microplate reader. The percentage of NO scavenging was measured through comparison with the absorbance values of the blank sample.

2.3.3 Superoxide radical scavenging assay

Superoxide (O_2^-) was generated using the enzymatic method. Briefly, the extracts were mixed with an equal volume of reaction reagent [2 mM Na_2 EDTA in phosphate buffer (50 mM KH_2PO_4/KOH, pH 7.4), 0.05 mM nitroblue tetrazolium chloride (NBT) in a buffer, and 1 mM hypoxanthine in 50 mM KOH]. The reaction was started by adding xanthine oxidase (XOD) in a buffer to the mixture (final XOD concentration was 0.05 U/ml). After 1 h of incubation at room temperature, scavenging activity was measured by absorbance, which was read using a microplate reader at 560 nm. Trolox and BHA, a stable antioxidant, were used as a reference control; SOD and allopurinol were used as a positive control. The NBT reduction (%) was calculated according to the following formula: % inhibition =

$(A0/AX)/A0 \times 100$, where $A0$ and AX are the absorbance values of the blank sample and the tested samples, respectively.

2.3.4 Determination of XOD-inhibitory activity

XOD-inhibitory activity was measured by detecting uric acid formation according to the method described by Puig et al. (1989) with slight modifications. First, the extracts and reaction reagent [2 mM Na_2 EDTA in a phosphate buffer (50 mM KH_2PO_4/KOH, pH 7.4) and 1 mM hypoxanthine in 50 mM KOH] were mixed in a 96-well microplate. The reaction was started by adding XOD in a buffer to the mixture (final XOD concentration was 0.05 U/ml). After 1 h of incubation at room temperature, uric acid production was measured by absorbance, which was read using a microplate reader at 295 nm. Trolox and BHA, a stable antioxidant, were used as a reference control. SOD and allopurinol were used as a positive control. Uric acid production was calculated according to the following formula: % inhibition = $(A0/AX)/A0 \times 100$, where $A0$ and AX are the absorbance values of the blank sample and the tested samples, respectively.

2.4 Cell culture

The RAW 264.7 murine macrophage cell line was obtained from the Korea Cell Line Bank (Seoul, Korea). Cells were cultured in 1% PS/DMEM containing 10% heat-inactivated FBS at 37°C in a 5% CO_2 incubator.

2.5 Cytotoxicity assay - MTT and LDH release assays

Cell viability and cytotoxicity were determined using a 3-*(4,5-dimethylthiazol-2-yl)*-2,5-diphenyltetrazolium bromide (MTT) cell viability assay and lactic dehydrogenase (LDH) release assay. Cells were seeded at a density of 5×10^4 cells/well into a 96-well flat-bottom cell culture plate in the presence or absence of the extracts. Mitochondrial enzyme activity, which is an indirect measure of the number of viable respiring cells, was determined using an MTT reagent after 40 h of treatment with methanol extract or its fractions. Absorbance was read using a microplate reader (Bio-Tek Instruments) at 595 nm. The effect of extracts on cell viability was evaluated as the relative absorbance compared to that of control cultures. LDH leakage is known to be a marker of damage to the cell membrane, and the LDH level was detected using the culture supernatants according to the LDH cytotoxicity detection kit instructions (Takara Shuzo Co.). Cytotoxicity was expressed as the percentage of released LDH (LDH released into the medium/maximal LDH release $\times$ 100). Maximal LDH release was measured after lysis of the cells with 0.5% Triton X-100.

2.6 Measurement of NO and PGE$_2$ production

The amount of nitrite was determined using a colorimetric assay (Green et al., 1982). Briefly, 100 µl of cell culture medium was mixed with an equal volume of Griess reagent (1% sulfanilamide and 0.1% naphthylethylenediamine in 5% phosphoric acid) and incubated at room temperature for 10 min. The absorbance at 540 nm was recorded using a microplate reader. Nitrite concentration was determined using extrapolation from a sodium nitrite standard curve. Concentration of prostaglandin E_2 (PGE$_2$) in the culture medium was quantified by enzyme-linked immunosorbent assay (ELISA) according to the manufacturer's instructions.

2.7 Measurement of iNOS enzyme activity

The activity of the iNOS enzyme in the cell lysate was measured as the L-arginine- and NADPH-dependent generation of nitrite. Briefly, 200 μg cell lysate was incubated for 180 min at room temperature in 100 μl of a reaction buffer containing 20 mM sodium phosphate buffer, 2 mM NADPH, 2 mM L-arginine, and 10 μm FAD at pH 6.7. The reaction was stopped by adding 10 U/ml LDH and 10 mM pyruvate. Next, the reaction mixture was incubated with an equal volume of Griess reagent. The absorbance at 540 nm was recorded using a microplate reader. Nitrite concentration was determined by extrapolation from a sodium nitrite standard curve.

2.8 Western blot analysis

Cells were washed twice with ice-cold PBS and collected. The cells were then treated with a lysis buffer [1× RIPA (Upstate Cell Signaling Solutions, Lake Placid, NY, USA), 1 mM phenylmethylsulfonyl fluoride (PMSF), 1 mM Na_3VO_4, 1 mM NaF, 1 μg/ml aprotinin, 1 μg/ml pepstatin, and 1 μg/ml leupeptin] and incubated on ice for 1 h. Cell debris was removed by centrifugation and then protein concentration was determined using a Bio-Rad protein assay reagent (Bio-Rad Laboratories, Hercules, CA, USA). Cell lysates were subjected to 7.5% or 10% SDS-polyacrylamide gel electrophoresis and transferred to polyvinylidene difluoride membranes. The membranes were blocked with a solution of 0.1% Tween 20/Tris-buffed saline containing 5% nonfat milk powder for 1 h at room temperature. After incubation overnight at 4°C with the indicated primary antibody, the membranes were incubated with a horseradish peroxidase-conjugated secondary antibody for 1 h at room temperature. Immunodetection was carried out using an ECL Western blotting detection reagent. The signal intensity of relative bands was determined using image acquisition and analysis software (LabWorks, Cambridge, UK).

2.9 RNA preparation and reverse transcription-polymerase chain reaction (RT-PCR)

Total cellular RNA was isolated using a Trizol reagent (Molecular Research Center, Cincinnati, OH, USA) according to the manufacturer's instructions. RNA concentration and purity were determined by measuring absorbance at 260 and 280 nm. A cDNA synthesis was performed using the ImProm-II™ Reverse Transcription System (Promega, Madison, WI, USA) with an oligo dT-15 primer, as recommended by the supplier. PCR analyses were then performed on aliquots of cDNA preparations using a thermal cycler. The reactions were carried out in a 25 μl volume containing (final concentration) 1 unit of Taq DNA polymerase, 0.2 mM dNTP, 10× reaction buffer, and 100 pmol primers (Table 1). The cycle number was optimized to ensure product accumulation in the exponential range. β-Actin was used as an internal control to normalize the RNA content of each sample. Amplification was initiated at 94°C for 5 min, followed by 18–27 cycles of denaturation at 94°C for 45 s, annealing at the appropriate primer-pair annealing temperature for 45 s, and extension at 72°C for 1 min, followed by a final extension of 10 min at 72°C. After amplification, portions of the PCR reactions were electrophoresed on 2% agarose gel and visualized using ethidium bromide staining and a UV transilluminator (SLB Mylmagger; UVP Inc., Upland, CA, USA). The signal intensity of relative bands was determined using image acquisition and analysis software (LabWorks).

Gene		Primer sequences
iNOS	Forward	5'-CCCTTCCGAAGTTTCTGGCAGCAGC-3'
	Reverse	5'-GGCTGTCAGAGCCTCGTGGCTTTGG-3'
COX-2	Forward	5'-CACTACATCCTGACCCACTT-3'
	Reverse	5'-ATGCTCCTGCTTGAGTATGT-3'
TNF-α	Forward	5'-TTGACCTCAGCGCTGAGTTG-3'
	Reverse	5'-CCTGTAGCCCACGTCGTAGC-3'
IL-1β	Forward	5'-CAGGATGAGGACATGAGCACC-3'
	Reverse	5'-CTCTGCAGACTCAAACTCCAC-3'
IL-6	Forward	5'-GTACTCCAGAAGACCAGAGG-3'
	Reverse	5'-TGCTGGTGACAACCACGGCC-3'
β-Actin	Forward	5'-AGGCTGTGCTGTCCCTGTATGC-3'
	Reverse	5'-ACCCAAGAAGGAAGGCTGGAAA-3

Table 1. The sequences of primers used in RT-PCR analysis.

2.10 Transient transfection and luciferase assay

Cells were seeded at a density of 5×10^3 cells/well into a 96-well flat-bottom cell culture plate and cultured for 18 h. RAW 264.7 cells were transiently transfected with or without a NF-κB-promoted luciferase reporter gene plasmid pNF-κB-Luc (Promega) and a Renilla luciferase reporter plasmid pRL-TK (Stratagene, La Jolla, CA, USA), to control for transfection efficiency using a FuGENE 6 transfection reagent (Roche, Indianapolis, IN, USA). At 24 h after the start of transfection, cells were incubated with LPS (100 ng/ml) in the presence or absence of the extracts for 24 h. Luciferase activity in the cell lysate was measured using a Dual-Luciferase Reporter Assay Kit (Promega) and a FLUOstar Optima (BMG Labtech, Offenburg, Germany). Luciferase activity was normalized to transfection efficiency, as monitored using a Renilla luciferase expression vector. The level of induced luciferase activity was determined as a ratio to the luciferase activity of unstimulated cells.

2.11 Statistical analysis

All experiments were conducted in triplicate, but only data from one representative trial are presented. Results are expressed as the mean ± standard deviation (SD). Treatment effects were analyzed using a paired t-test.

3. Results

3.1 Antioxidant activities of *S. quelpaertensis* leaf extracts

Table 2 summarizes the antioxidant activities of *S. quelpaertensis* leaf methanol extract and its fractions, represented by IC_{50}. The IC_{50} values for DPPH radical scavenging activity against MeOH extract, EtOAc, and BuOH fractions were 862.5, 288.9, and 166.4 µg/ml, respectively.

DPPH radical scavenging activity of the BuOH fraction was more potent than that of other tested samples. For NO scavenging activity, the IC_{50} value (259.4 µg/ml) was calculated only for the EtOAc fraction; other tested samples exhibited minimal NO scavenging activity. All tested samples (except the water fraction) exhibited XOD-inhibition activity and superoxide radical scavenging activity. XOD-inhibition activity occurred in the following (decreasing) order: EtOAc fraction > hexane fraction > MeOH extract > BuOH fraction. Superoxide radical scavenging activity occurred in the following (decreasing) order: EtOAc fraction > BuOH fraction > hexane fraction > MeOH extract > water fraction. The IC_{50} values for the EtOAc fraction on XOD-inhibition activity and superoxide radical scavenging activity assay were 32.4 and 21.9 µg/ml, respectively. As shown in Table 2, overall antioxidant activity was more potent in the EtOAc fraction than in any other tested samples.

Sample	IC_{50} (µg/ml) [a]			
	DPPH radical scavenging activity	Nitric oxide scavenging activity	Uric acid generation activity	Superoxide generation activity
Methanol extract	862.5 ± 6.4	*	352.9 ± 16.0	113.5 ± 13.4
Hexane fraction	*	*	238.4 ± 5.6	62.8 ± 4.3
EtOAc fraction	288.9 ± 12.7	259.4 ± 1.6	32.4 ± 1.6	21.9 ± 5.4
BuOH fraction	166.4 ± 9.4	*	473.5 ± 15.4	23.4 ± 5.9
Water fraction	*	*	-	305.2 ± 6.9
Trolox	3.49 ± 0.3	*	220.3 ± 12.3	32.5 ± 1.9
BHA [b]	7.6 ± 0.2	*	801.7 ± 11.7	*
Allopurinol	N/A	N/A	1.33 ± 0.1	5.1 ± 0.1
SOD [c]	N/A	N/A	*	4.9 ± 1.9

a) IC50 values were calculated from regression lines using five different concentrations in triplicate experiments.
b) Butylated hydroxyl anisole
c) Superoxide dismutase
N/A: Not assay
* : Can't calculate the value of IC50
- : < 5% xanthine oxidase inhibitory activity at maximum concentration used for assay.

Table 2. Antioxidant activities of the methanol extract and its various fractions from *Sasa quelplaertensis* leaf.

Sample	TC_{50}[a] (µg/ml)	IC_{50}[b] (µg/ml)	Selectivity index[c]
MeOH extract	>2000	1341.7 ± 4.9	>1.8
Hexane fraction	240.1 ± 19.8	175.0 ± 9.6	1.4
EtOAc fraction	465.2 ± 10.2	68.6 ± 0.1	6.8
BuOH fraction	>2000	>2000	-
Water fraction	>2000	>2000	-

a) TC_{50} is the concentration producing 50% toxicity in RAW 264.7 cells.
b) IC_{50} is the concentration producing 50% inhibition of NO production in RAW 264.7 cells.
c) Selectivity Index = TC_{50} / IC_{50}.

Table 3. Cell toxicity and the effects of the methanol extract and its fractions of Sasa quelpaetensis on LPS-induced NO production in RAW 264.7 cells.

Next, we compared the effects of *S. quelpaertensis* leaf extract on LPS-induced NO production in RAW 264.7 cells (see Table 3). Among the tested samples, the EtOAc fraction had the highest selectivity index (6.8), indicating it had potent anti-inflammatory properties. Thus, we focused on the anti-inflammatory effects of the EtOAc fraction using LPS-stimulated RAW 264.7 cells.

3.2 EtOAc fraction inhibits NO production and iNOS expression

The effects of the EtOAc fraction on NO production in LPS-stimulated RAW 264.7 cells were investigated by measuring the amount of nitrite released into the culture medium using a

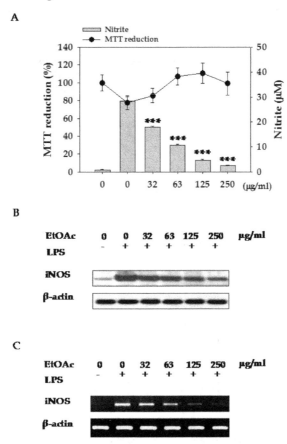

Fig. 1. Effect of EtOAc fraction on the NO production, iNOS protein and iNOS mRNA expression level in LPS-stimulated RAW 264.7 cells. (A) Cells were treated with LPS (100 ng/ml) alone or LPS plus the indicated concentrations of EtOAc fraction for 24 h. *** $P <$ 0.001 vs LPS alone-treated cells. Data are expressed in area density as the mean ± SD for three independent experiments. (B) Cells were treated with LPS (100 ng/ml) alone or LPS plus the indicated concentrations (μg/ml) of EtOAc fraction for 24 h. (C) Cells were co-treated with LPS (100 ng/ml) or LPS with EtOAc fraction at the indicated concentration for 6h. Total RNA was subjected to RT-PCR.

Griess reagent system. As shown in Fig. 1A, NO levels increased remarkably with LPS, up to 30 µM, but co-treatment with the EtOAc fraction significantly decreased NO levels in a dose-dependent manner. In addition, the EtOAc fraction did not affect the viability of RAW 264.7 cells at concentrations from 32 to 250 µg/ml.

To investigate whether the inhibition of NO production by the EtOAc fraction was a result of inhibition of the corresponding gene expression, we analyzed the expression of iNOS protein and mRNA using Western blotting and RT-PCR. LPS increased the levels of cellular iNOS protein and mRNA at 24 h and 6 h after treatment, respectively. However, co-treatment of the EtOAc fraction (32, 63, 125 and 250 µg/ml) with LPS decreased both LPS-induced protein (Fig. 1B) and iNOS mRNA (Fig. 1C) in a dose-dependent manner.

We also measured iNOS enzymic activity to investigate whether the EtOAc fraction affected enzymatic activity. As shown in Fig. 2, EtOAc treatment (32, 63, 125 and 250 µg/ml) did not affect iNOS protein enzyme activity. However, iNOS enzyme activity was inhibited by 1400 W, which was used as the positive control (data not shown). These results confirmed that the EtOAc fraction inhibited NO production in LPS-stimulated RAW 264.7 cells through the regulation of iNOS gene expression.

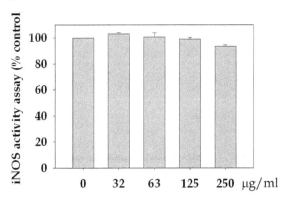

Fig. 2. Effect of EtOAc fraction on iNOS enzyme activity. The iNOS activity was measured as using L-arginine as substrate and NADPH-dependent generation of nitrite, the stable oxidation products of NO. The assay was performed by incubating with 200 µg of the cytosol protein from LPS-stimulated cells, in the absence or presence of EtOAc fraction, for 180 min at room temperature in 200 µl reaction buffer containing 20 mM Tris–HCl, pH 8.0, 2 mM NADPH, 2 mM L-arginine, 10 µM FAD. NO_3^- was reduced to NO_2^- by incubation at 37°C for 15 min with 0.1 U/ml nitrate reductase, 0.1 mM NADPH, 5 µM FAD.

3.3 EtOAc fraction inhibits PGE_2 production and COX-2 expression

PGE_2 is the major metabolite produced by COX-2 at inflammation sites. Therefore, we examined the effects of the EtOAc fraction on PGE_2 production and COX-2 expression. PGE_2 production increased remarkably with LPS (7,800 pg/ml), but co-treatment with the EtOAc fraction significantly decreased PGE_2 production in a dose-dependent manner (Fig. 3A).

To investigate whether the inhibition of PGE_2 production by the EtOAc fraction was due to inhibition of the corresponding gene expression, we analyzed the expression of COX-2 protein and mRNA using Western blotting and RT-PCR. As shown in Fig. 3B, COX-2 protein levels increased in response to LPS treatment, but co-treatment of the EtOAc fraction (32, 63, 125 and 250 µg/ml) with LPS decreased COX-2 protein levels in a dose-dependent manner. In addition, RT-PCR analysis revealed that the expression of COX-2 mRNA was correlated with its protein levels (Fig. 3C). These results indicate that the inhibitory effect of the EtOAc fraction on PGE_2 production involved regulation of COX-2 gene expression.

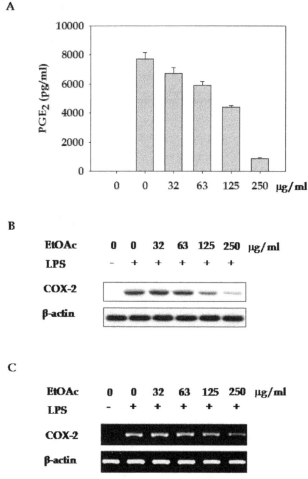

Fig. 3. Effect of EtOAc fraction on the PGE_2 production, COX-2 protein and mRNA expression level in LPS-stimulated RAW 264.7 cells. (A) Cells were treated with LPS (100 ng/ml) alone or LPS plus the indicated concentrations of EtOAc fraction for 24 h. *** $P <$ 0.001 vs LPS alone-treated cells. Data are expressed in area density as the mean ± SD for three independent experiments. (B) Cells were treated with LPS (100 ng/ml) alone or LPS plus the indicated concentrations (µg/ml) of EtOAc fraction for 24 h. (C) Cells were co-treated with LPS(100 ng/ml) or LPS with EtOAc fraction at the indicated concentration for 6 h. Total RNA was subjected to RT-PCR.

3.4 EtOAc fraction inhibits pro-inflammatory cytokine mRNA expression

Pro-inflammatory cytokines, such as IL-1β, IL-6, and TNF-α, are known to affect LPS-induced macrophage activation during immune responses. Therefore, we investigated the effects of the EtOAc fraction on the expression of TNF-α, IL-1β, and IL-6 mRNA in LPS-stimulated RAW 264.7 cells using RT-PCR analysis. The mRNA levels of these cytokines increased at 6 h (IL-1β and IL-6) or 4 h (TNF-α) after LPS treatment. However, co-treatment with the indicated concentrations of EtOAc fraction significantly decreased LPS-induced TNF-α, IL-1β, and IL-6 mRNA levels in a dose-dependent manner (Fig. 4); at a EtOAc fraction concentration of 125 μg/ml, mRNA levels of IL-1β, IL-6, and TNF-α decreased by 55%, 60%, and 45%, respectively (Fig. 4B).

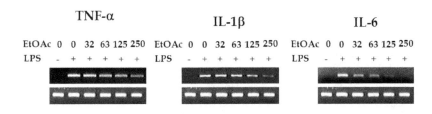

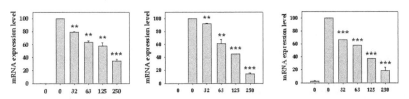

Fig. 4. Effect of EtOAc fraction on TNF-α, IL-1β and IL-6 mRNAs expression level in LPS-stimulated RAW 264.7 cells. (A) RT-PCR analysis of TNF-α, IL-1β and IL-6 mRNA expression using total RNA extracted RAW 264.7 macrophages stimulated with LPS (100 ng/ml) alone or LPS plus the indicated concentrations (μg/ml) of EtOAc fraction for 6 h (TNF-α for 4h). (B) Quantification of TNF-α, IL-1β, and IL-6 mRNA expression was performed by densitometric analysis of the RT-PCR products. The relative level was calculated as the ratio of pro-inflammatory mRNA expression to β-actin mRNA expression. *** $P < 0.001$, ** $P < 0.01$ vs LPS alone-treated cells.

3.5 EtOAc fraction suppresses NF-κB transcriptional activation

NF-κB regulated the expression of pro-inflammatory cytokines, iNOS, and COX-2. Therefore, we investigated the effect of the EtOAc fraction on NF-κB activation using a transient transfection assay with a NF-κB-promoted luciferase reporter gene plasmid (pNF-κB-Luc) in RAW 264.7 cells. The treatment group of EtOAc fraction alone exhibited activity similar to the unstimulated control group, confirming that the EtOAc fraction had no effect on NF-κB activation in the cells. However, LPS treatment (100 ng/ml, 24 h) increased luciferase activity 12-fold compared to the unstimulated control group. The EtOAc fraction significantly decreased LPS-induced luciferase activity in a dose-dependent manner (Fig. 5). At a concentration of 125 µg/ml, the EtOAc fraction decreased luciferase activity by approximately 70% compared to the LPS-stimulated control group. This finding suggests that the EtOAc fraction exerts anti-inflammatory effects by suppressing the NF-κB activation pathway.

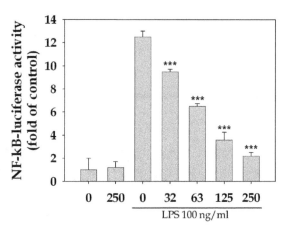

Fig. 5. Effect of EtOAc fraction on LPS-induced NF-κB transcriptional activation. Cells were treated with LPS (100 ng/ml) alone or LPS plus the indicated concentrations (µg/ml) of EtOAc fraction for 24 h. NF-κB activation detected by luciferase reporter assays. *** $P < 0.001$ vs LPS alone-treated cells.

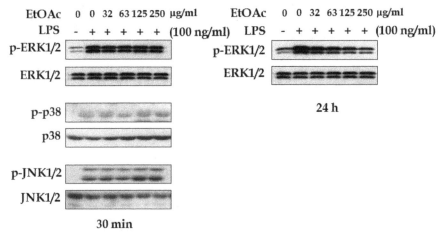

Fig. 6. Effect of EtOAc fraction on the phosphorylation of ERK1/2, p38, and JNK in LPS-stimulated RAW 264.7 cells. Cells were treated with LPS (100 ng/ml) alone or LPS plus the indicated concentrations (µg/ml) of EtOAc fraction for 30 min or 24 h. The protein levels were determined by Western blotting.

3.6 EtOAc fraction suppresses the phosphorylation of ERK1/2

Because some MAPKs are known to be stimulated by inflammatory mediators, we also investigated how the EtOAc fraction affected three MAPKs (ERK1/2, JNK1/2, and p38 MAPK) in LPS-stimulated RAW 264.7 macrophages. The phosphorylations of these three kinases were detected after cells were subjected to 30 min of LPS treatment. The activation of the three MAPKs by LPS treatment did not decrease with co-treatment of the EtOAc fraction, but the EtOAc fraction suppressed the phosphorylation of ERK1/2 at 24 h after LPS treatment (Fig. 6).

4. Discussion

In the human body, oxidative stress is associated with many diseases. Therefore, researchers are currently intensely focused on identifying antioxidant agents in plants that may protect against oxidative stress, including the *Sasa* species already used in alternative medicines (Jensen et al., 2008; Nakajima et al., 2003; Sood et al., 2009). This study evaluated the potential of using *S. quelpaertensis* leaf in nutraceuticals. As the first step toward identifying phytochemicals with beneficial health effects from *S. quelpaertensis* leaf extracts, we evaluated *in vitro* antioxidant capacities such as DPPH radical scavenging activity, NO scavenging activity, XOD-inhibitory activity, and superoxide radical scavenging activity.

Among the various fractions, the *n*-butanol soluble fraction exhibited the strongest DPPH radical scavenging activity (IC_{50} = 166.4 µg/ml). This result was consistent with the results of Park et al. (2007), who also found significant DPPH radical scavenging activity in the *n*-butanol soluble fraction among *n*-hexane, EtOAc, and aqueous extracts from *S. borealis*. However, the EtOAc fraction was the most potent in nitric oxide scavenging activity (IC_{50} = 259.4 µg/ml), superoxide scavenging activity (IC_{50} = 21.9 µg/ml), and xanthine oxidase inhibitory activity (IC_{50} = 32.4 µg/ml), suggesting its potential as an antioxidant agent.

Antioxidants such as vitamins C reportedly exhibit anti-inflammatory activity via suppression of NF-κB activation (Calfee-Mason et al., 2002; Muñoz et al., 1997). Therefore, we further investigated the anti-inflammatory potential of the EtOAc fraction, which exhibited the strongest antioxidant potential among various solvent fractions using the RAW 264.7 cell line.

NO is an essential bio-regulatory molecule within the nervous, immune, and cardiovascular systems (Bredt & Snyder, 1990; Gold et al., 1990; Palmer et al., 1987). However, increased levels of NO derived from iNOS can result in the formation of peroxynitrite after reaction with oxygen free radicals during inflammatory responses (Posadas et al., 2000). In the RAW 264.7 cell, NO production is closely associated with COX-2 expression (Salveminiet al., 1995), which produces PGE_2 and induces an inflammatory reaction (Bennett et al., 1977a, 1980b, 1982c; Rigas et al., 1993). iNOS and COX-2 are key enzymes regulating the production of NO and PGE_2, central mediators of inflammation (Possadas et al., 2000; Tsatsanis et al., 2006).

This study demonstrated that the EtOAc fraction inhibited NO production and iNOS expression, but it had no effect on iNOS enzyme activity. Additionally, PGE_2 production and COX-2 expression were attenuated by the EtOAc fraction in a dose-dependent manner. These results suggest that the EtOAc fraction from *S. quelpaertensis* leaves reduced NO and PGE_2 production via transcriptional regulation of iNOS and COX-2 genes.

Pro-inflammatory cytokines, such as IL-1β, IL-6, and TNF-α, interact with each other (Pålsson-McDermott & O'Neill, 2004) and affect LPS-induced macrophage activation during immune responses (Conti et al., 2004). Moreover, IL-1β, IL-6, and TNF-α secretion increases in patients with some inflammatory diseases, such as ulcerative colitis and Crohn's disease (Reinecker et al., 1993); these cytokines play an important role in particle-induced inflammation in the lung (Driscoll, 2000; Mansour & Levitz, 2002; Yucesoy et al., 2002). TNF-α is the main mediator of the LPS reaction and is involved in innate immune reactions and chronic inflammatory reactions (Lee et al., 2003). IL-1β is associated with T-cell activation, B-cell maturation, and NK cell activation (Delgado et al., 2003). Therefore, effective regulation of inflammatory mediators is essential (Driscoll, 2000; Hotamisligil, 2008; Hummasti & Hotamisligil, 2010). In this study, the EtOAc fraction significantly decreased LPS-induced TNF-α, IL-1β, and IL-6 mRNA levels. This finding suggests that the EtOAc fraction exerts a beneficial health effect by inhibiting the production of many inflammatory mediators.

NF-κB is an inducible eukaryotic transcription factor that can regulate the expression of numerous genes involved in proliferation, apoptosis, and the immediate–early steps of inflammatory and immune responses (Place et al., 2003). NF-κB activation in response to pro-inflammatory stimuli involves the degradation of inhibitor κB (IκB) by the IκB kinase (IKK) complex. NF-κB is subsequently released, translocates into the nucleus, and initiates expression of pro-inflammatory mediators such as cytokines, chemokines, adhesion molecules, iNOS, and COX-2 (Baeuerle & Baltimore, 1996; Hayden & Ghosh, 2004). Most anti-inflammatory drugs have been shown to suppress the expression of these genes by inhibiting the NF-κB activation pathway (Gilroy et al., 2004). Researchers have recently been working to identify an anti-inflammatory agent to suppress the NF-κB activation pathway (Le et al., 2009; Reddy & Reddanna, 2009). Thus, an NF-κB inhibitor may be useful in the development of therapeutic drugs to control the inflammation associated with human diseases in a clinical environment.

The other major extracellular signal transduction pathway stimulated by inflammatory mediators is the MAPK pathway (Guha & Mackman, 2001). Three major MAPK pathways are a highly conserved family of protein serine/threonine kinases and include the ERK1/2, the c-Jun NH_2-terminal kinase (JNK1/2), and the p38 mitogen-activated kinase (p38). These kinases can trigger the nuclear accumulation and activity of various transcription factors, such as NF-κB, ATF2, Elk1, c-fos, and c-jun, which can modulate cytokine and inflammatory mediator expression (Aga et al., 2004; Herlaar & Brown, 1999).

LPS produces inflammatory mediators by activating the NF-κB and MAPK pathways, and then induces inflammation in macrophages (Aga et al., 2004; Guha & Mackman, 2001; Zhang & Ghosh, 2000). On the basis of the inhibitory effect of the EtOAc fraction on the production of inflammatory mediators such as iNOS, COX-2, IL-1β, IL-6, and TNF-α, we examined the effect of the EtOAc fraction on NF-κB and MAPK activation in LPS-stimulated RAW 264.7 cells. The EtOAc fraction reduced the transcriptional activities of NF-κB, as well as the delayed phosphorylation of the ERK1/2 in LPS-stimulated RAW 264.7 cells. Taken together, these results suggest that the EtOAc fraction from *S. quelpaertensis* leaves exhibited at least some anti-inflammatory properties by suppressing NF-κB transcriptional activity and delaying ERK1/2 activation in LPS-stimulated RAW 264.7 cells.

Plants of the genus *Sasa* are known to biosynthesize various compounds such as triterpenoids, flavonoids, phenylpropanoids, and flavonolignans (Lee et al., 2007; Sultana &

Lee, 2009). In previous research, we demonstrated that a hot water extract of *S. quelpaertensis* leaves exhibited moderate anti-inflammatory activities in LPS-stimulated RAW 264.7 cells (Hwang et al., 2007). An ethanol/water extract of bamboo leaf mainly contains flavones, glycosides, phenolic acids, coumarin lactones, anthraquinones, and amino acids (Lu et al., 2005; Zhang & Ding, 1996). Thus, the moderate anti-inflammatory activity of the hot water extract may be due to water-soluble phytochemicals. The EtOAc fraction of *S. quelpaertensis* leaves, which contains mainly lipid-soluble compounds, has exhibited potent anti-proliferative effects via inducing apoptosis on human leukemia HL-60 cells (Jang et al., 2008). However, the bioactive compounds contained in the plant have not yet been identified (Sultana & Lee, 2010). We confirmed that the EtOAc extract contains various compounds, including tricin 7-O-β-D-glucopyranoside, two phenylpropanoids, p-hydroxy benzaldehyde, and p-coumaric acid, as we investigated the relationships between various compounds and their antioxidant or anti-inflammatory properties.

5. Conclusion

As an initial step to evaluate the beneficial health effects of *S. quelpaertensis*, we investigated the antioxidant activity and anti-inflammatory activity of *S. quelpaertensis* leaf extract. Among the various fractions, the *n*-butanol soluble fraction exhibited the strongest DPPH radical scavenging activity (IC_{50} = 166.4 µg/ml). The EtOAc soluble fraction had the strongest inhibitory effect in the NO scavenging activity, superoxide scavenging activity, and xanthine oxidase inhibitory activity assay (IC_{50} values were 259, 21.9, and 32.4 µg/ml, respectively). Next, we investigated the anti-inflammatory properties of the EtOAc fraction in LPS-stimulated RAW 274.7 cells. The EtOAc fraction inhibited production of NO, PGE_2, iNOS, and COX-2 in a dose-dependent manner. Additionally, pro-inflammatory cytokines, such as IL-1β, IL-6, and TNF-α, decreased after co-treatment with the EtOAc fraction compared to the LPS-treated group. These results indicate that the EtOAc fraction exhibits anti-inflammatory properties via the inhibition of many inflammatory mediators. Finally, on the basis of the inhibitory effect of the EtOAc fraction on inflammatory mediators, we examined how the EtOAc fraction affected the LPS-induced activation of the NF-κB and MAPK pathways. The EtOAc fraction inhibited the phosphorylation of ERK1/2 and the transactivation of NF-κB, suggesting that the EtOAc fraction suppresses the production of pro-inflammatory mediators via the inhibition of NF-κB transactivation and ERK 1/2 phosprorylation. Taken together, these results indicate that *S. quelpaertensis* leaf has potential for use as an antioxidant and anti-inflammatory agent.

6. Acknowledgement

This study was supported by the Grant of Regional Innovation System (B0012292)) of Ministry of Knowledge Economy (MKE), Republic of Korea.

7. References

Aga, M., Watters, JJ., Pfeiffer, ZA., Wiepz, GJ., Sommer, JA., & Bertics, PJ. (2004). Evidence for nucleotide receptor modulation of cross talk between MAP kinase and NF-kappa B signaling pathways in murine RAW 264.7 macrophages. *American Journal of Physiology - Cell Physiology*, Vol. 286, No. 4, (April, 2004), pp. (C923-930), 0363-6143

Bae, K. (2000). *The Medicinal plants of Korea*, Kyo-Hak Publishing Company, 8909056584, Seoul, Republic of Korea

Baeuerle, PA., & Baltimore, D. (1996). NF-kappa B: ten years after. *Cell*, Vol. 87, No. 1, (October, 1996), pp. (13-20), 0092-8674

Bennett, A., Carroll, MA., Stamford, IF., & Williams, F. (1982). Prostaglandins and human lung carcinomas. *British journal of cancer*, Vol. 46, No. 6, (December, 1982), pp. (888-893), 0007-0920

Bennett, A., Carter, L., & Stamford, IF. (1980) Prostaglandin-like material extracted from squamous cacinomas of the head and neck. *British journal of cancer*, Vol. 41, No. 2, (February, 1980), pp. (204-208), 007-0920

Bennett, A., Charlier, EM., McDonald, AM., Simpson, JS., Stamford, IF., & Zebro, T. (1977). Prostaglandins and breast cancer. *The Lancet*, Vol. 310, No. 8039, (September, 1977), pp. (624-626), 0099-5355

Bredt, DS., & Snyder, SH. (1990). Isolation of nitric oxide synthetase, a calmodulin-requiring enzyme. *Proceedings of the National Academy of Sciences of the United States of America*, Vol. 87, No. 2, (January, 1990), pp. (682-685), 0027-8424

Calfee-Mason, KG., Spear, BT., & Glauert, HP. (2002). Vitamin E inhibits hepatic NF-kappaB activation in rats administered the hepatic tumor promoter, phenobarbital. *Journal of Nutrition*, Vol. 132, No. 10, (October, 2002), pp (3178-3185), 0022-3166

Choi, YJ., Lim, HS., Choi, JS., Shin, SY., Bae, JY., Kang, SQ., Kang, IJ., & Kang, YH. (2008). Blockage of chronic high glucose-induced endothelial apoptosis by Sasa borealis bamboo extract. *Experimental Biology and Medicine*, Vol. 233, No. 5, (May, 2008), pp. (580-591), 1535-3702

Conti, B., Tabarean, I., Andrei, C., & Bartfai, T. (2004). Cytokines and fever. *Frontiers in bioscience*, Vol. 9, No 1, (May, 2004), pp. (1433-1449), 1093-9946

Delanty, N., & Dichter, MA. (1998). Oxidative injury in the nervous system. *Acta Neurologica Scandinavica*, Vol. 98, No. 3, (September, 1998), pp. (145-153), 0001-6314

Delgado, AV., McManus, AT., & Chambers, JP. (2003). Production of tumor necrosis factor-alpha, interleukin 1-beta, interleukin 2 and interleukin 6 by rat leukocyte subpopulations after exposure to substance. *Neuropeptides*, Vol. 37, No. 6, (December, 2003), pp. (355-361), 0143-4179

Driscoll, KE. (2000). TNF-alpha and MIP-2: role in particle-induced inflammation and regulation by oxidative stress. *Toxicology Letters*, Vol. 112-113, (March, 2000), pp. (177-183), 0378-4274

Feelisch, M., & Stamler, JS. (1st Ed.). (1996). *Methods in nitric oxide research*, John Wiley & Sons, 0471955248, Chichester, England

Gallin, JI., & Snyderman, R. (3rd Ed.). (1999). *Inflammation: Basic principles and Clinical Correlates*, Lippincott Williams & Wilkins, 9780397517596, Pennsylvania, United States of America

Gilroy, DW., Lawrence, T., Perretti, M., & Rossi, AG. (2004). Inflammatory Resolution: new opportunities for drug discovery. *Nature Reviews Drug Discovery*, Vol. 3, No. 5, (May 2004), pp. (401-416), 1474-1776

Gold, ME., Wood, KS., Byrns, RE., Fukuto, J., & Ignarro, LJ. (1990). NG-methyl-L-arginine causes endothelium-dependent contraction and inhibition of cyclic GMP formation in artery and vein. *Proceedings of the National Academy of Sciences of the United States of America*, Vol. 87, No. 1, (June, 1990), pp. (4430-4434), 0027-8424

Green, LC., Wagner, DA., Glogowski, J., Skipper, PL., Wishnok, JS., & Tannenbaum, SR. (1982). Analysis of nitrate, nitrite, and [15N] nitrate in biological fluids. *Analytical biochemistry*, Vol. 126, No. 1, (October, 1982), pp. (131-138), 0003-2697

Guha, M., & Mackman, N. (2001). LPS induction of gene expression in human monocytes. *Cellular Signalling*, Vol. 13, No. 2, (February, 2001), pp. (85-94), 0898-6568

Hasegawa, T., Tanaka, A., Hosoda, A., Takano, F., & Ohta, T. (2008). Antioxidant C-glycosyl flavones from the leaves of *Sasa kurilensis* var. *gigantea*. *Phytochemistry*, Vol. 69, No. 6, (April, 2008), pp. (1419-1424), 0031-9422

Hayden, MS., & Ghosh, S. (2004). Signaling to NF-kappaB. *Genes & Development*, Vol. 18, No. 18, (September, 2004), pp. (2195-2224), 0890-9369

Herlaar, E., & Brown, Z. (1999). p38 MAPK signalling cascades in inflammatory disease. *Molecular Medicine Today*, Vol. 5, No. 10, (October, 1999), pp. (439-447), 1357-4310

Hotamisligil, GS. (2008). Inflammation and endoplasmic reticulum stress in obesity and diabetes. *International journal of obesity (Lond)*, Vol. 32 (Suppl 7), (December, 2008), pp. (S52-S54), 0307-0565

Hummasti, S., & Hotamisligil, GS. (2010). Endoplasmic reticulum stress and inflammation in obesity and diabetes. *Circulation Research*, Vol. 107, No. 5, (September, 2010), pp. (579-591), 0009-7330

Hwang, JH., Choi, SY., Ko, HC., Jang, MG., Jin, YJ., Kang, SI., Park, JG., Chung, WS., & Kim, SJ. (2007). Anti-inflammatory Effect of the Hot Water Extract from Sasa quelpaertensis Leaves. *Food Science and Biotechnology*, Vol. 16, No. 5, pp. (728-733), 1226-7708

Jang, MG., Park, SY., Lee, SR., Choi, SY., Hwang, JH., Ko, HC., Park, JG., Chung, WS., & Kim, SJ. (2008). Sasa quelpaertensis leaf extracts induce apoptosis in human leukemia HL-60 cells. *Food Science and Biotechnology*, Vol. 17, No. 1, pp. (188-190), 1226-7708

Jeong, YH., Chung, SY., Han, AR., Sung, MK., Jang, DS., Lee, J., Kwon, Y., Lee, HJ. & Seo, EK. (2007). P-glycoprotein inhibitory activity of two phenolic compound, (-)-syrigaresinol and tricin from *Sasa borealis*. *Chemistry and Biodiversity*, Vol. 4, No. 1, pp. (12-16), 1612-1872

Jensen, GS., Wu, X., Patterson, KM., Barnes, J., Carter, SG., Scherwitz, L., Beaman, R., Endres, JR., & Schauss, AG. (2008). In vitro and in vivo antioxidant and anti-inflammatory capacities of an antioxidant-rich fruit and berry juice blend. Results of a pilot and randomized, double-blinded, placebo-controlled, crossover study. *Journal of Agricultural and Food Chemistry*, Vol. 56, No. 18, (September, 2008), pp. (8326-8333), 0021-8561

Kurokawa, T., Itagaki, S., Yamaji, T., Nakata, C., Nodo, T., Hirano, T. & Iseki, K. (2006). Antioxidant activity of a novel extract from bamboo grass (AHSS) against ischemia-reperfusion injury in rat small intestine. *Biological & Pharmaceutical Bulletin*, Vol.29, No.11, (November, 2006), pp. (2301-2303), 0918-6158

Lee, AK., Sung, SH., Kim, YC., & Kim, SG. (2003). Inhibition of lipopolysaccharide-inducible nitric oxide synthase, TNF-a and COX-2 expression by sauchinone effect in I-kBa phosphorylation, C/EBP and AP-1 avtivation. *British journal of pharmacology*, Vol. 139, No. 1, (May, 2003), pp. (11-20), 0007-1188

Lee, J., Jeong, YH., Jang, DS., & Seo, EK. (2007). Three terpenes and one phenolic compounds from Sasa borealis. *Journal of Applied Biological Chemistry*, Vol. 50, No. 1, (March, 2007), pp. (13-16), 1976-0442

Lee, TY., Lee, KC., Chen, SY., & Chang, HH. (2009). 6-Gingerol inhibits ROS and iNOS through the suppression of PKC-alpha and NF-kappaB pathways in lipopolysaccharide-stimulated mouse macrophages. *Biochemical and Biophysical Research Communications*, Vol. 382, No. 1, (April, 2009), pp. (134-139), 0006-291X

Lu, B., Wu, X., Tie, X., Zhang, Y., & Zhang, Y. (2005). Toxicology and safety of anti-oxidant of bamboo leaves. Part 1: Acute and subchronic toxicity studies on anti-oxidant of bamboo leaves. *Food and Chemical Toxicology*, Vol. 43, No. 5, (May, 2005), pp. (783-792), 0278-6915

Mansour, MK., & Levitz, SM. (2002). Interactions of fungi with phagocytes. *Current Opinion in Microbiology*, Vol. 5, No. 4, (August, 2002), pp. (359-365), 1369-5274

Martínez, JA. (2006). Mitochondrial oxidative stress and inflammation: an slalom to obesity and insulin resistance. *Journal of physiology and biochemistry*, Vol. 62, No. 4, (December, 2006), pp. (303-306), 1138-7548

Muñoz, E., Blázquez, MV., Ortiz, C., Gomez-Díaz, C., & Navas, P. (1997). Role of ascorbate in the activation of NF-kappaB by tumour necrosis factor-alpha in T-cells. *Biochemical Journal*, Vol. 325, No. Pt 1, (July 1997), pp. (23-28), 0264-6021

Nakajima, Y., Yun, YS., & Kunugi, A. (2003). Six new flavonolignans from Sasa veitchii (Carr.) Rehder. *Tetrahedron*, Vol. 59, No. 40, (September, 2003), pp. (8011-8015), 0040-4020

Okabe, S., Takeuchi, K., Takagi, K., & Shibata, M. (1975). Stimulatory effect of the water extract of bamboo grass (Folin solution) on gastric acid secretion in pylorus-ligated rats. *Japanese Journal of Pharmacology*, Vol. 25, No. 5, (October, 1975), pp. (608-609), 0021-5198

Palmer, RM., Ferrige, AG., & Moncada, S. (1987). Nitric oxide release accounts for the biological activity of endothelium-derived relaxing factor. *Nature*, Vol. 327, No. 6122, (June, 1987), pp. (524-526), 0028-0836

Pålsson-McDermott, EM., & O'Neill, LA. (2004). Signal transduction by the lipopolysaccharide receptor, Toll-like receptor-4. *Immunology*, Vol. 113, No. 2, (October, 2004), pp. (153-162), 0019-2805

Park, HS., Lim, JH., Kim, HJ., Choi, HJ., & Lee, IS. (2007). Antioxidant flavones glycosides from the leaves of Sasa borealis. *Archives of Pharmacal Research*, Vol. 30, No. 2, (February, 2007), pp. (161-166), 0253-6269

Place, RF., Haspeslagh, D., & Giardina, C. (2003). Induced stabilization of IkappaBalpha can facilitate its re-synthesis and prevent sequential degradation. *Journal of Cellular Physiology*, Vol. 195, No. 3, (June, 2003), pp. (470-478), 0021-9541

Posadas, I., Terencio, MC., Guillén, I., Ferrándiz, ML., Coloma, J., Payá, M., & Alcaraz, MJ. (2000). Co-regulation between cyclo-oxygenase-2 and inducible nitric oxide synthase expression in the time-course of murine inflammation. *Naunyn-Schmiedeberg's Archives of Pharmacology*, Vol. 361, No. 1, (January, 2000), pp. (98-106), 0028-1298

Puig, JG., Mateos, FA., & Diaz, VD. (1989). Inhibition of xanthine oxidase by allopurinol: a therapeutic option for ischaemia induced pathological processes?. *Annals of the rheumatic diseases*, Vol. 48, No. 11, (November, 1989), pp. (883-888), 0003-4967

Raidaru, G., Ilomets, T., Mottus, A. & Maser, M. (1997). Isolation of polysaccharides with antitumor activity from Sasa kurilensis(Fr. et Sar.). *Experimental Oncology*, Vol. 20, No. 4, pp. (34-39), 1812-9269

Reddy, DB., & Reddanna, P. (2009). Chebulagic acid (CA) attenuates LPS-induced inflammation by suppressing NF-kappaB and MAPK activation in RAW 264.7 macrophages. *Biochemical and Biophysical Research Communications*, Vol. 381, No. 1, (March, 2009), pp. (112-117), 0006-291X

Reinecker, HC., Steffen, M., Witthoeft, T., Pflueger, I., Schreiber, S., MacDermott, RP., & Raedler, A. (1993). Enhanced secretion of tumour necrosis factor-alpha, IL-6, and IL-1 beta by isolated lamina propria mononuclear cells from patients with ulcerative colitis and Crohn's disease. *Clinical & Experimental Immunology*, Vol. 4, No. 1, (October, 1993), pp. (174-181), 0009-9104

Ren, M., Reilly, RT., & Sacchi, N. (2004). Sasa health exerts a protective effects on Her2/NeuN mammary tumorigenesis. *Anticancer Research*, Vol. 24, No. 5A, (September-October, 2004), pp. (2879-2884), 0250-7005

Rigas, B., Goldman, IS., & Levine, L. (1993). Altered eicosanoid levels in human colon cancer. *The Journal of laboratory and clinical medicine*, Vol. 122, No. 5, (November, 1993), pp. (518-523), 0022-2143

Salvemini, D., Manning, PT., Zweifel, BS., Seibert, K., Connor, J., Currie, MG., Needleman, P., & Masferrer, JL. (1995). Dual inhibition of nitric oxide and prostaglandin production contributes to the antiinflammatory properties of nitric oxide synthase inhibitors. *The Journal of clinical investigation*, Vol. 96, No. 1, (July, 1995), pp. (301-308), 0021-9738

Seki, T., Morimura, S., Ohba, H., Tang, Y., Shigematsu, T., Maeda, H., & Kida, K. (2008). Immunostimulation-mediated antitumor activity by preconditioning with rice-shochu distillation residue against implanted tumor in mice. *Nutrition & Cancer*, Vol. 60, No. 6, (2008), pp. (776-783), 0163-5581

Shibata, M., Yamatake, M., Sakamoto, M., Kanamori, K., & Takagi, K. (1975). Phamacological studies on bamboo grass (1). Acute toxicity and anti-inflammatory and antiulcerogenic activities of water-soluble fraction(Folin) extracted from Sasa albomarginata Makino et Shibata. *Nippon Yakurigaku Zasshi*, Vol. 71, No. 5, (July, 1975), pp. (481-485), 0015-5691

Shibata, M., Fujii, M., & Yamaguchi, R. (1979). Pharmacological studies on bamboo grass. IV. Toxicological and pharmacological effects of the extract (FIII) obtained from Sasa albomarginata Makino et Shibata (author's transl). *Nippon Yakurigaku Zasshi*, Vol. 99, No. 6, (June, 1979), pp. (663-668), 0015-5691

Sood, S., Arora, B., Bansal, S., Muthuraman, A., Gill, NS., Arora, R., Bali, M., & Sharma, PD. (2009). Antioxidant, anti-inflammatory and analgesic potential of the Citrus decumana L. peel extract. *Inflammopharmacology*, Vol. 17, No. 5, (October, 2009), pp. (267-274), 0925-4692

Sultana, N., & Lee, NH. (2010). A new alkene glycoside from the leaves of Sasa quelpaertensis Nakai. *Bulletin of the Korean Chemical Society*, Vol. 31, No. 4, (April, 2010), pp. (1088-1090), 0253-2964

Sultana, N., & Lee, NH. (2009). New phenylpropanoids from Sasa quelpaertensis Nakai with Tyrosinase inhibition acitivities. *Bulletin of the Korean Chemical Society*, Vol. 30, No. 8, (August, 2009), pp. (1729-1732), 0253-2964

Suzuki, S., Saito, T., Uchiyama, M., & Akiya, S. (1968). Studies on the anti-tumor activity of polysaccharides. I. Isolation of hemicelluloses from Yakushima-bamboo and their growth inhibitory activity against sarcoma-180 solid tumor. *Chemical & Pharmaceutical Bulletin*, Vol. 16, No. 10, (October, 1968), pp. (2032-2039), 0918-6158

Tateyama, C., Ohta, M. & Uchiyama, T. (1997). Free radical scavenging activities of flower petals extracts. *Journal of the Japanese Society of Food Science and Technology*, Vol. 44, No. 9, (June, 1998), pp. (640–646), 1341-027X

Tracey, KJ. (2002). The inflammatory reflex. *Nature*, Vol. 420, No. 6917, (December, 2002), pp. (853-859), 0028-0836

Tsatsanis, C., Androulidaki, A., Venihaki, M., & Margioris, AN. (2006). Signalling networks regulating cyclooxygenase-2. *The International Journal of Biochemistry & Cell Biology*, Vol. 38, No. 10, (April, 2006), pp. (1654-1661), 1357-2725

Tsunoda, S., Yamamoto, K., Skamoto, S., Inoue, H., & Nagasawa, H. (1998). Effects of Sasa Health, extract of bamboo grass leaves, on spontaneous mammary tumourigenesis in SHN mice. Anticancer Research, Vol, 18, No. 1A, (January-February, 1998), pp. (153-158), 0250-7005

Valko, M., Leibfritz, D., Moncol, J., Cronin, MT., Mazur, M., & Telser, J. (2007). Free radicals and antioxidants in normal physiological functions and human disease. *The International Journal of Biochemistry & Cell Biology*, Vol. 39, No. 1, (August, 2006), pp. (44-84), 1357-2725

Victor, VM., & Rocha, M. (2007). Targeting antioxidants to mitochondria: a potential new therapeutic strategy for cardiovascular diseases. *Current Pharmaceutical Design*, Vol. 13, No. 8, (March, 2007), pp. (845-863), 1381-6128

Winrow, VR., Winyard, PG., Morris, CJ., & Blake, DR. (1993). Free radicals in inflammation: second messengers and mediators of tissue destruction. *British Medical Bulletin*, Vol. 49, No. 3, (July, 1993), pp. (506-522), 0007-1420

Yang, JH., Lim, HS., & Heo, YR. (2010). *Sasa borealis* leaves extract improves insulin resistance by modulating inflammatory cytokine secretion in high fat diet-induced obese C57/BL6J mice. *Nutrition Research and Practice*, Vol. 4, No. 2, (April, 2010), pp. (99-105), 1976-1457

Yamafuji, K., & Murakami, H. (1968). Antitumor potency of lignin and pyrocatecol and their action on deoxyribonucleic acid. *Enzymologia*, Vol. 35, No. 3, (September, 1968), pp. (139-153), 0013-9424

Yucesoy, B., Vallyathan, V., Landsittel, DP., Simeonova, P., & Luster, MI. (2002). Cytokine polymorphisms in silicosis and other pneumoconioses. *Molecular and Cellular Biochemistry*, Vol. 234-235, No. 1-2, (May-June, 2002), pp. (219-224), 0300-8177

Zhang, G., & Ghosh, S. (2000). Molecular mechanisms of NF-kappaB activation induced by bacterial lipopolysaccharide through Toll-like receptors. *Journal of Endotoxin Research*, Vol. 6, No. 6, (2000), pp. (453-457), 0968-0519

Zhang, Y., & Ding, XL. (1996). Studies on anti-oxidative fraction in bamboo leaves and its capacity to scavenge active oxygen redicals. *Journal of Bamboo Research*, Vol. 15, No. 3, (1996), pp. (17-24), 1000-6567

8

Antioxidant and Anti-Proliferative Capacity of a Dichloromethane Extract of *Dicerocaryum senecioides* Leaves

Leseilane J. Mampuru[1,*], Pirwana K. Chokoe[1], Maphuti C. Madiga[1],
Annette Theron[2], Ronald Anderson[2] and Matlou P. Mokgotho[1]

[1]*Department of Biochemistry, Microbiology and Biotechnology,
Faculty of Science and Agriculture, University of Limpopo, Sovenga,
[2]Medical Research Council Unit for Inflammation and Immunity,
Department of Immunology, Faculty of Health Sciences, University of Pretoria and
Tshwane Academic Division of the NHLS, Pretoria,
South Africa*

1. Introduction

Plant derivatives have been used over the years to treat a wide variety of ailments, from microbial infections to various forms of neoplastic growth. The isolation and characterisation of novel compounds that might serve as leads for the development of new and effective drugs from medicinal plants has now become an area of much interest worldwide (de las Heras et al., 1998; de Mesquita et al., 2009, 2011; Russo et al., 2010; Suffness & Pezzuto, 1990; Taylor et al., 2001). To this end, plants have been shown to have very high anti-oxidative activity that makes them potential anti-proliferative, anti-invasive and pro-apoptotic agents. Indeed, in drug discovery or drug assessment using cell lines, researchers endeavour to find compounds that lead to the triggering of apoptosis or programmed cell death in diseased cells such as cancer or HIV infected cells (Cragg et al., 1993; Cragg & Newman, 2000; de Mesquita et al., 2011; Huerta-Reyes et al., 2004; Klos et al., 2009). A candidate drug is, therefore, introduced to the cells and its effects ascertained. The most ideal is a compound that is potent at low concentrations and discriminates between diseased and normal cells (Cochrane et al., 2008; Wang, 1998).

The chemopreventive effects of vegetables and fruits are attributed to a combined effect of various phenolic phytochemicals which are generally antioxidant in nature, along with vitamins, dietary fibers, sulforophanes (in broccoli), selenium, carotenes, lycopenes, indoles, and isoflavones (Gurib-Fakim, 2006). These polyphenolic compounds possess known properties which include free radical scavenging, inhibition of hydrolytic and oxidative enzymes, as well as anti-proliferative and anti-inflammatory actions, anti-bacterial, and anti-viral activities to some extent (Frankel, 1995; Pinmai et al., 2008). Subsequently, the intake of herbal remedies and some common dietary supplements rich in antioxidants and micronutrients has been associated with reduced risks of cancer, diabetes and other degenerative disorders associated with inflammation and ageing (Bandera et al., 2007; Liu et al, 2008; de Mesquita et al., 2009; Parsons et al., 2008). Despite the many concerns regarding the degree of bioavailability and biotransformation of these phytochemicals in *in vivo* experimental settings, as compared to the *in vitro* situations, this wide group of natural molecules nonetheless represents a promising class as anticancer drugs, due to their multiple targets in cancer cells and their limited toxic effect on normal cells (Manach et al., 2005). In fact, many of the plant-derived phytochemicals have already been isolated, characterised and incorporated into the pharmaceutical industry for generation of potent chemotherapeutic drugs (Russo et al., 2010).

Dicerocaryum senecioides subsp. *transvaalense* (Klotzsch) J. Abels [family: Pedaliaceae], is a creeping perennial widely used both as a traditional medicinal plant and a nutritional source in many parts of southern Africa. The plant has been identified in our laboratory as a potential repository for anti-oxidant, anti-proliferative and anti-inflammatory agents. *Dicerocaryum senecioides* (vernacular: *malala 'a kwaetše or lempati*) grows widely in sandy soils of the veld in southern Africa. The sprawling stems grow vigorously in summer and less for the rest of the year. The plant covers an area of up to 10 m², and the stems bear distinctive fruit with two spines on the upper side. The small, hairy leaves of *D. senecioides* like those of related family members, *D. zanguebarium* (Lour.) Merrill and *D. eriocarpum* (Decne.) are used not only as food, but also in folk medicine for treating measles, as a hair shampoo, treatment of wounds, and to facilitate births in domestic animals and humans (Barone et al., 1995; Benhura & Marume 1992; Luseba et al., 2007). Nevertheless, the therapeutic mechanisms of action of *D. senecioides* have not been established. Recent findings in our laboratory have demonstrated that a dichloromethane extract of *D. senecioides* leaves exhibit strong anti-inflammatory (Madiga et al., 2009) and noticeable anti-proliferative properties against various cancer cell lines tested (unpublished data). These activities are assumed to be due to the plant's inherent anti-oxidative capacity, thought to be related to an abundance of phenolic compounds and flavonoids.

Exposure to potentially damaging reactive oxidants occurs unrelentingly throughout life because of the continuous endogenous generation of these agents by physiological processes, particularly mitochondrial respiration (Circu & Aw, 2010). Exogenous sources of reactive oxidants include cigarette smoke and other atmospheric pollutants, as well as certain pharmacological agents and chemicals. In addition to these, the phagocytic cells of the innate host immune system are also major producers of toxic oxidants. Neutrophils and macrophages are known to recruit and play vital roles in acute and chronic inflammation, respectively (Kasama et al., 1993). During inflammation, a marked recruitment and activation of inflammatory cells including neutrophils is noted. Activation of these phagocytes leads to the generation and release of reactive oxygen species (ROS) such as superoxide anion radical, hydrogen peroxide and hypochlorous acid (Weiss & Lobuglio, 1982). Depending on their concentration, ROS can be beneficial or damaging to cells and tissues. At physiological levels, ROS function as "redox messengers" in intracellular signaling and regulation, whereas excess ROS induce oxidative modification of cellular macromolecules, inhibit protein function, and promote cell death (Circu & Aw, 2010). Moreover, the generated ROS can influence the carcinogenic process by oxidatively damaging DNA and promoting malignant transformation in bystander cells in tissue culture (Jackson et al., 1989).

Since the identification of oxidant and antioxidant compounds is imperative for predicting and reducing health risks (Tunón et al., 1995), while the identification and development of useful and safe cancer treatment agents from herbal medicines is a well-recognised strategy in drug development (de Mesquita et al., 2009, 2011), this study was designed to investigate potential antioxidant and anti-proliferative activities of the leaf extracts of *D. senecioides* in order to corroborate its indigenous medicinal usage and the supposed indigenous exploit as a nutritional supplement.

2. Materials and methods

2.1 Materials used

All reagents were supplied by Sigma-Aldrich Chemical Company (St. Louis, MO, USA), unless otherwise stated. All other reagents were of high quality and were obtained from reputable suppliers.

2.2 Methods

2.2.1 Extraction and fractionation

Fresh leaves of *D. senecioides* were collected, during the rainy season (January to April), from the grounds of the University of Limpopo, South Africa and dried for three days in an oven at 40°C. The dried leaves were then pulverised into a fine powder using pestle and mortar. The powder (46.15 g) was then extracted with absolute methanol (0.10 g/ml) by shaking for 72 h at room temperature. After the debris had settled, the green supernatant was filtered with a Whatman no.1 filter paper and concentrated to dryness under reduced pressure at 40°C using a Büchi Rotavapor R-200/205 (Büchi, Switzerland). The crude residue (14.79 g) was resuspended in ethanol: water (30:10, v/v). The ethanol: water extract was further fractionated by solvent-solvent extraction using *n*-hexane (D1 fraction), dichloromethane (D2 fraction), *n*-butanol (D3 fraction) and water (D4 fraction). The fractions were concentrated on a Büchi Rotavapor R-200/205 and the resultant residues (D1, 0.9 g; D2, 0.96 g; D3, 1.89 g; and D4, 5.4 g) were dissolved to an appropriate concentration in either acetone (for TLC) or dimethylsulphoxide (DMSO) (for anti-proliferative experiments) and stored in dark bottles at -20°C until required. A schematic representation of the fractionation procedure is illustrated in Fig. 1.

2.2.2 Phytochemical analysis

Chemical constituents of the extracts were analysed by thin layer chromatography (TLC). Ten microliters of each stock solution (10 mg/ml in acetone) from crude, D1, D2, D3 and D4 fractions were loaded individually onto the baseline of the Merck silica gel 60-F_{254} TLC plate (Macherey-Nagel, Düren, Germany) and the components were then separated with either chloroform: ethyl acetate: formic acid, CEF (10:8:2, v/v/v) (intermediate polarity/acidic) or butanol: acetic acid: water, BAW (4:1:5, v/v/v) (acidic/polar) or ethyl acetate: methanol: water, EMW (10:1.35:1, v/v/v) (polar/neutral) depending upon the nature of the fraction components. Chromatograms were visualised and circled under UV light at 254 nm and 365 nm for quenching and fluorescing compounds, respectively. The constituent phytochemicals were detected with vanillin-sulphuric acid reagent spray (0.1 g vanillin: 28 ml methanol: 1 ml sulphuric acid), followed by heating at 110°C in an oven for 3 min for optimal colour development.

2.2.3 Antioxidant activity analyses

The role of free radical reactions in disease pathology (e.g., in atherosclerosis, inflammation, ageing, ischemic heart diseases, neurodegenerative diseases, etc.) is well established, suggesting that these reactions are necessary for normal metabolism but can be detrimental to health as well. In this study, the antioxidant and free radical scavenging activities of the leaf extracts of *D. senecioides* were evaluated both qualitatively and quantitatively using the 2, 2-diphenyl-1-picrylhydrazyl (DPPH) chemical antioxidant assay.

2.2.3.1 TLC-DPPH antioxidant screening

The TLC-DPPH antioxidant assay is a qualitative method generally used for the screening of the anti-oxidative potential of plant extracts. It involves the chromatographic separation of the fractions, after which the chromatogram is sprayed with a purple/violet coloured radical solution, 0.2% DPPH (in absolute methanol). When DPPH interacts with antioxidant compounds, it accepts either electrons or hydrogen atoms, and this neutralises its free radical character. In the process, the purple/violet diphenyl-picrylhydrazyl colour is changed to a yellow diphenyl-picrylhydrazine colour in the presence of an antioxidant compound. The R_f values of the antioxidant compounds can thus be determined on the chromatogram. In this experiment, the TLC was run to separate the constituent compounds in the fractions, as described in section 2.2.2, and the plate was later stained with 0.2% DPPH solution to identify compounds that possess antioxidant activity.

2.2.3.2 DPPH radical scavenging effect

This is a quantitative assay method. Used as a reagent, DPPH offers a convenient and accurate method for titrating the oxidisable groups of natural or synthetic antioxidants. The 2, 2-diphenyl-1-picrylhydrazyl radical scavenging activities of the crude, D1, D2, D3 and D4 fractions were determined according to the method described by Katsube et al. (2004). The assay involves the measurement of the disappearance of the coloured free radical, DPPH, by spectrophotometric determination. A 1000 µg/ml stock solution of the plant extract was serially diluted and pipetted (10 µl) into a 96-well plate. An equivalent amount of 100x diluted ascorbic acid (vitamin C) was used as a positive control. One hundred and eighty five microliters of a 0.2% DPPH solution (in absolute methanol and further dissolved in a 50% ethanol solution) was added to each well and the plate gently shaken for 5 min at room temperature. The change in absorbance at 550 nm was measured using a microtiter plate reader (DTX 880 multimode detector, Beckman Coulter, Fullerton, CA, USA). The percentage of scavenging activity was measured as:

$$\% \text{ inhibition} = \frac{[\text{absorbance of blank sample} - \text{test sample}]}{[\text{absorbance of blank sample}]} \times 100$$

Where, the blank sample contained only DMSO and DPPH.

2.2.4 Reducing power

Reducing powers of the crude, D1, D2, D3 and D4 fractions were measured using a spectrophotometric method. Briefly, various concentrations of the fractions (0-250 µg/ml) were prepared in 100 µl of dH_2O; vitamin C (100 µl of 100x dilute) was used as a positive control. Two hundred and fifty microliters of 0.2 M phosphate buffer (pH 6.6) and 1% (w/v) potassium ferricyanide [$K_3Fe(CN)_6$] were added to each sample. The test samples were incubated at 50°C for 20 min. Two hundred and fifty microliters of 10% (w/v) TCA were later added to each tube and centrifuged at 900 x g for 10 min. Subsequently, 250 µl of the upper layer from each test sample was aspirated and transferred into clean Eppendorf tubes, and then diluted with an equal volume of dH_2O. An additional 50 µl of 0.1% (w/v) ferric chloride ($FeCl_3$) was added to each tube, mixed and 200 µl of this mixture transferred into a microtiter plate and the absorbance measured at 700 nm using a microtiter plate reader (DTX 880 multimode detector, Beckman Coulter, Fullerton, CA, USA).

2.2.5 Neutrophil isolation

In order to assess the selective inhibitory ability of the D2 fraction for the transformed cell lines, its cytotoxic effect was evaluated against the normal human neutrophil cells. Neutrophils were isolated from heparinised venous blood (5 units of preservative-free heparin per ml of blood) from healthy adult volunteers. The neutrophils were separated from mononuclear leukocytes by centrifugation on Histopaque-1077 (Sigma Diagnostics) cushions at 400 x g for 25 min at room temperature. The resultant pellet was suspended in phosphate-buffered saline (PBS, 0.15 M, pH 7.4) and sedimented with 3% gelatine to remove most of the erythrocytes. Following centrifugation (280 x g at 10°C for 10 min), residual erythrocytes were removed by selective lysis with 0.83% ammonium chloride at 4°C for 10 min. The neutrophils, which were routinely of high purity (>90%) and viability (>95%), as determined by light microscopy and fluorescence microscopy (exclusion of ethidium bromide) respectively, were resuspended to (1 x 10^7 cells/ml) in PBS, pH 7.4, and held on ice until used.

2.2.6 Neutrophil viability

Isolated neutrophils (1x10^7 cells/ml) were exposed to the D2 fraction (0, 100, 200, 400, 600 and 800 µg/ml) for 0, 15 and 30 min at 37°C before addition of propidium iodide (PI). The percentage cells, whose cell membrane integrity was compromised (PI positive), were determined by using an Epics® Altra™ Flow Cytometer (Beckman Coulter Inc., Fullerton, CA, USA) fitted with a water-cooled Enterprise laser. PI intercalates into the DNA, and cannot enter the cell if the cell membrane is intact; therefore all PI positive cells have a disrupted cell membrane, indicating that these cells are not viable.

2.2.7 Cell culture

A murine macrophage cell line, Raw 264.7 (ATCC, Rockville, USA), was routinely cultured in RPMI-1640 growth medium (Gibco, Auckland, New Zealand) supplemented with 10% (v/v) fetal bovine serum, FBS (Hyclone, Cramlington, UK) and 1% (v/v) penicillin, streptomycin, neomycin (PSN) antibiotic cocktail (Gibco, Auckland, New Zealand) at 37°C in a humidified 5% CO_2/95% atmosphere.

2.2.8 MTT cytotoxicity assay

Cell viability of D2-treated Raw 264.7 cells was determined by the MTT [3-(4, 5-dimethylthiazol-2-yl)-2, 5-diphenyltetrazolium bromide] assay. Experimental cells were seeded at 2 x 10^5 cells/ml in a 96-well cell culture plate (Nunc™, Roskilde, Denmark) and incubated at 37°C overnight to allow the cells to attach. The cells were then exposed to various concentrations (0, 50, 100, 200, and 250 µg/ml) of the D2 fraction dissolved in DMSO. A mock sample (cells, RPMI-1640 and 0.05% DMSO) served as a negative control. The plates were incubated at 37°C for 0, 24, 48 and 72 h after which 40 µl of 5 mg/ml MTT was added to each well. Following incubation at 37°C for 3 h, the medium was aspirated and the remaining cells were washed once with pre-warmed PBS, pH 7.4. The reduced MTT was then dissolved in 50 µl DMSO and the absorbance was measured at 595 nm using a Model 550 microtiter-plate multimode detector (Bio-Rad Laboratories, California, USA). The percentage of viable cells was calculated as follows:

$$\% \text{ viability } = \frac{[A_{595}\text{of control } - A_{595}\text{of sample}]}{A_{595}\text{of control}} \times 100$$

2.2.9 Cell proliferation by real time cell analysis

The effect of the D2 fraction on cell proliferation was also assessed by real time cell analysis in which RAW 264.7 mouse macrophages were cultured for 24 h at 37°C in a 16-well E-plate 16 docked in a real time cell analysis dual plate (RTCA-DP) analyser (ACEA Biosciences, Inc., California, USA). After 24 h of growing, the cells were then treated with the D2 fraction as described in section 2.2.8 and cell densities of the treated cells were quantitatively monitored for 48 h at 37°C and represented as cell-index values.

2.2.10 Morphological analysis of apoptosis

The effects of the D2 fraction were evaluated for pro-apoptotic potential by microscopic analysis of the chromosomal DNA of the D2-treated Raw 264.7 cells. Apoptotic nuclei are identified by condensed chromatin gathering at the periphery of the nuclear membrane or totally fragmented apoptotic bodies. Briefly, cells were exposed to various concentrations of the D2 fraction (0, 50, 100, 200, and 250 µg/ml) for 24 h and washed with PBS, pH 7.4. The cells were then stained with 4', 6-diamidino-2-phenylindole (DAPI), which forms fluorescent complexes with double-stranded DNA by binding in the minor groove of the nucleic acid backbone. Cells were viewed and recorded under a Nikon Eclipse Ti inverted fluorescence microscope fitted with a camera (Nikon, Japan).

2.2.11 Statistical analysis

The results of each series of experiments are expressed as the mean values ± standard error of the mean (SEM). Levels of the statistical significance are calculated using the paired student t-test when comparing two groups, or by analysis of variance (ANOVA). The p-values of ≤ 0.05 were considered significant.

3. Results

3.1 Extraction and fractionation

The schematic representation of the extraction and the sequential (solvent-solvent) fractionation of the crude methanolic leaf extract of D. senecioides, using different solvents, are represented in Fig. 1.

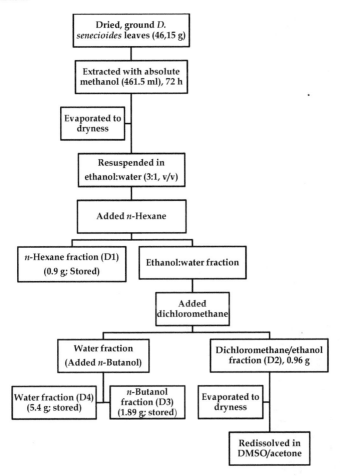

Fig. 1. The schematic representation of the fractionation of the crude methanolic leaf extract of *D. senecioides*.

3.2 TLC-DPPH free radical scavenging activity

TLC was used for the qualitative detection of constituent compounds in *D. senecioides*. As shown in Fig. 2A, the D2 fraction showed the most constituent components with strong intensities using the CEF (10:8:2, v/v/v), EMW (10:1.35:1, v/v/v) and BAW (4:1:5, v/v/v) solvent systems followed by the crude, and then the D3 fraction. Both the D1 and D4 fractions did not exhibit any noticeable antioxidant activity on the TLC plate. Since the antioxidant activity of plant extracts cannot be evaluated by only one method because of the complex nature of phytochemicals, it was thus imperative to use several assays to evaluate the antioxidant activity of of *D. senecioides* leaf extracts. The TLC-DPPH method of qualitative antioxidant detection revealed that crude, D2 and D3 fractions all possessed antioxidant activities which were manifested by a bright yellow colour. The three fractions exhibited a similar R_f value (R_f = 0.78) when resolved on the BAW solvent system.

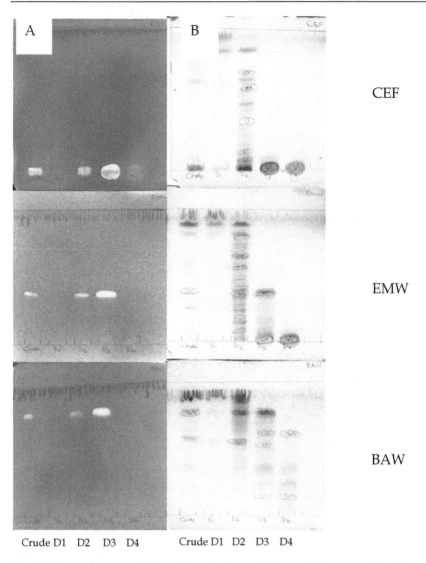

Crude D1 D2 D3 D4   Crude D1 D2 D3 D4

Fig. 2. Chromatograms of the various fractions of *D. senecioides* sprayed with vanillin/
sulphuric acid reagent (A) to show compounds extracted with methanol (crude), *n*-hexane
(D1), dichloromethane (D2), *n*-butanol (D3) and water (D4); and 0.2% DPPH solution (B) to
indicate compound(s) with antioxidant activity. Note the high antioxidant activity displayed
by the D3 fraction, and the moderate amounts in the crude and D2 fractions. Both D1 and
D4 fractions exhibited no detectable antioxidant activity.

The D3 fraction, in particular, had the strongest scavenging activity (Fig. 2B). These
observations demonstrate the presence of antioxidant compounds in *D. senecioides*. Because
this is a qualitative method, a quantitative assay was also used to evaluate the abilities of the
fractions to scavenge DPPH.

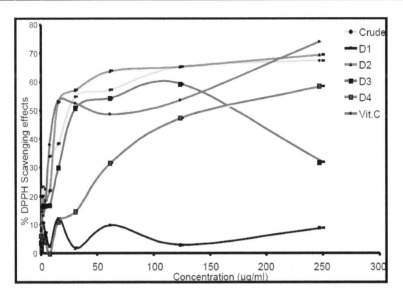

Fig. 3. DPPH radical scavenging capacities of methanol (crude), *n*-hexane (D1), dichloromethane (D2), *n*-butanol (D3) and water (D4) fractions.

3.2 DPPH free radical scavenging activity

The anti-oxidative potential of the D2 fraction was also evaluated quantitatively using the DPPH free radical scavenging activity assay. As shown in Fig. 3, the D2 fraction possessed a high DPPH-scavenging activity from 62.5 µg/ml (63.8%) to 250 µg/ml (69.5%) as compared to the other fractions; the order of potency in descending order was D2> crude> D3> D4> D1 (Fig. 3). Vitamin C (diluted 100x) was used as a positive control. DMSO, as a negative control, showed no scavenging activity. The reducing powers of the fractions were also evaluated.

3.3 Reducing ability

The reducing potentials of the different fractions were determined by their ability to reduce ferric ions. The presence of antioxidants with reducing potential causes the reduction of the Fe^{3+}-ferricyanide complex to the ferrous (Fe^{2+}) form. Therefore, Fe^{2+} can be monitored by measuring the formation of Perl's Prussian blue at 700 nm (Öztürk et al., 2006). Fig. 4 shows the reducing power of *D. senecioides* fractions and vitamin C (positive control) using the potassium ferricyanide reduction method. The reducing power of the fractions increased with increasing concentrations. The D2 fraction showed a higher reducing power than the other fractions in a dose-dependent fashion. However, its reducing power was less than that of vitamin C which was diluted 100x.

3.4 Neutrophil viability

Since the D2 fraction displayed the most potent anti-oxidative activity, it warranted further assessment on the possible anti-proliferative activity against cancer cells. Thus, its selective cytotoxicity for the transformed cell lines was investigated against freshly isolated human blood neutrophils, used as normal control cells. The neutrophils, treated with the D2 fraction for 15 min, showed a significant decrease in viability at a concentration of 400 µg/ml with 91% viable cells; while after 30 min, a significant decrease was observed at 600 µg/ml with 89% viable cells (Fig. 5). However, the experimental concentrations used (0-250 µg/ml) were found not to be cytotoxic to the normal, control neutrophil cells.

3.5 Anti-proliferative effect of D2 fraction on RAW 264.7 cells

The effect of the D2 fraction on proliferation of RAW 264.7 cells was analysed by determining viability and growth of treated cells using the MTT assay and real time cell analysis, respectively. The D2 fraction decreased cell viability (Fig. 6) and growth (Fig. 7) in a time- and dose-dependent manner.

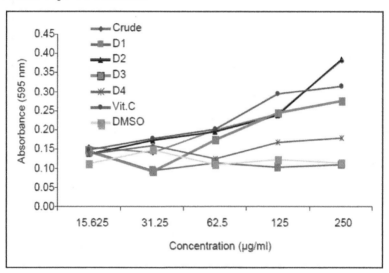

Fig. 4. Reducing powers of methanol (crude), n-hexane (D1), dichloromethane (D2), n-butanol (D3) and water (D4) fractions, vitamin C (positive control, 100x diluted) and DMSO (negative control, less than 0.1%).

3.6 Apoptotic morphology

Treated cells were shown to die through apoptosis when stained with DAPI nucleic acid stain (Fig. 8). The DAPI stain is sensitive to DNA conformation and the state of chromatin in cells, and is thus used to grade nuclear damage. Cells dying through apoptosis displayed nuclei that stained bright blue as their chromatin was condensed, whilst those that had reached advanced stages of apoptosis showed totally fragmented morphology of nuclear (apoptotic) bodies that also stained bright blue (Fig. 8).

4. Discussion

The objective of this study was to investigate the anti-oxidative and anti-proliferative potentials of leaf extracts of *D. senecioides*. TLC serves as a qualitative, screening method to characterise the phytochemical constituents of plants. It also enables comparison of the chemical composition of different fractions using different solvents; high quality resolution is based on the polar/nonpolar nature of the constituent compounds. TLC separation of the fractions showed that the D2 fraction contains more compounds when sprayed with vanillin than the other fractions (Fig. 2A).

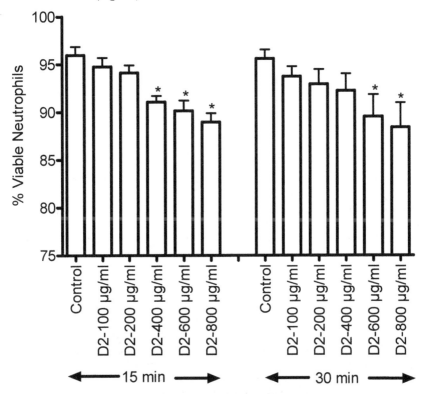

Fig. 5. Viability of normal human neutrophils after exposure to various concentrations of the D2 fraction for 0, 15 and 30 min at 37°C before addition of propidium iodide (PI). The results represent five different experiments expressed as mean values ± SEM. *Statistically significant (P<0.05).

Subsequent investigations were focused on the anti-oxidative potential of the D2 fraction. Oxygen-derived free radicals and other reactive oxygen species (ROS) generated endogenously and exogenously are associated with the pathogenesis of various diseases such as atherosclerosis, diabetes, cancer, arthritis and the ageing process (Halliwell & Gutteridge, 1999). Many natural products are available as chemoprotective agents against common cancers worldwide, and many of these are powerful antioxidants. These natural products, many of which are phenolic compounds, are found in vegetables, fruits, plant extracts and herbs. Although the mechanism of their protective effects is unclear, the fact that the consumption of fruits and vegetables lowers the incidence of carcinogenesis is broadly supported (Reddy et al., 2003). Certainly, anti-oxidative properties are generally considered to confer beneficial, chemopreventive properties on a molecule.

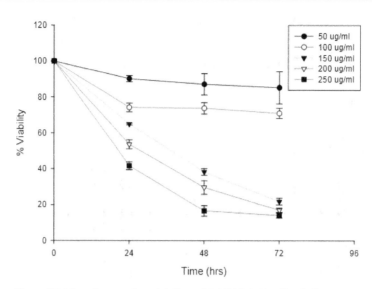

Fig. 6. The effect of D2 fraction on the viability of RAW 264.7 cells. Cells were treated with increasing concentrations of the D2 fraction for 0, 24, 48 and 72 h, followed by viability determination by the MTT assay. Viability was calculated as percentage of untreated control cells. The results represent the mean of two independent experiments, each done in duplicate ± SEM.

The antioxidant activities of the various fractions were measured using qualitative TLC-DPPH and a quantitative DPPH spectrophotometric assay based on the scavenging of the stable DPPH free radical, while the Fe^{3+}-Fe^{2+} reductive method was used to determine the reducing potentials of the fractions. Different antioxidant assays are used to facilitate the screening and identification of the anti-oxidative activity of plant fractions in comparison with that of known, stable antioxidants. Because antioxidants can act by different mechanisms, and more than one mechanism can be involved, it is possible for an antioxidant to protect in one system, but fail in another. Evidently, the understanding of mechanisms and dynamics of the antioxidant action is essential for designing appropriate experimental methods and proper interpretation of the results. Therefore, antioxidant activity must be evaluated using different test methods on the basis of the mechanisms and dynamics of antioxidant action (Arouma, 2003; Niki, 2010).

Consequently, the free radical scavenging activities of the plant fractions were evaluated according to their abilities to scavenge synthetic DPPH. This assay provides useful information on the reactivity of the compounds with stable free radicals. Vitamin C was used for comparison because it is known to be the most abundant and effective water-soluble antioxidant in the body. The qualitative TLC-DPPH antioxidant method was used to screen fractions in order to indicate which of these had potential antioxidant activity which merited further investigation. After the plates were sprayed with the DPPH solution, unique bands with strong and characteristic intense yellow colour appeared (Fig. 2B). The D3 fraction showed a strong yellow colour followed by D2> crude> D1> D4 fractions. The intensity of the yellow colour depends on the quantity and nature of the compound present at that area.

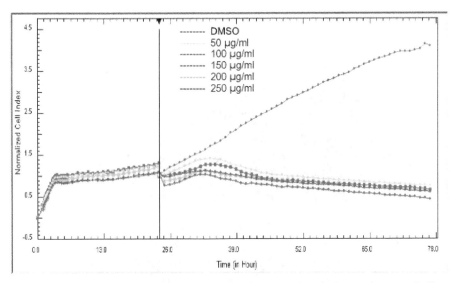

Fig. 7. Real time cell analysis plot of RAW 246.7 cells treated with the D2 fraction. Cells were cultured for 24 h and then followed by treatment with various concentrations of the D2 fraction for a further 48 h. Cell proliferation was measured by continuously monitoring cell indices using an RTCA-DP analyser. Cell indices were normalised at 24 h and then treated with the extract (see arrow head). The final DMSO concentration was 0.05%.

The quantitative DPPH spectrophotometric assay method was also used to quantify the antioxidant activities of the crude, D1, D2, D3 and D4 fractions. This is a rapid and low cost method commonly used in antioxidant studies. An antioxidant molecule present in plant extracts can quench the DPPH free radicals by either providing a hydrogen atom or by donating an electron (Bondet et al., 1997). The results of the quantitative DPPH assay suggest that the D2 fraction possesses an impressive antioxidant scavenging activity in comparison to D1, D3, and D4 (Fig. 3). Comparison of these results showed a contradictory relationship between the activities measured by the qualitative TLC-DPPH screening method and the quantitative DPPH spectrophotometric assay. The D3 fraction showed stronger scavenging activity in the qualitative TLC-DPPH assay (Fig. 2B) than the other fractions, while in the quantitative DPPH assay (Fig. 3), the D2 fraction displayed the strongest anti-oxidative activity (found to be comparable to the crude extract), possibly because of the synergistic behaviour of compounds present in the D2 fraction.

The aforementioned methods focused on the radical scavenging activities of antioxidants extracted from the fractions. However, the antioxidant activities of natural antioxidants may also result from their reducing powers, because the constituent compounds may act by donating electrons to free radicals and convert them to more stable products. The reducing power of a compound may serve as a significant indicator of its potential antioxidant activity (Rajeshwar et al., 2005). The D2 fraction showed significant reducing power when assayed using the potassium ferricyanide test (Fig. 4). This fraction also demonstrated the ability to convert $FeCl_3$ from the ferric to the ferrous state, a feature indicative of hydrogen-donating potential (Rajeshwar et al., 2005). The D2 fraction was therefore found to have various radical scavenging activities that could be due to the presence of a number of phenolic compounds. Clearly, further work needs to be undertaken to confirm the antioxidant property of this fraction by using other antioxidant assessment methods, as well as to characterise and identify the active agent or agents.

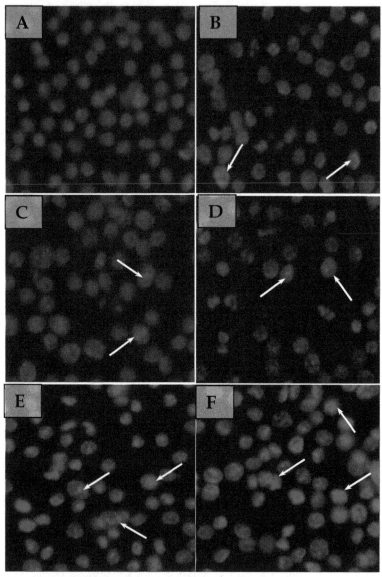

Fig. 8. DAPI nucleic acid staining demonstrating apoptotic morphology in RAW 264.7 cells after exposure to various concentrations of D2 fraction for 24 h. Cells were photographed under an inverted fluorescence microscope at 40x magnification. A = DMSO control, B = 50 μg/ml, C = 100 μg/ml, D = 150 μg/ml, E = 200 μg/ml and F = 250 μg/ml. Arrows indicate nuclear shrinkage and chromatin condensation.

The D2 fraction was further evaluated for anti-proliferative activity by analysis of its effect on the growth and viability of Raw 264.7 cells, a murine-derived macrophage cell line, using real time cell analysis and MTT assay, respectively. The MTT assay demonstrated that the D2 fraction induced a time- and concentration-dependent decrease in cell viability (Fig. 6). Fig. 7 showed that the D2 fraction resulted in a decrease in the cell index, a unit-less, quantitative measure of the number of cells present in a given E-plate 16 well. The measurement of cell proliferation using an RTCA-DP analyser allowed constant monitoring of cell death in real-time without interfering with cell behaviour. Further, evaluation of the effect of the D2 fraction in normal human neutrophil cells demonstrated a degree of specific and selective cytotoxicity to cancer cells. This was so because the viability of the normal neutrophil cells was unaffected by the experimental concentration range (0-250 µg/ml) used. However, these cells were found to be moderately susceptible to the toxic D2 concentrations (600 and 800 µg/ml) used (Fig. 5).

Furthermore, Raw 264.7 cells were shown to die through apoptosis as indicated by the staining of the treated cells with DAPI nucleic acid stain. Cells undergoing apoptosis are characterised by cytoplasmic shrinkage, chromatin condensation, membrane blebbing and formation of apoptotic bodies (Wyllie et al., 1980). Indeed, these hallmark features of apoptosis were observed in Raw 264.7 cells treated with various concentrations of the D2 fraction for 24 h (Fig. 8). In contrast, the chromatin of untreated cells remained intact and unaffected after 24 h, as indicated by the evenly spread DAPI nucleic acid stain and granular morphological appearance of the stained nuclei (Fig. 8). The pro-apoptotic activity of the D2 fraction and the prevention of excess free radical production by the D2 fraction illustrate a commendable chemoprotective and chemotherapeutic potential, as this ability allows the fraction to induce cancer cell death without eliciting the inflammatory response often associated with necrotic cell death.

Since bioactive compounds within plant extracts are often blended with other ineffectual constituents, and the activity of the compound of interest is frequently dampened or masked by these unwanted compounds, plant extracts require further purification in order to isolate the active ingredients in their pure form, and/or to trim down the redundant, interfering components. In this study, the D2 fraction was found to possess both anti-oxidative and selective anti-proliferative properties. It is, therefore, essential to fractionate and purify the D2 fraction and to evaluate the anti-oxidative and the anti-proliferative potentials of the resultant bioactive principles against positively tested anticancer compounds (such as doxorubicin) that are currently available in the market.

5. Conclusion

The D2 fraction of D. senecioides displayed properties of an ideal anti-oxidative and anti-proliferative agent. The fraction showed impressive antioxidant activity both as a free-radical scavenger and a reducing agent. Moreover, the induction of apoptosis in the macrophage lineage used suggests that the fraction has the potential to combat chronic inflammation at three stages: i.e., inhibiting initial free radical production, mopping up excess free radicals and eradicating macrophages responsible for the over-production of reactive oxygen species. Furthermore, the pro-apoptotic activity of the D2 fraction has the ability to induce cancer cell death without eliciting the inflammatory response observed in necrotic cell death. Future investigations should, therefore, focus not only on unravelling the actual anti-oxidative and anti-proliferative mechanisms of action, but also on molecular and chemical characterisation of the active components of the D2 fraction. Irrespective of the underlying mechanism(s) of action and precise identification of the active chemical entities present in the D2 fraction, the results of the current study have established a promising anti-oxidative and anticancer potential of the D2 fraction of *D. senecioides*. Considering chemoprevention of cancer, as well as other disorders, particularly chronic inflammatory diseases, this represents a particularly attractive and promising combination of biological activities. Certainly, a full understanding of the redox control of apoptotic initiation and execution could also underpin the development of therapeutic intervention strategies targeted at other oxidative stress-associated disorders.

6. Acknowledgements

This work was made possible by grants from the National Research Foundation (NRF) of South Africa (GUN 2069108) and the University of Limpopo Senate Research Fund (SENRC 03/057-072) awarded to LJM. PKC and MCM were recipients of postgraduate scholarships from NRF and Medical Research Council (MRC) of South Africa, respectively.

7. References

Arouma, O.I. (2003). Methodological considerations for characterizing potential antioxidant action of bioactive components in plant foods. *Mutation Research* 52, 9-20.

Bandera, E.V., Kushi, L.H., Moore, D.F., Gifkins, D.M., & McCullough, M.L. (2007). Fruits and vegetables and endometrial cancer risk: A systematic literature review and meta-analysis. *Nutrition and Cancer* 58(1): 6-21.

Benhura, M.A.N., & Marume, M. (1992). The mucilaginous polysaccharide material isolated from *ruredzo (Dicerocaryum zanguebarium)*. *Journal of Food Chemistry* 46: 7-11.

Bondet, V., Brand-Williams, W., & Berset, C. (1997). Kinetics and mechanisms of antioxidant activity using the DPPH free radical method. *LWT* 30: 609-615.

Circu, M.L., & Aw, T.Y. (2010). Reactive oxygen species, cellular redox systems, and apoptosis. *Free Radical Biology & Medicine* 48: 749-762.

Cochrane, B.C., Nair, P.K.R., Melnick, S.J., Resek, A.P., & Ramachandran, C. (2008). Anticancer effects of *Annona glabra* plant extracts in human leukaemia cell lines. *Journal of Anticancer Research* 28: 965-972.

Conner, E.M., & Grisham, M.B. (1996). Inflammation, free radicals and antioxidants. *Nutrition* 12: 274-277.

Cragg, G.M, Schepartz, S.A., Suffness, M., & Grever, M.R. (1993). The taxol supply crisis. New NCI policies for handling the large-scale production of novel natural product anticancer and anti-HIV agents. *Journal of Natural Products* 56: 1657-1668.

Cragg, G.M., & Newman, D.J. (2000). Antineoplastic agents from natural sources: achievements and future directions. *Expert Opinion on Investigational Drugs* 9: 1-15.

De las Heras, B., Slowing, K., Benedi, J., Carretero, E., Ortega, T., Toledo, C., Bermejo, P., Iglesias, I., Abad, M.J., Gomez-Serranillos, P., Liso, P.A., Villar, A., & Chiriboga, X. (1998). Anti-inflammatory and antioxidant activity of plants used in traditional medicine in Ecuador. *Journal of Ethnopharmacology* 61: 161-166.

De Mesquita, M.L., De Paula, J.E., Pessoa, C., De Moraes, M.O., Costa-Lotufo, L.V., Grougnet, R., Michel, S., Tellequin, F., & Espindola, L.S. (2009). Cytotoxic activity of

Brazilian Cerrado plants used in traditional medicine against cancer cell lines. *Journal of Ethnopharmacology* 123: 439-445.

De Mesquita, M.L., Araujo, R.M., Bezerra, D.P., Filho, R.B., De Paula, J.E., Silveira, E.R., Pessoa, C., De Moraes, M.O., Costa-Lotufo, L.V., & Espindola, L.S. (2011). Cytotoxicity of δ-tocotrienols from Kielmeyera coriacea against cancer cell lines. *Bioorganic & Medicinal Chemistry* 19: 623-630.

Gurib-Fakim, A. (2006). Medicinal plants: Traditions of yesterday and drugs of tomorrow. *Molecular Aspects of Medicine* 27: 1-93.

Halliwell, B., & Gutteridge, J.M.C. (1999). *Free Radicals in Biology and Medicine*, Oxford University Press, New Yolk, pp. 688-689.

Huerta-Reyes, M., Basualdo, M., Del.C., Abe, F., Jimenez-Estrada, M., Soler, C., & Reyes-Chilpa, R. (2004). HIV-1 inhibitory compounds from Calophyllum brasiliense leaves. *Biological & Pharmaceutical Bulletin* 27: 1471-1475.

Jackson, J.H., Gajewski, E., Schraufstatter, I.U., Hyslop, P.A., Fuciarelli, A.F., Cochrane, G.C., & Dizdaroglu, M. (1989). Damage to the bases in DNA induced by stimulated human neutrophils. *Journal of Clinical Investigation* 84: 1644-1649.

Kasama, T., Strieter, R.M., Standiford, T.J., Burdick, M.D., & Kunkel, S.L. (1993). Expression and regulation of human neutrophil-derived macrophage inflammatory protein-1 alpha. *Journal of Experimental Medicine* 178, 63-72.

Klos, M., van der Venter, M., Mline, P.J., Traore, H.N., Meyer, D., & Oosthuizen, V. (2009). *In vitro* anti-HIV activity of 5 selected South African medicinal plant extracts. *Journal of Ethnopharmacology* 124: 182-188.

Liu, H., Qui, N., Ding, H.H., & Yao, R.Q. (2008). Polyphenols contents and antioxidant capacity of 68 Chinese herbals suitable for medical or food uses. *Food Research International* 41: 363-370.

Madiga, M.C., Cockeran, R., Mokgotho, M.P., Anderson, R., & Mampuru, L.J. (2009). Dichloromethane extract of *Dicerocaryum senecioides* leaves exhibits remarkable anti-inflammatory activity in human T-lymphocytes. *Natural Product Research* 23(11): 996-1006.

Manach, C., Williamson, G., Morand, C., Scalbert, A., & Remesy, C. (2005). Bioavailability and bioefficacy of polyphenols in humans. I. Reveiw of 97 bioavailability studies. *American Journal of Clinical Nutrion* 81: 230S-242S.

Öztürk, M., Aydogmus- Öztürk., F., Dury., M.E., & Topcu G. (2006). Antioxidant activity of stem and root extracts of Rhubarb (*Rheum ribes*): an edible medicinal plant. *Journal of Food Chemistry* 80: 112-116.

Niki, E. (2010). Assessment of antioxidant capacity *in vitro* and *in vivo*. *Free Radical Biology & Medicine* 49: 503-515.

Parsons, J.K., Newman, V.A., Mohler, J.L., Pierce, J.P., Flatt, S., & Marshall, J. (2008). Dietary modification in patients with prostate cancer on active surveillance. A randomized, multicenter feasibility study. *BJU International* 101(10): 1227-1231.

Pinmai, S., Chunlaratthanabhorn, S., Ngamkitidechakul, C., Soonthornchareon, N., & Hahnvajanawong, C. (2008). Synergistic growth inhibitory effects of *Phyllanthus emblica* and *Terminalia bellerica* extracts with conventional cytotoxic agents in human hepatocellular carcinoma and lung cancer cells. *World Journal of Gastroenterology* 14: 1491-1497.

Rajeshwar, Y., Senthil-Kumar, G.P., Gupta, M., & Mazumder, U.K. (2005). Studies on *in vitro* antioxidant activities of methanol extract of *Mucuna pruriens* (Fabaceae) seeds. *European Bulletin on Drug Research* 13: 33-39.

Reddy, L., Odhav, B., & Bhoola, K.D. (2003). Natural products for cancer prevention: a global perspective. *Pharmacology and Therapeutics* 99: 1-13.

Russo, M., Spagnuolo, C., Tedesco, I., & Russo, G.L. (2010). Phytochemicals in cancer prevention and therapy: truth or dare? *Toxins* 2: 517-551.

Suffness, M., & Pezzuto, J.M. (1990). Assays related to cancer drug discovery. In: Hostettman, K. (Ed.). *Methods in Plant Biochemistry: Assays for Bioactivity,* 6. Academic Press, London, pp. 71-133.

Tunón, H., Olavsdotter, C., & Bohlin L. (1995). Evaluation of anti-inflammatory activity of some Swedish medicinal plants. Inhibition of prostaglandin biosynthesis and PAF-induced exocytosis. *Journal of Ethnopharmacology* 48: 61-76.

Wang, H.K. (1998). Plant-derived anticancer agents currently in clinical use or clinical trials. *The Investigation Drugs Journal* 1: 92-102.

Weiss, S.J., & Lobuglio, A.F. (1982). Phagocyte-generated oxygen metabolites and cellular injury. *Laboratory Investigations* 4: 5-18.

Weitzman, S.A., Weitberg, A.B., Clack, E.P., & Stossel, T.P. (1985). Phagocytes as carcinogens: malignant transformation produced by human neutrophils. *Science* 227: 1231-1233.

9

Plant Polyphenols as Antioxidants Influencing the Human Health

Sanda Vladimir-Knežević, Biljana Blažeković,
Maja Bival Štefan and Marija Babac
University of Zagreb, Faculty of Pharmacy and Biochemistry,
Croatia

1. Introduction

Widely distributed in plant kingdom and abundant in our diet plant polyphenols are today among the most talked about concerning the classes of phytochemicals. There are several thousand plant-derived compounds of biogical interest that have more than one phenolic hydroxyl group attached to one or more benzene rings, thus qualifying as polyphenols. In recent years, polyphenols have gained a lot of importance because of their potential use as prophylactic and therapeutic agents in many diseases, and much work has been presented by the scientific community which focuses on their antioxidant effects. Traditionally, herbal medicines with antioxidant properties have been used for various purposes and epidemiological data also point at widespread acceptance and use of these agents. Plant polyphenols have been studied with intention to find compounds protecting against a number of diseases related to oxidative stress and free radical-induced damage, such as cardiovascular and neurodegenerative diseases, cancer, diabetes, autoimmune disorders and some inflammatory diseases. In order to evaluate the efficacy of polyphenols as antioxidants as well as to elucidate the mode of their action, researchers today are using a wide range of experimental models, from the simplest chemical antioxidant assays through the biologically more relevant cellular-based assays to the most accurate animal models, and ultimately clinical studies in humans. The latest scientific knowledge offers a more detailed understanding of the biological effects of polyphenols and their role in human health promotion and disease prevention.

This chapter is focused on plant polyphenols, taking into consideration aspects relative to their biosynthesis, structure, botanical sources, chemical analysis, evaluation of antioxidant action, bioavailability as well as their potential health benefits.

2. Biosynthesis, classification and distribution of plant polyphenols

Phenolic compounds are ubiquitous in the plant species but their distribution at the plant tissue, cellular and subcellular levels is not uniform. Insoluble phenolics are found in cell walls, while the soluble phenolics are present within the vacuoles. They are essential to the plant's physiology being involved in diverse functions such as structure, pigmentation, pollination, pathogen and herbivore resistance, as well as growth and development. Insoluble phenolics, linked to various cell components, contribute to the mechanical strength of cell walls and play a regulatory role in the plant growth and morphogenesis. Phenolics from cell inside take a part in response to stress and pathogens. An enhancement of phenylpropanoid metabolism and the amount of phenolic compounds can be observed under different environmental factors and stress conditions (Dewick, 2001; Korkina, 2007). The most plant phenolics are derived from trans-cinnamic acid, which is formed from L-phenylalanine by the action of L-phenylalanine ammonia-lyase (PAL), the branch point enzyme between primary (shikimate pathway) and secondary (phenylpropanoid pathway) metabolism. The shikimate pathway provides an alternative route to the formation of aromatic compounds particularly the aromatic amino acids. L-Phenylalanine, as C_6C_3 building block, is precursor for a wide range of natural products. In plants, frequently the first step is the elimination of ammonia from the side chain to generate cinnamic acid which is later modified to hydroxycinnamic acid (p-coumaric acid). Other related derivatives are obtained by further hydroxylation and methylation reactions sequentially building up substitution patterns typical of shikimate pathway metabolites. Loss of two carbons from the side chain of hydroxycinnamic derivatives leads to formation of hydroxybenzoic acids. Flavonoids are biosynthesized via a combination of the shikimic acid and acylpolymalonate pathways. The crucial biosynthetic reaction is the condensation of one molecule p-coumaroyl-CoA with three molecules malonyl-CoA to a calcone intermediate that consists of two phenolic groups which are connected by an open three carbon bridge. Plants collectively synthesize several thousand known different phenolic compounds and the number of these fully characterised is continually increasing. They can be considered as the most abundant plant secondary metabolites with highly diversified structures, ranging from simple molecules such as phenolic acids to highly polymerized substances such as tannins. The common feature of plant phenolic compounds is the presence of a hydroxy-substituted benzene ring within their structure. They may be classified into different groups as a function of the number of phenol rings contained and the structural elements that bind these rings to one another. Distinctions are thus made between the flavonoids, phenolic acids, stilbenes and lignans. These compounds occur primarily in conjugated form, with one or more sugar residues linked to hydroxyl groups, although direct linkages of the sugar unit to an aromatic carbon atom also exist. Associations with other compounds, such as organic acids, amines and lipids, and linkages with other phenols are also common (Dewick, 2001; Boudet, 2007; Martens & Mithöfer, 2005).

Flavonoids comprise the most abundant class of plant polyphenols with more than 6000 structures which have been identified. They share a carbon skeleton of diphenyl propanes, two benzene rings (A and B) joined by a linear three carbon chain ($C_6C_3C_6$). This central chain usually forms a closed pyran ring (C) with one of the benzene rings. Based on the variation in the type of heterocycle involved, flavonoids may be divided into six subclasses: flavones, flavonols, flavanones, flavanols, anthocyanidins and isoflavonoids. This subdivision is primarily based on the presence (or absence) of a double bond on position 4 of the C (middle) ring, then a double bond between carbon atoms 2 and 3 of the C ring, and hydroxyl groups in the B ring (Table 1). Flavones are characterized by the presence of a double bond between C2 and C3 in the heterocycle of the flavan skeleton. The B ring is attached to C2 and usually no substituent is present at C3. This exactly represents the difference to the flavonols where a hydroxyl group can be found at that C3 position while flavanones have a saturated three-carbon chain. Flavanols contain a saturated three-carbon chain with a hydroxyl group in the C3. Anthocyanidins are positively charged at acidic pH

Class	Main structure	Compound	Plant source	Reference
Flavone		apigenin 4',5,7-OH	*Matricaria recutita* *Achillea millefolium*	(Švehlíková & Repčák, 2006; Trumbeckaite et al., 2011)
		luteolin 3',4',5,7-OH	*Cynara scolymus* *Thymus vulgaris*	(Mulinacci et al., 2004; Bazylko & Strzelecka, 2007)
Flavonol		quercetin 3',4',3,5,7-OH	*Sambucus nigra* *Betula pendula*	(Keinänen & Julkunen-Tiitto, 1998; Verberic et al., 2009)
		kaempferol 4',3,5,7-OH	*Ginkgo biloba* *Moringa oleifera*	(Beek & Montoro, 2009; Verma et al., 2009)
Flavanone		naringenin 4',5,7-OH	*Citrus paradisi* *Humulus lupulus*	(Kanaze et al., 2003; Helmja et al., 2007)
		hesperetin 3',5,7-OH 4'-OCH₃	*Citrus limon* *Citrus sinensis*	(González-Molina et al., 2010; Khan et al., 2010)
Flavanol		catechin 4',5',3,5,7-OH	*Quercus petraea* *Potentilla erecta*	(Vivas et al., 2006; Tomczyk & Latté, 2009)
		gallocatechin 3',4',5',3,5,7-OH	*Hamamelis virginiana* *Camellia sinensis*	(Dauer et al., 2003; Ashihara et al., 2010)
Anthocyanidin		cyanidin 3',4',3,5,7-OH	*Vaccinium myrtillus* *Cenaturea cyanus*	(Du et al., 2004; Takeda et al., 2005)
		pelargonidin 4',3,5,7-OH	*Pelargonium sp.* *Fragaria ananassa*	(Mitchell et al., 1998; Fossen et al., 2004)
Isoflavonoid		daidzein 4',7-OH	*Glycine max* *Trifolium pratense*	(Beck et al., 2005; Peng et al., 2004)
		genistein 4',5,7-OH	*Glycine max* *Genista tinctoria*	(Rimbach et al., 2008; Rigano et al., 2009)

Table 1. Classification of some common flavonoids indicating their major plant sources.

and this equilibrium form is called flavylium cation (2-phenylbenzopyrylium). In the flavonoid structure, a phenyl group is usually substituted at the 2-position of the pyran ring. In isoflavonoids the substitution is at the 3-position (Harborne & Williams, 2000; Dewick, 2001; Middleton et al., 2000). Individual differences within each group arise from variation in number and arrangement of the hydroxyl groups and their extent of alkylation and/or glycosylation. Flavonoids occur both in the free form and as glycosides, most are O-glycosides but a considerable number of flavonoid C-glycosides are also known. The O-glycosides have sugar substituents bound to a hydroxyl group of the aglycone, usually located at position 3 or 7, whereas the C-glycosides have sugar groups bound to a carbon of the aglycone, usually C6 or C8. The most common carbohydrates are rhamnose, glucose, galactose and arabinose. Flavonoid-diglycosides are also frequently found. Two very common disaccharides contain glucose and rhamnose, 1→6 linked in neohesperidose and 1→2 linked in rutinose. An interesting combination of flavonoid and lignan structure is found in a group of compounds called flavonolignans. They arise by oxidative coupling process between flavonoid and a phenylpropanoid, usually coniferyl alcohol. Additionally, the flavanols exist as oligomers and polymers referred to as condensed tannins or proanthocyanidins (Harborne & Williams, 2000; de Rijke et al., 2006). Table 1 summarizes the chemical structures of the most common flavonoids and their botanical sources.

Class	Main structure	Compound	Plant source	Reference
Phenolic acid	Hydroxycinnamic acid (HCA)	ferulic acid 4–OH; 3–OCH₃	*Citrus sinensis* *Pinus maritima*	(Swatsitang et al., 2000; Virgili et al., 2000)
		caffeic acid 3,4–OH	*Ocimum basilicum* *Helianthus annuus*	(Kwee & Niemeyer, 2011; Weisz et al., 2009)
		chlorogenic acid (5-O-caffeoylquinic acid)	*Coffea arabica* *Ilex paraguariensis*	(Koshiro et al., 2007; Marques & Farah, 2009)
		rosmarinic acid (α-O-caffeoyl-3,4-dihydroxyphenyl-lactic acid)	*Rosmarinus officinalis* *Melissa officinalis*	(Petersen & Simmonds, 2003; Weitzel & Petersen, 2011)
	Hydroxybenzoic acid (HBA)	p-HBA 4–OH	*Daucus carota* *Vitex negundo*	(Sircar & Mitra, 2009; Guha et al., 2010)
		gallic acid 3, 4, 5–OH	*Quercus robur* *Hamamelis virginiana*	(Mämmelä et al., 2000; Wang et al., 2003)
Stilbene		resveratrol 3,5,4'-OH	*Vitis vinifera* *Polygonum cuspidatum*	(Pascual-Martí et al., 2001; Chen et al., 2001)
		piceatannol 3,5,3',4'-OH	*Vitis vinifera* *Euphorbia lagascae*	(Kim et al., 2009; Duarte et al., 2008)
Lignan		secoisolariciresinol 4,9,4',9'-OH 3,3'-OCH₃	*Linum usitatissimum* *Secale cereale*	(Li et al., 2008; Smeds et al., 2009)
		isotaxiresinol 4,3',4'-OH 3-OCH₃	*Taxus yunnanensis* *Taxus wallichiana*	(Banskota et al., 2004; Chattopadhyay et al., 2003)

Table 2. Some typical non-flavonoid phenolic compounds of various structures and their plant source.

Phenolic acids are the most common non-flavonoid naturally occurring phenolics which contain two distinguishing constitutive carbon frameworks: the hxydroxycinnamic (C_6C_3) and hydroxybenzoic (C_6C_1) structure. Although the basic skeleton remains the same, the numbers and position of hydroxyl and methoxyl groups on the benzene rings create the variety (Table 2). Only a minor fraction of phenolic acids exists in the free form. Instead, the majority are linked through ester, ether or acetal bonds either to structural components of the plant, larger polyphenols or smaller organic molecules (e.g., glucose, quinic acid). These linkages give rise to a vast array of derivatives (Robbins, 2003). Hydroxybenzoic acids are found in the free form as well as combined into esters of glycosides. Some of them are constituents of hydrolysable tannins which are compounds containing a central core of glucose or another polyol esterified with gallic acid or its dimer hexahydrohydiphenic acid, also called gallotannins and ellagitannins (Dai & Mumper, 2010).

Stilbenes (1,2-diarylethenes) belong to a relatively small group of non-flavonoid class of phenolic compounds found in a wide range of plant sources. Ring A usually carries two hydroxyl groups in the m-position, while ring B may be substituted by hydroxyl and methoxyl groups in various position (Table 2). Stilbenes exist as stereoisomers and naturally occurring stilbenes are overwhelmingly present in the *trans* form. They occur in free and glycosylated forms and as dimeric, trimeric and polymeric stilbenes, the so-called viniferins. One of the most relevant and extensively studied stilbene is *trans*-resveratrol found largely in grapes (Cassidy et al., 2000).

Lignans also constitute a group of non-flavonoid phenolics that are structurally characterized by the coupling of two phenylpropanoid units by a bond between the β-positions in the propane side chains (Table 2). According to recent nomenclature recommendations the units are treated as propylbenzene units, giving the positions 8 and 8' to these linked carbon atoms. When the phenylpropane units are linked by another carbon-carbon bond, the compound class is named as neolignan. Lignans comprise a whole class of compounds with a similar basic skeleton, but with large variations in substitution patterns. They are mostly present in the free form, while their glycoside derivatives are only a minor form (Willför et al., 2006).

3. Phytochemical characterization of polyphenols

The biological properties of polyphenols and their health benefits have intensified research efforts to discover and utilise methods for the extraction, separation and identification of these compounds from natural sources. Despite a great number of investigations, the separation and quantification of various polyphenolics remain difficult, especially the simultaneous determination of their different structural groups. Quantification of phenolic compounds in plant materials is influenced by their chemical nature, the extraction method employed, sample particle size, storage time and conditions, as well as assay method, selection of standards and presence of interfering substances such as waxes, fats, terpenes and chlorophylls. A number of spectrophotometric methods have been developed for quantification of plant phenolics. These assays are based on different principles and can be classified as either those which determine total phenolic content or those quantifying a specific group of class of phenolic compounds (Ignat et al., 2011; Naczk & Shahidi, 2006). The Folin–Ciocalteu assay is widely used for determination of total phenolics. This assay relies on the transfer of electrons in alkaline medium from phenolic compounds to phosphomolybdic/phosphotungstic acid reagent to form blue coloured complexes that are determined spectrophotometrically at 760 nm (Dai & Mumper, 2010; Singleton et al., 1999). Tannins are capable of binding proteins to form water-insoluble substances. The absorbance corresponding to non-tannins is measured after precipitation of tannins with hide powder or casein, and the tannin content is than calculated by the difference (EDQM, 2006; Jurišić Grubešić et al., 2005). Vanillin and proanthocyanidin assays are usually used to estimate total procyanidinidins (condensed tannin), while hydrolysable tannins can be quantified by the potassium iodate method (Dai & Mumper, 2010; Hartzfeld et al., 2002). Determination of phenolic acids can be performed by the method described in European Pharmacopoeia using nitrite-molybdate reagent of Arnow which forms complexes with ortho-diphenols (Blažeković et al., 2010; EDQM, 2006). On the other hand, complexation of the phenolics with Al(III) is the principle of spectrophotometric assay used for quantification of total flavonoids (Jurišić Grubešić et al., 2007; Vladimir-Knežević et al., 2011). Determination of anthocyanins is based on their characteristic behaviour under acidic conditions causing the transformation of anthocyanins to red-coloured flavylium cation (Ignat et al., 2011). The above mentioned spectrophotometric assays give an estimation of the total phenolic contents, while various chromatographic techniques are employed for separation, identification and quantification of individual phenolic compounds.

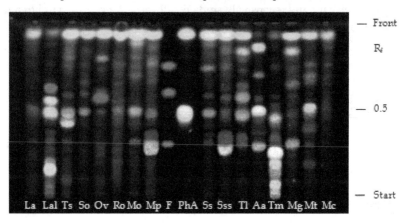

Experimental conditions: HPTLC silica gel 60 F_{254} plate; ethyl acetate - formic acid - water 8:1:1 (V/V/V) as mobile phase; NST/PEG for detection, UV 365 nm. Tracks: F (Flavonoids) - rutin (R_f=0.30), isoquercitrin (R_f=0.59), quercitrin (R_f=0.74) and PhA (Phenolic acids) - chlorogenic acid (R_f=0.48), rosmarinic acid (R_f=0.92) as references; La - *Lavandula angustifolia* Mill., Lal - *Lamium album* L., Ts - *Thymus serpyllum* L., So - *Salvia officinalis* L., Ov - *Origanum vulgare* L., Ro - *Rosmarinus officinalis* L., Mo - *Melissa officinalis* L., Mp - *Mentha* x *piperita* L., Ss - *Salvia sclarea* L., Sss - *Satureja subspicata* Bartl. ex Vis., Tl - *Thymus longicaulis* C. Presl, Aa - *Acinos arvensis* (Lam.) Dandy, Tm - *Teucrium montanum* L., Mg - *Micromeria graeca* (L.) Benth. ex Reich., Mt - *Micromeria thymifolia* (Scop.) Fritsch, Mc - *Micromeria croatica* (Pers.) Schott.

Fig. 1. HPTLC chromatogram of flavonoids and phenolic acids in metanolic extracts of various Lamiaceae species originating from Croatia.

Thin layer chromatography (TLC) is useful for a rapid screening of plant extracts for phenolic substances prior to detailed analysis by instrumental techniques especially because many samples can be analysed simultaneously (Fig. 1). The separation of phenolic compounds is mainly achieved by using silica gel as stationary phase and various mobile phases with UV monitoring or following specific spray reagents (de Rijke et al., 2006). High performance liquid chromatographic technique (HPLC) is now most widely used for both separation and quantification of phenolic compounds. The chromatographic conditions of the HPLC methods include the use of, almost exclusively, a reversed-phase C18 column, UV–Vis diode array detector, and a binary solvent system containing acidified water (solvent A) and a polar organic solvent (solvent B). Reversed phase (RP) HPLC has become a dominating analytical tool for the separation and determination of polyphenols with different detection systems, such as diode array detector (DAD), mass or tandem mass spectrometry. Liquid chromatography–mass spectrometry (LC–MS) techniques are nowadays the best analytical approach to study polyphenols from different biological sources, and are the most effective tool in the study of the structure of phenolic compounds. Tandem-MS detection has largely replaced single-stage MS operation because of much better selectivity and the wider-ranging information that can be obtained. Capillary electrophoresis (CE), which is an alternative separation technique to HPLC, is especially suitable for the separation and quantification of low to medium molecular weight polar and charged compounds, the resultant separations being often faster and more efficient than the corresponding HPLC separations. Gas chromatography (GC) is another technique that has been employed for separation and identification of different phenolic compounds. GC methods developed for the analysis of polyphenols require the derivatisation to volatile compounds by methylation, trifluoroacetylation, conversion to trimethylsilyl derivatives and mass-spectrometric detection (Ignat et al., 2011; Naczk & Shahidi, 2006; de Rijke et al., 2006).

4. Antioxidant effectiveness of plant polyphenols

Oxidative stress is defined as an imbalance between production of free radicals and reactive metabolites, so-called oxidants or reactive oxygen species (ROS), and their elimination by protective mechanisms, referred to as antioxidants. This imbalance leads to damage of important biomolecules and cells, with potential impact on the whole organism. Oxidative stress can damage lipids, proteins, carbohydrates and DNA in cells and tissues, resulting in membrane damage, fragmentation or random cross linking of molecules like DNA, enzymes and structural proteins and even lead to cell death induced by DNA fragmentation and lipid peroxidation. These consequences of oxidative stress construct the molecular basis in the development of cardiovascular diseases, cancer, neurodegenerative disorders, diabetes and autoimmune disorders. ROS are products of a normal cellular metabolism and play vital roles in the stimulation of signalling pathways in cells in response to changes in intra- and extracellular environmental conditions. Most ROS are generated in cells by the mitochondrial respiratory chain. During endogenous metabolic reactions, aerobic cells produce ROS such as superoxide anion ($O_2^{\bullet-}$), hydroxyl radical ($OH^{\bullet}$), hydrogen peroxide (H_2O_2) and organic peroxides as normal products of the biological reduction of molecular oxygen. The electron transfer to molecular oxygen occurs at the level of the respiratory chain, and the electron transport chains are located in the membranes of the mitochondria. Under hypoxic conditions, the mitochondrial respiratory chain also produces nitric oxide (NO), which can generate reactive nitrogen species (RNS). ROS/RNS can further generate other reactive species by inducing excessive lipid peroxidation. In order to combat and neutralize the deleterious effects of ROS/RNS, various antioxidant strategies have involved either the increase of endogenous antioxidant enzyme defences (e.g., superoxide dismutase, glutathione peroxidase, glutathione reductase and catalase) or the enhancement of non-enzymatic defences (e.g., glutathione, vitamins) through dietary or pharmacological means. Antioxidants can delay, inhibit or prevent the oxidation of oxidizable substrate by scavenging free radicals and diminishing oxidative stress. However, in disease conditions, the defence against ROS is weakened or damaged and the oxidant load increases. In such conditions, external supply of antioxidants is essential to countervail the deleterious consequences of oxidative stress (Ratnam et al., 2006; Reuter et al., 2010). It has been proposed that polyphenols can act as antioxidants by a number of potential mechanisms. The free radical scavenging, in which the polyphenols can break the free radical chain reaction, as well as suppression of the free radical formation by regulation of enzyme activity or chelating metal ions involved in free radical production are reported to be the most important mechanisms of their antioxidant activity. The interaction between polyphenolic compounds with other physiological antioxidants is another possible antioxidant pathway for these compounds (Fraga et al., 2010; Perron & Brumaghim, 2009).

In order to evaluate the efficacy of polyphenols as antioxidants as well as to elucidate the mode of their action, researchers today are using a wide range of experimental models, from the simplest chemical antioxidant assays through the biologically more relevant cellular-based assay to the most accurate animal models, and ultimately clinical studies in humans. Taking into account all known advantages and limitations, each currently employed method provides useful information at certain level of biological organization.

4.1 Chemical-based antioxidant assays

Widely used for initial antioxidant screening, chemical-based assays are the most popular methods for an evaluation of antioxidant properties of plant extracts as well as their bioactive constituents. Due to the implication of redox mechanisms in the pathogenesis of numerous human diseases, the vast majority of the available *in vitro* approaches to polyphenolic antioxidant research are based on the redox-linked colorimetric assays. Although it has been established that polyphenols exert antioxidant effects via different modes of action, free radical scavenging abilities seems to be the most important. Namely, polyphenolic compounds possess ideal structure chemistry for free radical neutralization because they have: (i) phenolic hydroxyl groups that are prone to donate a hydrogen atom or an electron to a free radical; (ii) extended conjugated aromatic system to delocalize an unpaired electron (Dai & Mumper, 2010). Among widely employed antioxidant assays, scavenging capacity assays against stable, non-biological radicals (e.g., DPPH$^\bullet$ and ABTS$^{\bullet+}$) and assays against specific ROS/RNS can be distinguished. Especially popular DPPH assay is a convenient and accurate method which provides a simple and rapid way to evaluate free radical-scavenging ability. This assay uses a stable and commercially available organic radical 2,2-diphenyl-1-picrylhydrazyl (DPPH$^\bullet$). Interaction of this purple-coloured radical with an antioxidant agent, which is able to neutralize its free radical character, leads to the formation of yellow-coloured diphenylpicrylhydrazine (Fig. 2) and resulting colour change, proportional to the effect, can be quantified spectrophotometrically. Based on the DPPH free radical scavenging effectiveness, it has been established that numerous polyphenolic compounds of different classes are strong antioxidants (Okawa et al., 2001; Villaño et al., 2007; Vladimir-Knežević et al., 2011). Also frequently used colorimetric method is Trolox equivalent antioxidant capacity (TEAC) assay, which is based on scavenging of blue-green ABTS radical cation by antioxidants present in sample (Nenadis et al., 2004).

Oxygen radical absorbance capacity (ORAC), deoxyribose assays as well as superoxide anion scavenging capacity are usually used to predict scavenging abilities of plant polyphenols against biologically relevant peroxyl, hydroxyl and superoxide radicals, respectively (Cano et al., 2002; Kang et al., 2010). Reducing properties of polyphenols are also very important in terminating free radical-induced chain reactions and are mainly studied in terms of iron(III)-iron(II) transformation abilities. For that purpose ferric reducing antioxidant power (FRAP) assay or potassium ferricyanide reducing method are used (Firuzi et al., 2005; Vladimir-Knežević et al., 2011). In the context of the methods appropriate for quantification of polyphenol total antioxidant capacity, the phosphomolybdenum assay based on the ability to reduce Mo(VI) to Mo(V) is also worth of mention (Blažeković et al.,

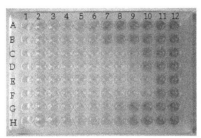

Experimental: The DPPH scavenging activities of ethanolic extract of *Micromeria croatica* (Pers.) Schott (A, B), polyphenolic constituents rosmarinic acid (C, D), and quercetin (E, F), as well as referent antioxidant butylated hydroxyanisole (G, H) were evaluated by mixing seral dilution of samples (concentration range 200-0.20 μg/mL; 1-11) with ethanolic solution of DPPH (100 μM), with regard to DPPH control (12). After incubation for 30 min, absorbance was measured at 490 nm using microplate reader.

Fig. 2. Application of DPPH assay on *Micromeria croatica* extract and polyphenolic constituents.

2010). Another important antioxidative mechanism of polyphenols arises from their capability to chelate transition metals, such as iron and copper, through multiple hydroxyl groups and the carbonyl moiety, when present (Leopoldini et al., 2011). Iron(II) is a primary cause of the ROS generation *in vivo* and plays a pivotal role in contributing to oxidative stress, DNA damage, and cell death, so it has been the target of many antioxidant therapies. By removing and neutralising prooxidative metals, polyphenols may prevent oxidative damage of important biomolecules due to highly reactive hydroxyl radicals generated by the Fenton reaction which is catalysed by Fe^{2+} or Cu^+ ions (Mladenka et al., 2011; Perron & Brumaghim, 2009). Moreover, polyphenols may also act as preventive antioxidants through the inhibition of prooxidative enzymes, like xanthine oxidase (Selloum et al., 2001) which is a physiological source of superoxide anions in eukaryotic cells. Among all biologically important macromolecules, unsaturated membrane lipids are particularly prone to oxidative damage. Therefore, the *in vitro* models of lipid peroxidation, as a well-established mechanism of cellular injury, can be used as an indicator of oxidative stress in cells and tissues. Polyphenols were proved to inhibit chain reaction of oxidative degradation of polyunsaturated fatty acids integrated in micelles, emulsions, liposomes, low-density lipoproteins (LDL) and animal tissues, which was previously induced by different prooxidans (hydroxyl radicals, iron(II) ions, UV radiation). The extent of lipid peroxidation was mostly evaluated spectrophotometrically, in terms of quantification of thiobarbituric acid-reactive substances as end products - TBARS assay (Blažeković et al., 2010; T. Miura et al., 2000).

4.2 Cell-based antioxidant assays

Since the biological systems are much more complex than the simple chemical mixtures and antioxidant compounds may operate via multiple mechanisms, the studies employing complex cellular testing systems provide a more useful approach towards understanding the *in vitro* antioxidant capacities of polyphenols and their behaviours in living cells to reduce oxidative damage (Niki, 2010). The cellular antioxidant activity assay (CAA), developed by Wolfe & Liu (2007), centres on dichlorofluorescin, a probe molecule trapped within cells that can be easily oxidised to produce fluorescence. The test uses 2,2'-azobis(2-amidinopropane) dihydrochloride-generated peroxyl radicals to oxidise dichlorofluorescin, and the ability of antioxidant compounds to inhibit this process in HepG2 human hepatocarcinoma cells. The study has suggested that polyphenols can act at the cell membrane and break peroxyl radical chain reactions at the cell surface, or they can be taken up by the cell and react with ROS intracellularly. Therefore, the efficiency of cellular uptake and/or membrane binding combined with the radical scavenging activity likely dictates the antioxidative effectiveness of different polyphenols. Blasa et al. (2011) consider that red blood cells represent the cheapest and easily available cell type and their ability to cope with ROS/RNS is relevant in the body.

4.3 *In vivo* animal studies

To overcome differences between *in vitro* test systems and the whole organism, as well as the obvious constraints of human clinical studies, animal studies are widely applied in antioxidant research (Mortensen et al., 2008). The capacity and efficacy of antioxidants *in vivo* may be assessed most accurately due to their effect on the level of oxidation in biological fluids and tissues, thus animal studies of polyphenols are mainly focused on serum total antioxidant capacity, lipid peroxidation and antioxidant enzymes activity measurements. Hepatoprotective studies with animal models use exogenously administered hepatotoxin such as carbon tetrachloride (CCl_4), a free radical generating compound that induce an oxidative stress, and related damage of biomolecules and cell death. Polyphenols were found to be able to protect the liver against cellular oxidative damage and maintenance of intracellular level of antioxidant enzymes (Amat et al., 2010; Fernandez-Martinez et al., 2007). Neuroprotective properties of polyphenolic antioxidant compound curcumin were reported based on its ability to inhibit homocysteine (Hcy) neurotoxicity and related Hcy-induced lipid peroxidation in animals' hippocampi (Ataie et al., 2010). Studies performed in apolipoprotein E-deficient mice proved that polyphenols from wine and tea can prevent the development and/or reduce progression of atherosclerosis, probably due to their potent antioxidative activity and ability to protect LDL against oxidation (Hayek et al., 1997; Y. Miura et al., 2001).

4.4 Human studies

At present there is a big gap between the knowledge of *in vitro* and *in vivo* effectiveness of polyphenols as antioxidants, and human studies are still scarcer than those on animals. Oxidative damage and antioxidant protection by polyphenols have been studied in healthy people (preventive effect) or those suffering from certain disease (therapeutic effect). The available human studies of polyphenols can be divided into intervention studies, which are under defined circumstances (such as clinical trials) applying nutritional intervention and measuring the biological outcome (effect), and observational epidemiological studies. Various epidemiological studies have shown an inverse association between the consumption of polyphenols or polyphenol-rich foods and the risk of cardiovascular diseases. In this context, strong epidemiological evidences indicate that moderate consumption of wine is associated with a significant reduction of cardiovascular events. However, the respective contribution of wine polyphenols and alcohol to these effects was not well clarified (Hansen et al., 2005; Manach et al., 2005). Additionally, recent clinical trials on resveratrol, as the main antioxidant in wine, have been largely focused on characterizing its pharmacokinetics and metabolism as well as the potential role in the management of diabetes, obesity, Alzheimer's disease and cancer (Patel et al., 2011). Considering the lack of relevant data, the future clinical trials should be aimed at identifying the cardiovascular benefits of resveratrol. In order to verify the polyphenols as antioxidants in *in vivo* conditions there is still a lot of scientific research to be done. The emerging findings suggest that continued research through well-designed and adequately powered human studies that undoubtedly verify health-promoting antioxidant activity of polyphenols in *in vivo* conditions are more than welcome.

5. Bioavailability of polyphenols

Bioavailability is usually defined as the fraction of an ingested nutrient or compound that reaches the systemic circulation and the specific sites where it can exert its biological activity (Porrini & Riso, 2008). To establish conclusive evidence for the effectiveness of dietary polyphenols in disease prevention and human health improvement, it is useful to better define the bioavailability of polyphenols. The health effects of polyphenols in human and in animal models depend on their absorption, distribution, metabolism and elimination. The chemical structure of polyphenols determines their rate and extent of absorption as well as the nature of the metabolites present in the plasma and tissues. The most common polyphenols in human diet are not necessarily the most active within the body, either because they have a lower intrinsic activity or because they are poorly absorbed from the intestine, highly metabolized, or rapidly eliminated (Manach et al., 2004). Evidence of their absorption trough the gut barrier is given by the increase in the antioxidant capacity of plasma after intake of plant polyphenols. More direct evidence on the bioavailability of phenolic compounds has been obtained by measuring the concentration in plasma and urine after the ingestion of either pure compounds or plant extracts with the known content of the compounds of interest (Baba et al., 2005; Koutelidakis et al., 2009).

Polyphenols are present in plants as aglycones, glycosides, esters or polymers. Aglycones can be absorbed from the small intestine, while glycosides, esters and polymers must be hydrolyzed by intestinal enzymes, or by the colonic microflora, before they can be absorbed (Fig. 3). Although this can be considered as a general rule, some exceptions occur like unchanged anthocyanin glycosides detected in human plasma and urine (Kay et al., 2004). The absorption of plant flavonoids which are predominantly bound to different sugars mostly occurs in the small intestine. There are two possible routes by which the glycosides could be hydrolysed and the first one involves the action of lactase phlorizin hydrolase (LPH) in the brush-border of the small intestine epithelial cells. The released aglycone may then enter epithelial cells by passive diffusion due to increased lipophilicity. The second mechanism includes cytosolic β-glucosidase (CBG) within the epithelial cells where the polar glucosides are transported through the active sodium-dependent glucose transporter 1 (SGLT1). On the other hand, SLGT1 was reported not to transport flavonoids and, moreover, those glycosylated flavonoids, and some aglycones, have the capability to inhibit the glucose transporter. It has been observed that polyphenols differ in site of their absorption. Data on absorption of quercetin-4'-glucoside and quercetin-3-rutinoside illustrate the major impact of structural differences on the site of absorption. Quercetin-4'-glucoside is absorbed in the small intestine after hydrolysis, while the quercetin-3-rutinoside is absorbed in the colon as free and metabolised forms produced by the microflora (Crozier et al., 2010). Hydroxicinnamic acids, when ingested in the free form, are rapidly absorbed from the stomach or the small intestine. However, in plants these compounds mainly occur as esters and therefore a release of free form is required before absorption. For example, ferulic acid, the main phenolic compound present in cereals, is esterified to arabinoxylans of the grain cell walls. Although it has been shown that esterases are present throughout the entire gastrointestinal tract, the release of ferulic acid mainly occurs in the colon after the hydrolysis by microbial xylanase and esterase (Poquet et al., 2010). Proanthocyanidins as the most widespread polyphenols in plants are very poorly absorbed due to their polymeric nature and high molecular weight. Since their concentrations can be much higher in the lumen of gastrointestinal tract then in plasma or other body tissues, proanthocyanidins may have direct effects on the intestinal mucosa, which are important because the intestine is particularly exposed to oxidizing agents and may be affected by inflammation and numerous diseases such as cancer. Polyphenols that are not absorbed in the stomach or small intestine will be carried to the colon where they undergo substantial structural modifications. Those absorbed in the upper part of the gastrointestinal tract, metabolized in the liver and excreted in the bile or directly from the enterocyte back to the small intestine will also reach the colon but in a different form (e.g. glucuronide conjugates). The colonic microflora hydrolyzes glycosides into aglycones and extensively metabolizes the aglycones into simpler compounds, such as phenolic acids (Fig. 3). Conjugated metabolites secreted in bile can also be hydrolised by β-glucuronidases of microbial origin. The released aglycones can be reabsorbed and undergo enterohepatic cycling, as indicated by a second plasma peak. Some microbial metabolites exert biological activity, such as equol produced from daidzein having better phytoestrogenic properties than the original isoflavone. Inter-individual variations in formation of active metabolites caused by different composition of colonic microflora are also observed (Del Rio et al., 2010; Manach et al., 2004).

The absorption of polyphenols is followed by extensive conjugation and metabolism. Phenolic compounds are conjugated in the intestinal cells and later in the liver that restricts their potential toxic effects and facilitates their biliary and urinary excretion by increasing their hydrophilicity. This process mainly includes glucuronidation, sulfation and methylation catalyzed by following enzymes: UDP glucuronosyl transferase (UDPGT), phenol sulfotransferase (SULT) and cathel-O-methyltransferaze (COMT), respectively (Scalbert & Williamson, 2000). The conjugation mechanisms of polyphenols are highly efficient, and free aglycones are generally either absent or present in low concentrations in plasma after the consumption of nutritional doses. Green tea catechins, whose aglycones can constitute a significant proportion of the total amount in plasma, present an exception (Lee et al., 2002). Rosmarinic acid, partly absorbed in unchanged form and partly metabolized by microflora in the colon, is found to be present in plasma as conjugated and/or methylated forms accompanied by the conjugated forms of its metabolites (caffeic, ferulic and m-coumarinic acid). In the same study, looking at the metabolites formed from rosmarinic acid between rats and humans large differences are observed and attributed to the differences in the enzyme location, affinity of substances and the characteristics of the enzymatic reactions, which corresponds to data for epicatechin and quercetin (Baba et al., 2005).

Generally, it is important to identify the circulating metabolites of polyphenols because the nature and position of the conjugating groups can affect their biological properties (Day et al., 2000). The accumulation of polyphenol metabolites in the target tissues where they exert biological activities is the most important phase of polyphenol metabolic pathway, however, a few studies reported on their concentrations in human tissues. Isoflavones were found to accumulate in breast and prostate tissues (Hong et al., 2002; Maubach et al., 2003). Tea polyphenols and theaflavins were detected in the prostate, and their tissue bioavailability was greater in humans than in animals (Henning et al., 2006). Since, polyphenols are extensively modified and the forms appearing in the blood and tissues are usually different from the forms found in plants, greater attention should be focused on exploring the potential biological activity of polyphenol metabolites. In understanding bioavailability of plant polyphenols, the differences between animal models and human should be taken into account.

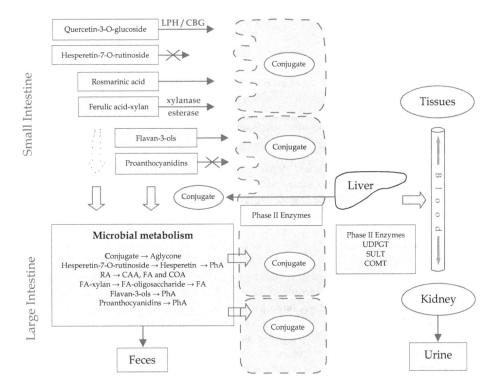

CAA – Caffeic acid, CBG - Cytosolic β-glucosidase, COA - m-Coumarinic acid, COMT - Cathel-O-methyltransferaze, FA – Ferulic acid, LPH - Lactase phlorizin hydrolase, PhA – Phenolic acids, RA – Rosmarinic acid, SULT - Phenol sulfotransferase, UDPGT - UDP glucuronosyl transferase.

Fig. 3. Pathway of absorption and metabolism of selected polyphenols.

6. Polyphenols in aging and oxidative stress-related diseases

Aging is a natural process that is defined as a progressive deterioration of biological functions after the organism has attained its maximal reproductive competence; it leads to the disabilities and diseases that limit normal body functions. Major hypotheses of aging include altered proteins; DNA damage and less efficient DNA repair; inappropriate crosslinking of proteins, DNA and other structural molecules; a failure of neuroendocrine secretion; cellular senescence in the cell culture system; an increase in free radical-mediated oxidative stress and changes in the order of gene expression (T. Farooqui & A.A. Farooqui, 2009). It has been pointed out that oxidative stress experienced during normal metabolism has primary contribution to aging. Today much attention is given to the therapeutic effects of polyphenols, which have been shown to mitigate age-associated phenomena such as oxidative stress, chronic inflammation, and toxin accumulation (Queen & Tollefsbol, 2010). Plant polyphenols are serious candidates in explanations of the protective effects of vegetables and fruits against various diseases. Epidemiologic studies are useful for evaluation of the human health effects of long-term exposure to physiologic concentrations of polyphenols, but reliable data on polyphenol contents of food are still scarce (Arts & Holman, 2005). With respect to cardiovascular health, polyphenols may alter lipid metabolism, inhibit low-density lipoprotein (LDL) oxidation, reduce atherosclerotic lesion formation, inhibit platelet aggregation, decrease vascular cell adhesion molecule expression, improve endothelial function and reduce blood pressure. Polyphenols have also been shown to exert beneficial cognitive effects, to reverse specific age-related neurodegeneration and to exert a variety of anti-carcinogenic effects including an ability to induce apoptosis in tumour cells (Vauzour et al., 2010), inhibit cancer cell proliferation (Walle et al., 2007), prevent angiogenesis (Mojzis et al., 2008) and tumour cells invasion (Weng & Yen, 2011).

Cardiovascular disease (CVD) is one of the leading causes of death in many economically developed nations. Some of the major risk factors for CVD can not be changed (age, sex, genetic predisposition), but diet and lifestyle are modifiable risk factors (Leifert & Abeywardena, 2008). Accordingly, current knowledge favours the notion that risk factors other than raised plasma cholesterol play an important role in the development of CVD, such as oxidative stress, vascular inflammation and endothelial dysfunction (Zalba et al., 2007). Many human studies have demonstrated that altered oxygen utilization and/or increased formation of reactive oxygen species (ROS) contribute to atherogenesis, hypertension and progression of other CVD. For example, olive oil polyphenols increased the level of oxidized LDL autoantibodies (OLAB) which have protective role in atherosclerosis. In a crossover, controlled trial 200 healthy men were randomly assigned to 3-week sequences of 25 mL/day of three olive oils with high (366 mg/kg), medium (164 mg/kg) and low (2.7 mg/kg) phenolic contents. OLAB concentrations increased in a dose-dependent manner with the polyphenol content of the administered olive oil (Castañer et al., 2011). Phytoestrogen genistein was tested on sixty healthy postmenopausal women in a double blind, placebo controlled, randomized study where participants received either genistein (54 mg/day) or placebo. After six months of genistein therapy, the ratio between nitric oxide and endothelin-1 was increased and flow-mediated endothelium-dependent vasomotion in postmenopausal women improved (Sqadrito et al., 2002). Medina-Remón et al. (2011) confirmed that intake of polyphenols is negatively correlated with hypertension (Table 3). Human studies have also showed an association of moderate intake of alcoholic drinks containing polyphenols with a reduced risk of cardiovascular disease. The intake of these drinks decreased Nuclear factor-kappa B (redox sensitive transcription factor implicated in the pathogenesis of atherosclerosis) activation (Blanco-Colio et al., 2007). These observations have been proposed to explain the French paradox: the coexistence of relative high fat intake and the lower rate of cardiovascular disease in France, due to regular intake of drinks containing polyphenols.

Sample	Participants/Study	Effect	Reference
Diet rich in polyphenols	589 participants; blood pressure measured; total polyphenol excretion determined in urine	Polyphenol intake negatively associated with blood pressure levels and prevalence of hypertension	Medina-Remón et al., 2011
Grape antioxidant dietary fibre – 5.25 g dietary fibre, 1.4 g polyphenols per day	34 participants; 16 weeks supplementation with grape antioxidant dietary fibere; blood pressure and LDL levels measured	Significant reduction of total cholesterol, LDL level, systolic and diastolic blood pressures	Pérez-Jiménez et al., 2008
Alcoholic drinks with polyphenols; 2660 mg/L red wine 357 mg/L rum, and 89 mg/L brandy	16 volunteers; 16 g/m² of ethanol during 5 days; fat-enriched diet; examined NF-kappa B activation and circulating MCP-1 levels	Decreased NF-kappa B activation and MCP- 1 levels	Blanco-Colio et al., 2007
Green and black tea (EGCG)	21 postmenopausal healthy woman; flow-mediated dilation and nitro-mediated dilation measured before and 2 h after consumption of tea	Significant increase of endothelium-dependent flow-mediated dilation	Jochmann et al., 2008
Flavonoids from food	10054 participants; flavonoid intake estimated on the basis of the flavonoid concentrations in food; the incident cases of the diseases identified from national public health registers	Total cancer incidence lower at higher quercetin (mainly lung cancer); prostate cancer risk lower at higher myricetin; breast cancer risk lower at higher quercetin intake	Knekt et al., 2002
Regular diet	Patients afflicted with cancer of the oral cavity, pharynx, larynx and esophagus	Favonoid intake associated with a reduction in risk of incidence of cancer	De Stefani et al., 1999
Quercetin	51 patients with confirmed cancer no longer amenable to the standard therapy	Tyrosine kinase inhibited; CA 125 level decreased; α-fetoprotein level decreased	Ferry et al., 1996
Fruit and vegetable juices containing a high concentration of polyphenols	Population-based prospective study of 1836 Japanese Americans	Hazard ratio for Alzheimer's disease 0.24 for subjects who drank juices at least 3 times per week; 0.84 for subjects who drank juices 1 to 2 times per week	Dai et al., 2006
Functional drink rich in polyphenols	100 participants; plasmatic level of tHcy determined	Decrease of tHcy plasmatic level in Alzheimer patients	Morillas-Ruiz et al., 2010
Coffee and tea	200 participants, pure ethnic Chinese	Dose-dependent protective effect of Parkinson's disease in coffee and tea drinkers	Tan et al., 2003

CA 125 - Tumour marker present in greater concentration in ovarian cancer, EGCG - Epigallocatechin-3-gallate, LDL – Low-density lipoprotein, MCP-1 - Monocyte chemoattractant protein-1, NF-kappa B - Nuclear factor-kappa B, tHcy – total Homocysteine.

Table 3. Overview of the selected human studies.

A multi-stage process such as cancer development is characterised by the cumulative action of multiple events occurring in a single cell and can be described by three stages (initiation, promotion and progression) and ROS can act in all these stages of carcinogenesis (Valko et al., 2006). The reported data imply that growth factor-stimulated ROS generation can mediate intracellular signalling pathways by activating protein tyrosine kinases, inhibiting protein tyrosine phosphatase, and regulating redox-sensitive gene expression (Aslan & Özben, 2003). Different clinical and epidemiological studies presented in Table 3 have confirmed negative correlation between intake of polyphenols and incidence of cancer (Knekt et al., 2002; De Stefani et al., 1999; Ferry et al., 1996).

Among the most common neurologic diseases are neurodegenerative disorders, such as Alzheimer's disease (AD), Parkinson's disease (PD), and amyotrophic lateral sclerosis (ALS). The risk factors that have been identified for these diseases are mitochondrial dysfunction and oxidative damage which play important roles in the slowly progressive neuronal death (Esposito et al., 2002). The growing evidence suggests that the oxidative damage caused by the β-amyloid peptide in the pathogenesis of AD may be hydrogen peroxide mediated. The polyphenols from apple and citrus juices, such as quercetin, are able to cross the blood-brain barrier and show neuroprotection against hydrogen peroxide (Dai et al., 2006). The increased serum total homocysteine (tHcy) is identified as a risk factor for the development of AD. As the thiol group of homocysteine undergoes auto-oxidation in the plasma and generates ROS, polyphenols have preferences for the preventive-therapeutic use in AD (Morillas-Ruiz et al., 2010). The characteristic of PD is the selective degeneration of dopamine neurons in the nigrostriatal system where increased total iron has been found (Esposito et al., 2002). The protective effect of tea catehins against neuronal diseases may involve its radical scavenging and iron chelating activity and/or regulation of antioxidant protective enzymes (Weinreb et al., 2004) which was confirmed by Tan et al. (2003). Human studies considering neurodegenerative diseases are presented in Table 3.

Human studies suggest that plant polyphenols may reduce the risk of various chronic diseases, but there is a need for more studies to provide definitive proofs of their protective role. Further epidemiological studies should identify proper biomarkers of disease risk and demonstrate they are influenced by the consumption of plant polyphenols (Schalbert et al., 2005). There is also lack of validated biomarkers of polyphenol intake since polyphenol family encompasses very diverse compounds with highly different bioavailabilities, so the results obtained for one polyphenol compound cannot be generalized to others (Manach et al., 2005). Nevertheless, epidemiological studies are useful tool to study the health effects of polyphenols, providing us with information about significant differences among groups of people who have different lifestyles and have been exposed to different environmental factors.

7. References

Amat, N.; Upur, H. & Blažeković, B. (2010). *In vivo* hepatoprotective activity of the aqueous extract of *Artemisia absinthium* L. against chemically and immunologically induced liver injuries in mice. *Journal of Ethnopharmacology*, Vol.131, No.2, pp. 478-484, ISSN 0378-8741

Arts, I.C.W. & Hollman, P.C.H. (2005). Polyphenols and disease risk in epidemiologic studies. *The American Journal of Clinical Nutrition*, Vol.81, No.1, pp. 317S–325S, ISSN 1938-3207

Ashihara, H.; Deng, W.W.; Mullen, W. & Crozier, A. (2010). Distribution and biosynthesis of flavan-3-ols in *Camellia sinensis* seedlings and expression of genes encoding biosynthetic enzymes. *Phytochemistry*, Vol.71, No.5-6, pp. 559-566, ISSN 0031-9422

Aslan, M. & Özben, T. (2003). Oxidants in receptor tyrosine kinase signal transduction pathways. *Antioxidants & Redox Signaling*, Vol.5, No.6, pp. 781-788, ISSN 1557-7716

Ataie, A.; Sabetkasaei, M.; Haghparast, A.; Moghaddam, A.H. & Kazeminejad, B. (2010). Neuroprotective effects of the polyphenolic antioxidant agent, curcumin, against homocysteine-induced cognitive impairment and oxidative stress in the rat. *Pharmacology Biochemistry and Behavior*, Vol.96, No.4, pp. 378-385, ISSN 0091-3057

Baba, S.; Osakabe, N.; Natsume, M.; Yasuda, A.; Muto, Y.; Hiyoshi, K.; Takano, H.; Yoshikawa, T. & Terao, J. (2005). Absorption, metabolism, degradation and urinary excretion of rosmarinic acid after intake of *Perilla frutescens* extract in humans. *European Journal of Nutrition*, Vol.44, No.1, pp. 1–9, ISSN 1436-6207

Banskota, A.H.; Nguyen, N.T.; Tezuka, Y.; Tran, Q.L.; Nobukawa, T.; Kurashige, Y; Sasahara, M. & Kadota, S. (2004). Secoisolariciresinol and isotaxiresinol inhibit tumor necrosis factor-α-dependent hepatic apoptosis in mice. *Life Sciences*, Vol.74, No.22, pp. 2781-2792, ISSN 0024-3205

Bazylko, A. & Strzelecka, H. (2007). A HPTLC densitometric determination of luteolin in *Thymus vulgaris* and its extracts. *Fitoterapia*, Vol.78, No.6, pp. 391-395, ISSN 0367-326X

Beck, V.; Rohr, U. & Jungbauer, A. (2005). Phytoestrogens derived from red clover: An alternative to estrogen replacement therapy? *The Journal of Steroid Biochemistry and Molecular Biology*, Vol.94, No.5, pp. 499-518, ISSN 0960-0760

Beek, T.A. & Montoro, P. (2009). Chemical analysis and quality control of *Ginkgo biloba* leaves, extracts, and phytopharmaceuticals. *Journal of Chromatography A*, Vol.1216, No.11, pp. 2002-2032, ISSN 0021-9673

Blanco-Colio, L.M.; Muñoz-García, B.; Martín-Ventura, J.L.; Alvarez-Sala, L.A.; Castilla, M.; Bustamante, A.; Lamuela-Raventós, R.M.; Gómez-Gerique, J.; Fernández-Cruz, A.; Millán, J. & Egido, J. (2007). Ethanol beverages containing polyphenols decrease nuclear factor kappa-B activation in mononuclear cells and circulating MCP-1 concentrations in healthy volunteers during a fat-enriched diet. *Atherosclerosis*, Vol.192, No.2, pp. 335–341, ISSN 0021-9150

Blasa, M.; Angelino, D.; Gennari, L. & Ninfali, P. (2011). The cellular antioxidant activity in red blood cells (CAA-RBC): A new approach to bioavailability and synergy of phytochemicals and botanical extracts. *Food Chemistry*, Vol.125, No.2, pp. 685-691, ISSN 0308-8146

Blažeković, B.; Vladimir-Knežević, S.; Brantner, A. & Bival Štefan, M. (2010). Evaluation of antioxidant potential of *Lavandula* x *intermedia* Emeric ex Loisel. 'Budrovka': a comparative study with *L. angustifolia* Mill.. *Molecules*, Vol.15, No.9, pp. 5971-5987, ISSN 1420-3049

Boudet, A.M. (2007). Evolution and current status of research in phenolic compounds. *Phytochemistry*, Vol. 68, No.22-24, pp. 2722-2735, ISSN 0031-9422

Cano, A.; Arnao, M.B.; Williamson, G. & Garcia-Conesa, M.T. (2002). Superoxide scavenging by polyphenols: effect of conjugation and dimerization. *Redox Report*, Vol.7, No.6, pp. 379-383, ISSN 1743-2928

Cassidy, A.C.; Hanley, B. & Lamuela-Raventos, R.M. (2000). Isoflavones, lignans and stilbenes – origins, metabolism and potential importance to human health. *Journal of the Science of Food and Agriculture*, Vol.80, No.7, pp. 1044-1062, ISSN 0022-5142

Castañer, O.; Fitó, M.; López-Sabater, M.C.; Poulsen, H.E.; Nyyssönen, K.; Schröder, H.; Salonen, J.T.; De la Torre-Carbot, D.; Zunft, H.F.; De la Torre, R.; Bäumler, H.; Gaddi, V.A.; Saez, G.T.; Tomás, M. & Covas, M.I. for the EUROLIVE Study Group (2011). The effect of olive oil polyphenols on antibodies against oxidized LDL. A randomized clinical trial. *Clinical Nutrition*, Vol.30, No.4, pp. 490–493, ISSN 0261-5614

Chattopadhyay, S.K.; Kumar, T.R.; Maulik, P.R.; Srivastava, S.; Garg, A.; Sharon, A.; Negi, A.S. & Khanuja, S.P. (2003). Absolute configuration and anticancer activity of taxiresinol and related lignans of *Taxus wallichiana*. *Bioorganic and Medicinal Chemistry*, Vol.11, No.1, pp. 4945–4948, ISSN 0968-0896

Chen, L.; Han, Y.; Yang, F. & Zhang, T. (2001). High-speed counter-current chromatography separation and purification of resveratrol and piceid from *Polygonum cuspidatum*. *Journal of Chromatography A*, Vol.907, No.1-2, pp. 343-346, ISSN 0021-9673

Crozier, A.; Del Rio, D. & Clifford, M.N. (2010). Bioavailability of dietary flavonoids and phenolic compounds. *Molecular Aspects of Medicine*, Vol.31, No.6, pp. 446-467, ISSN 0098-2997

Dai, J. & Mumper, R.J. (2010). Plant phenolics: extraction, analysis and their antioxidant and anticancer properties. *Molecules*, Vol.15, No.10, pp. 7313-7352, ISSN 1420-3049

Dai, Q.; Borenstein, A.R.; Wu, Y.; Jackson, J.C. & Larson, E.B. (2006). Fruit and vegetable juices and Alzheimer's disease: the *Kame* project. *The American Journal of Medicine*, Vol.119, No.9, pp. 751-759, ISSN 0002-9343

Dauer, A.; Rimpler, H. & Hensel, A. (2003). Polymeric proanthocyanidins from the bark of *Hamamelis virginiana*. *Planta Medica*, Vol.69, No.1, pp. 89-91, ISSN 0032-0943

Day, A.J.; Bao, Y.; Morgan, M.R. & Williamson, G. (2000). Conjugation position of quercetin glucuronides and effect on biological activity. *Free Radical Biology and Medicine*, Vol.29, No.12, pp. 1234-1243, ISSN 0891-5849

de Rijke, E.; Out, P.; Niessen, W.M.; Ariese, F.; Gooijer, C. & Brinkman, U.A. (2006). Analytical separation and detection methods for flavonoids. *Journal of Chromatography A*, Vol.1112, No.1-2, pp. 31-63, ISSN 0021-9673

Del Rio, D.; Costa, L.G.; Lean, M.E. & Crozier, A. (2010). Polyphenols and health: what compounds are involved? *Nutrition, metabolism, and cardiovascular diseases*, Vol.20, No.1, pp. 1-6, ISSN 1590-3729

De Stefani, E.; Ronco, A.; Mendilaharsu, M. & Deneo-Pellegrini, H. (1999). Diet and risk of cancer of the upper aerodigestive tract - II. Nutrients. *Oral Oncology*, Vol.35, No.1, pp. 22-26, ISSN 1368-8375

Dewick, P.M. (2001). *Medicinal natural products: a biosynthetic approach*, John Wiley & Sons, ISBN 0-471-49641-0, 122-166, West Sussex, United Kingdom

Du, O.; Jerz, G. & Winterhalter, P. (2004). Isolation of two anthocyanin sambubiosides from bilberry (*Vaccinium myrtillus*) by high-speed counter-current chromatography. *Journal of Chromatography A*, Vol.1045, No.1-2, pp. 59-63, ISSN 0021-9673

Duarte, N.; Kayser, O.; Abreu, P. & Ferreira, M.J. (2008). Antileishmanial activity of piceatannol isolated from *Euphorbia lagascae* seeds. *Phytotherapy Research*, Vol.22, No.4, pp. 455-457, ISSN 0951-418X

Esposito, E.; Rotilio, D.; Di Matteo, V.; Di Giulio, C.; Cacchio, M. & Algeri, A. (2002). A review of specific dietary antioxidants and the effects on biochemical mechanisms related to neurodegenerative processes. *Neurobiology of Aging*, Vol.23, No.5, pp. 719-735, ISSN 0197-4580

EDQM (European Directorate for the Quality of Medicines and Health Care). (2006). European Pharmacopoeia, 5th ed., Council of Europe, ISBN 92-871-5646-8, Strasbourg, France

Farooqui, T. & Farooqui, A.A. (2009). Aging: an important factor for the pathogenesis of neurodegenerative diseases. *Mechanisms of Ageing and Development*, Vol.130, No.4, pp. 203-215, ISSN 0047-6374

Fernandez-Martinez, E.; Bobadilla, R.A.; Morales-Rios, M.S.; Muriel, P. & Perez-Alvarez, V.M. (2007). Trans-3-phenyl-2-propenoic acid (cinnamic acid) derivatives: structure-activity relationship as hepatoprotective agents. *Medicinal Chemistry*, Vol.3, No.5, pp. 475-479(5), ISSN 1573-4064

Ferry, D.R.; Smith, A.; Malkhandi, J.; Fyfe, D.W.; deTakats, P.G.; Anderson, D.; Baker, J. & Kerr, D.J. (1996). Phase I clinical trial of the flavonoid quercetin; pharmacokintetics and evidence for in vivo tyrosine kinase inhibition. *Clinical Cancer Research*, Vol.2, No.4, pp. 659-668, ISSN 1557-3265

Firuzi, O.; Lacanna, A.; Petrucci, R.; Marrosu, G. & Saso, L. (2005). Evaluation of the antioxidant activity of flavonoids by "ferric reducing antioxidant power" assay and cyclic voltammetry. *Biochimica et Biophysica Acta (BBA) - General Subjects*, Vol.1721, No.1-3, pp. 174-184, ISSN 0304-4165

Fossen, T.; Rayyan, S. & Andersen, Ø.M. (2004). Dimeric anthocyanins from strawberry (*Fragaria ananassa*) consisting of pelargonidin 3-glucoside covalently linked to four flavan-3-ols. *Phytochemistry*, Vol.65, No.10, pp. 1421-1428, ISSN 0031-9422

Fraga, C.G.; Galleano, M.; Verstraeten, S.V. & Oteiza, P.I. (2010). Basic biochemical mechanisms behind the health benefits of polyphenols. *Molecular Aspects of Medicine*, Vol.31, No.6, pp. 435-445, ISSN 0098-2997

González-Molina, E.; Domínguez-Perles, R.; Moreno, D.A. & García-Viguera, C. (2010). Natural bioactive compounds of *Citrus limon* for food and health. *Journal of Pharmaceutical and Biomedical Analysis*, Vol.51, No.2, pp. 327-345, ISSN 0731-7085

Guha, G.; Rajkumar, V. & Ashok, R. (2010). Polyphenolic constituents of methanolic and aqueous extracts of *Vitex negundo* render protection to Hep3B cells against oxidative cytotoxicity. *Food and Chemical Toxicology*, Vol.48, No.8-9, pp. 2133-2138, ISSN 0278-6915

Hansen, A.S.; Marckmann, P.; Dragsted, L.O.; Finne Nielsen, I.L.; Nielsen, S.E. & Gronbak, M. (2005). Effect of red wine and red grape extract on blood lipids, haemostatic factors, and other risk factors for cardiovascular disease. *European Journal of Clinical Nutrition*, Vol.59, No.3, pp. 449-455, ISSN 0954-3007

Harborne, M. & Williams, R. (2000). Advances in flavonoid research since 1992. *Phytochemistry*, Vol.55, No.6, pp. 481-504, ISSN 0031-9422

Hartzfeld, P.W.; Forkner, R.; Hunter, M.D. & Hagerman, A.E. (2002). Determination of hydrolyzable tannins (gallotannins and ellagitannins) after reaction with potassium iodate. *Journal of Agricultural and Food Chemistry*, Vol.50, No.7, pp. 1785-1790, ISSN 0021-8561

Hayek, T.; Fuhrman, B.; Vaya, J.; Rosenblat, M.; Belinky, P.; Coleman, R.; Elis, A. & Aviram, M. (1997). Reduced progression of atherosclerosis in apolipoprotein E-deficient mice following consumption of red wine, or its polyphenols quercetin or catechin, is associated with reduced susceptibility of LDL to oxidation and aggregation. *Arteriosclerosis, Thrombosis, and Vascular Biology*, Vol.17, No.11, pp. 2744-2752, ISSN 1524-4636

Helmja, K.; Vaher, M.; Püssa, T.; Kamsol, K.; Orav, A. & Kaljurand, M. (2007). Bioactive components of the hop strobilus: comparison of different extraction methods by capillary electrophoretic and chromatographic methods. *Journal of Chromatography A*, Vol.1155, No.2, pp. 222-229, ISSN 0021-9673

Henning, S.M.; Aronson, W.; Niu, Y.; Conde, F.; Lee, N.H.; Seeram, N.P.; Lee, R.P.; Lu, J.; Harris, D.M.; Moro, A.; Hong, J.; Pak-Shan, L.; Barnard, R.J.; Ziaee, H.G.; Csathy, G.; Go, V.L.; Wang, H. & Heber, D. (2006). Tea polyphenols and theaflavins are present in prostate tissue of humans and mice after green and black tea consumption. *Journal of Nutrition*, Vol.136, No.7, pp. 1839–1843, ISSN 0022-3166

Hong, S.J.; Kim, S.I.; Kwon, S.M.; Lee, J.R. & Chung, B.C. (2002). Comparative study of concentration of isoflavones and lignans in plasma and prostatic tissues of normal control and benign prostatic hyperplasia. *Yonsei Medical Journal*, Vol.43, No.2, pp. 236-241, ISSN 0513-5796

Ignat, I.; Volf, I. & Popa, V.I. (2011). A critical review of methods for characterisation of polyphenolic compounds in fruits and vegetables. *Food Chemistry*, Vol.126, No.4, pp. 1821-1835, ISSN 0308-8146

Jochmann, N.; Lorenz, M.; von Krosigk, A.; Martus, P.; Böhm, V.; Baumann, G.; Stangl, K. & Stangl, V. (2008). The efficacy of black tea in ameliorating endothelial function is equivalent to that of green tea. *British Journal of Nutrition*, Vol.99, No.4, pp. 863–868, ISSN 1475-2662

Jurišić Grubešić, R.; Vuković, J.; Kremer, D. & Vladimir-Knežević, S. (2005). Spectrophotometric method for polyphenols analysis: prevalidation and application on *Plantago* L. species. *Journal of Pharmaceutical and Biomedical Analysis*, Vol.39, No.3-4, pp. 837-842, ISSN 0731-7085

Jurišić Grubešić, R.; Vuković, J.; Kremer, D. & Vladimir-Knežević, S. (2007). Flavonoid content assay: prevalidation and application on *Plantago* L. species. *Acta Chimica Slovenica*, Vol.54, pp. 397–406, ISSN 1318-0207

Kanaze, F.I.; Gabrieli, C.; Kokkalou, E.; Georgarakis, M. & Niopas, I. (2003). Simultaneous reversed-phase high-performance liquid chromatographic method for the determination of diosmin, hesperidin and naringin in different citrus fruit juices and pharmaceutical formulations. *Journal of Pharmaceutical and Biomedical Analysis*, Vol.33, No.2, pp. 243-249, ISSN 0731-7085

Kang, J.; Li, Z.; Wu, T.; Jensen, G.S.; Schauss, A.G. & Wu, X. (2010). Anti-oxidant capacities of flavonoid compounds isolated from acai pulp (*Euterpe oleracea* Mart.). *Food Chemistry*, Vol.122, No.3, pp. 610-617, ISSN 0308-8146

Kay, C.D.; Mazza, G.; Holub, B.J. & Wang, J. (2004). Anthocyanin metabolites in human urine and serum. *British Journal of Nutrition*, Vol.91, No.6, pp. 933–942, ISSN 0007-1145

Keinänen, B. & Julkunen-Tiitto, C.A. (1998). High-performance liquid chromatographic determination of flavonoids in *Betula pendula* and *Betula pubescens* leaves. *Journal of Chromatography A*, Vol.793, No.2, pp. 370-377, ISSN 0021-9673

Khan, M.K.; Abert-Vian, M.; Fabiano-Tixier, A.S.; Dangles, O. & Chemat, F. (2010). Ultrasound-assisted extraction of polyphenols (flavanone glycosides) from orange (*Citrus sinensis* L.) peel. *Food Chemistry*, Vol.110, No.2, pp. 851-858, ISSN 0308-8146

Kim, E.J.; Park, H.; Park, S.J.; Jun, J.G. & Park, J.H. (2009). The grape component piceatannol induces apoptosis in DU145 human prostate cancer cells via the activation of extrinsic and intrinsic pathways. *Journal of Medicinal Food*, Vol.12, No.5, pp. 943-951, ISSN 1096-620X

Knekt, P.; Kumpulainen, J.; Järvinen, R.; Rissanen, H.; Heliövaara, M.; Reunanen, A.; Hakulinen, T. & Aromaa, A. (2002). Flavonoid intake and risk of chronic diseases. *The American Journal of Clinical Nutrition*, Vol.76, No.3, pp. 560-568, ISSN 1938-3207

Korkina, L.G. (2007). Phenylpropanoids as naturally occurring antioxidants: from plant defence to human health. *Cellular and Molecular Biology*, Vol.53, No.6, pp. 15-25, ISSN 0270-7306

Koshiro, Y.; Jackson, M.C.; Katahira, R.; Wang, M.L.; Nagai, C. & Ashihara, H. (2007). Biosynthesis of chlorogenic acids in growing and ripening fruits of *Coffea arabica* and *Coffea canephora* plants. *Zeitschrift für Naturforschung C*, Vol.62, No.9-10, pp. 731-742, ISSN 0939-5075

Koutelidakis, A.; Argiri, A.; Serafini, M.; Proestos, C.; Komaitis, M.; Pecorari, M. & Kapsokefalou, M. (2009). Green tea, white tea, and *Pelargonium purpureum* increase the antioxidant capacity of plasma and some organs in mice. *Nutrition*, Vol.25, No.4, pp. 453-458, ISSN 0899-9007

Kwee, E.M. & Niemeyer, E.D. (2011). Variations in phenolic composition and antioxidant properties among 15 basil (*Ocimum basilicum* L.) cultivars. *Food Chemistry*, Vol.128, No.4, pp. 1044-1050, ISSN 0308-8146

Lee, M.J.; Maliakal, P.; Chen, L.; Meng, X.; Bondoc, F.Y.; Prabhu, S.; Lambert, G.; Mohr, S. & Yang, C.S. (2002). Pharmacokinetics of tea catechins after ingestion of green tea and (−)-epigallocatechin-3-gallate by humans: formation of different metabolites and individual variability. *Cancer Epidemiology, Biomarkers & Prevention*, Vol.11, No.10, pp. 1025-1032, ISSN 1055-9965

Leifert, W.R. & Abeywardena, M.Y. (2008). Cardioprotective actions of grape polyphenols. *Nutrition Research*, Vol.28, No.11, pp. 729-737, ISSN 0271-5317

Leopoldini, M.; Russo, N. & Toscano, M. (2011). The molecular basis of working mechanism of natural polyphenolic antioxidants. *Food Chemistry*, Vol.125, No.2, pp. 288-306, ISSN 0308-8146

Li, X.; Yuan, J.P.; Xu, S.P.; Wang, J.H. & Liu, X. (2008). Separation and determination of secoisolariciresinol diglucoside oligomers and their hydrolysates in the flaxseed extract by high-performance liquid chromatography. *Journal of Chromatography A*, Vol.1185, No.2, pp. 223-232, ISSN 0021-9673

Mämmelä, P.; Savolainen, H.; Lindroos, L.; Kangas, J. & Vartiainen, T. (2000). Analysis of oak tannins by liquid chromatography-electrospray ionisation mass spectrometry. *Journal of Chromatography A*, Vol.891, No.1, pp. 75-83, ISSN 0021-9673

Manach, C.; Mazur, A. & Scalbert, A. (2005). Polyphenols and prevention of cardiovascular diseases. *Current Opinion in Lipidolgy*, Vol.16, No.1, pp. 77-84, ISSN 1473-6535

Manach, C.; Scalbert, A.; Morand, C.; Rémésy, C. & Jiménez, L. (2004). Polyphenols: food sources and bioavailability. *American Journal of Clinical Nutrition*, Vol.79, No.5, pp. 727-747, ISSN 0002-9165

Marques, V. & Farah, A. (2009). Chlorogenic acids and related compounds in medicinal plants and infusions. *Food Chemistry*, Vol.113, No.4, pp. 1370-1376, ISSN 0308-8146

Martens, S. & Mithöfer, A. (2005). Flavones and flavone synthases. *Phytochemistry*, Vol.66, No.20, pp. 2399-2407, ISSN 0031-9422

Maubach, J.; Bracke, M.E.; Heyerick, A.; Depypere, H.T.; Serreyn, R.F.; Mareel, M.M. & De Keukeleire, D. (2003). Quantitation of soy-derived phytoestrogens in human breast tissue and biological fluids by high-performance liquid chromatography. *Journal of Chromatography B*, Vol.784, No.1, pp. 137-144, ISSN 1570-0232

Medina-Remón, A.; Zamora-Ros, R.; Rothés-Ribalta, M.; Andres-Lacueva, C.; Martínez-Gonzáles, M.A.; Covas, M.I.; Corella, D.; Salas-Salvadó, J.; Gómez-Garsia, E.; Ruiz-Gutiérrez, V.; García de la Corte, F.J.; Fiol, M.; Pena, M.A.; Saez, G.T.; Ros, E.; Serra-Majem, L.; Pinto, X.; Warnberg, J.; Estruch, R. & Lamuela-Raventos, R.M. (2011). Total polyphenol excretion and blood pressure in subjects at high cardiovascular risk. *Nutrition, Metabolism & Cardiovascular Diseases*, Vol.21, No.5, pp. 323-331, ISSN 0939-4753

Middleton, E.; Kandaswami, C. & Theoharides, T.C. (2000). The effects of plant flavonoids on mammalian cells: implications for inflammation, heart disease, and cancer. *Pharmacological Reviews*, Vol.52, No.4, pp. 673-751, ISSN 0031-6997

Mitchell, K.A.; Markham, K.R. & Boase, M.R. (1998). Pigment chemistry and colour of *Pelargonium* flowers. *Phytochemistry*, Vol.47, No.3, pp. 355-361, ISSN 0031-9422

Miura, T.; Muraoka, S.; Ikeda, N.; Watanabe, M. & Fujimoto, Y. (2000). Antioxidative and prooxidative action of stilbene derivatives. *Pharmacology & Toxicology*, Vol.86, No.5, pp. 203-208, ISSN 1600-0773

Miura, Y.; Chiba, T.; Tomita, I.; Koizumi, H.; Miura, S.; Umegaki, K.; Hara, Y., Ikeda, M. & Tomita, T. (2001). Tea catechins prevent the development of atherosclerosis in apoprotein E-deficient mice. *The Journal of Nutrition*, Vol.131, No.1, pp. 27-32, ISSN 1541-6100

Mladenka, P.; Macáková, K.; Filipský, T.; Zatloukalová, L.; Jahodár, L.; Bovicelli, P.; Silvestri, I.P.; Hrdina, R. & Saso, L. (2011). *In vitro* analysis of iron chelating activity of flavonoids. *Journal of Inorganic Biochemistry*, Vol.105, No.5, pp. 693-701, ISSN 0162-0134

Mojzis, J.; Varinska, L.; Mojzisova, G.; Kostova, I. & Mirossay, L. (2008). Antiangiogenic effects of flavonoids and chalcones. *Pharmacological research*, Vol.57, No.4, pp. 259-265, ISSN 1043-6618

Morillas-Ruiz, J.M.; Rubio-Perez, J.M.; Albaladejo, M.D.; Zafrilla, P.; Parra, S. & Vidal-Guevara, M.L. (2010). Effect of an antioxidant drink on homocysteine levels in Alzheimer's patients. *Journal of the Neurological Sciences*, Vol.299, No.1-2, pp. 175-178, ISSN 0022-510X

Mortensen, A.; Sorensen, I.K.; Wilde, C.; Dragoni, S.; Mullerová, D.; Toussaint, O.; Zloch, Z.; Sgaragli, G. & Ovesná, J. (2008). Biological models for phytochemical research: from cell to human organism. *The British Journal of Nutrition*, Vol.99E, Suppl1, pp. ES118-126, ISSN 1475-2662

Mulinacci, N.; Prucher, D.; Peruzzi, M.; Romani, A.; Pinelli, P.; Giaccherini, C. & Vincieri, F.F. (2004). Commercial and laboratory extracts from artichoke leaves: estimation of caffeoyl esters and flavonoidic compounds content. *Journal of Pharmaceutical and Biomedical Analysis*, Vol.34, No.2, pp. 349-357, ISSN 0731-7085

Naczk, M. & Shahidi, F. (2006). Phenolics in cereals, fruits and vegetables: occurrence, extraction and analysis. *Journal of Pharmaceutical and Biomedical Analysis*. Vol.41, No.5, pp. 1523-1542, ISSN 0731-7085

Nenadis, N.; Wang, L.F.; Tsimidou, M. & Zhang, H.Y. (2004). Estimation of scavenging activity of phenolic compounds using the ABTS$^{\bullet+}$ assay. *Journal of Agricultural and Food Chemistry*, Vol.52, No.15, pp. 4669-4674, ISSN 1520-5118

Niki, E. (2010). Assessment of antioxidant capacity *in vitro* and *in vivo*. *Free Radical Biology & Medicine*, Vol.49, No.4, pp. 503-515, ISSN 0891-5849

Okawa, M.; Kinjo, J.; Nohara, T. & Ono, M. (2001). DPPH (1,1-diphenyl-2-picrylhydrazyl) radical scavenging activity of flavonoids obtained from some medicinal plants. *Biological & Pharmaceutical Bulletin*, Vol.24, No.10, pp. 1202-1205, ISSN 1347-5215

Patel, K.R.; Scott, E.; Brown, V.A.; Gescher, A.J.; Steward, W.P. & Brown, K. (2011). Clinical trials of resveratrol. *Annals of the New York Academy of Sciences*, Vol.1215, No.1, pp. 161-169, ISSN 1749-6632

Pascual-Martí, M.C.; Salvador, A.; Chafer, A. & Berna, A. (2001). Supercritical fluid extraction of resveratrol from grape skin of *Vitis vinifera* and determination by HPLC. *Talanta*, Vol.54, No.4, pp. 735–740, ISSN 0039-9140

Peng, Y.; Chu, Q; Liu, F. & Ye, J. (2004). Determination of isoflavones in soy products by capillary electrophoresis with electrochemical detection. *Food Chemistry*, Vol.87, No.1, pp. 135-139, ISSN 0308-8146

Pérez-Jiménez, J.; Serrano, J.; Tabernero, M.; Arranz, S.; Díaz-Rubio, M.E.; García-Diz, L.; Goñi, I. & Saura-Calixto, F. (2008). Effects of grape antioxidant dietary fiber in cardiovascular disease risk factors. *Nutrition*, Vol.24, No.7-8, pp. 646–653, ISSN 0899-9007

Perron, N.R. & Brumaghim, J.L. (2009). A review of the antioxidant mechanisms of polyphenol compounds related to iron binding. *Cell Biochemistry and Biophysics*, Vol.53, No.2, pp. 75-100, ISSN 1085-9195

Petersen, M. & Simmonds, M.S.J. (2003). Rosmarinic acid. *Phytochemistry*, Vol.62, No.2, pp. 121-125, ISSN 0031-9422

Poquet, L.; Clifford, M.N. & Williamson, G. (2010). Bioavailability of flavanols and phenolic acids, In: *Plant Phenolics and Human Health: Biochemistry, Nutrition and Pharmacology*, C.G. Fraga, (Ed.), 51-90, John Wiley & Sons, ISBN 978-0-470-28721-7, New Jersey, USA

Porrini, M. & Riso, P. (2008). Factors influencing the bioavailability of antioxidants in foods: a critical appraisal. *Nutrition, Metabolism and Cardiovascular Diseases*, Vol.18, No.10, pp. 647–650, ISSN 0939-4753

Queen, B. & Tollefsbol, T.O. (2010). Polyphenols and aging. *Current Aging Science*, Vol.3, No.1, pp. 34–42, ISSN 1874-6128

Ratnam, D.V.; Ankola, D.D.; Bhardwaj, V.; Sahana, D.K. & Kumar, M.N. (2006). Role of antioxidants in prophylaxis and therapy: a pharmaceutical perspective. *Journal of Controlled Release*, Vol.113, No.3, pp. 189-207, ISSN 0168-3659

Reuter, S.; Gupta, S.C.; Chaturvedi, M.M. & Aggarwal, B.B. (2010). Oxidative stress, inflammation, and cancer: how are they linked? *Free Radical Biology & Medicine*, Vol.49, No.11, pp. 1603-1616, ISSN 0891-5849

Rigano, D.; Cardile, V.; Formisano, V.; Maldini, M.T.; Piacente, S.; Bevilacqua, J.; Russo, A. & Senatore, F. (2009). *Genista sessilifolia* DC. and *Genista tinctoria* L. inhibit UV light and nitric oxide-induced DNA damage and human melanoma cell growth. *Chemico-Biological Interactions*, Vol.180, No.2, pp. 211-219, ISSN 0009-2797

Rimbach, G.; Boesch-Saadatmandi, C.; Frank, J.; Fuchs, D.; Wenzel, U.; Daniel, H.; Hall, W.L. & Weinberg, P.D. (2008). Dietary isoflavones in the prevention of cardiovascular disease – A molecular perspective. *Food and Chemical Toxicology*, Vol.46, No.4, pp. 1308-1319, ISSN 0278-6915

Robbins, R.J. (2003). Phenolic acids in foods: an overview of analytical methodology. *Journal of Agricultural and Food Chemistry*, Vol.51, No.10, pp. 2866–2887, ISSN 0021-8561

Scalbert, A. & Williamson, G. (2000). Dietary intake and bioavailability of polyphenols. *Journal of Nutrition*, Vol.130, No.8, pp. 2073S–2085S, ISSN 0022-3166

Scalbert, A.; Manach, C.; Morand, C.; Rémésy, C. & Jiménez, L. (2005). Dietary polyphenols and the prevention of diseases. *Critical Reviews in Food Science and Nutrition*, Vol.45, No.4, pp. 287-306, ISSN 1040-8398

Selloum, L.; Reichl, S.; Müller, M.; Sebihi, L. & Arnhold, J. (2001). Effects of flavonols on the generation of superoxide anion radicals by xanthine oxidase and stimulated neutrophils. *Archives of Biochemistry and Biophysics*, Vol.395, No.1, pp. 49-56, ISSN 1096-0384

Singleton, V.L.; Orthofer, R. & Lamuela-Raventós, R.M. (1999). Analysis of total phenols and other oxidation substrates and antioxidants by means of Folin-Ciocalteu reagent. *Methods in Enzymology*, Vol.299, pp. 152-178, ISSN 0076-6879

Sircar, D. & Mitra, A. (2009). Accumulation of p-hydroxybenzoic acid in hairy roots of *Daucus carota* 2: Confirming biosynthetic steps through feeding of inhibitors and precursors. *Journal of Plant Physiology*, Vol.177, No.166, pp. 1370-1380, ISSN 0176-1617

Smeds, A.I.; Jauhiainen, L.; Tuomola, E. & Peltonen-Sainio, P. (2009). Characterization of variation in the lignan content and composition of winter rye, spring wheat, and spring oat. *Journal of Agricultural and Food Chemistry*, Vol.57, No.13, pp. 5837–5842, ISSN 0021-8561

Squadrito, F.; Altavilla, D.; Morabito, N.; Crisafulli, A.; D'Anna, R.; Corrado, F.; Ruggeri, P.; Campo, G.M.; Calapai, G.; Caputi, A.P. & Squadrito, G. (2002). The effect of the phytoestrogen genistein on plasma nitric oxide concentrations, endothelin-1 levels and endothelium dependent vasodilation in postmenopausal women. *Atherosclerosis*, Vol.163, No.2, pp. 339-347, ISSN 0021-9150

Švehlíková, V. & Repčák, M. (2006). Apigenin chemotypes of *Matricaria chamomilla* L.. *Biochemical Systematics and Ecology*, Vol.34, No.8, pp. 654-657, ISSN 0305-1978

Swatsitang, P.; Tucker, G.; Robards, K. & Jardine, D. (2000). Isolation and identification of phenolic compounds in *Citrus sinensis*. *Analytica Chimica Acta*, Vol.417, No.2, pp. 231-240, ISSN 0003-2670

Takeda, K.; Osakabe, A.; Saito, S.; Furuyama, D.; Tomita, A.; Kojima, Y.; Yamadera, M. & Sakuta, M. (2005). Components of protocyanin, a blue pigment from the blue flowers of *Centaurea cyanus*. *Phytochemistry*, Vol.66, No.13, pp. 1607-1613, ISSN 0031-9422

Tan, E.K.; Tan, C.; Fook-Chong, S.M.C.; Lum, S.Y.; Chai, A.; Chung, H.; Shen, H.; Zhao, Y.; Teoh, M.L.; Yih, Y.; Pavanni, R.; Chandran, V.R. & Wong, M.C. (2003). Dose-dependent protective effect of coffee, tea, and smoking in Parkinson's disease: a study in ethnic Chinese. *Journal of the Neurological Sciences*, Vol.216, No.1, pp. 163-167, ISSN 0022-510X

Tomczyk, M. & Latté, K.P. (2009). Potentilla – A review of its phytochemical and pharmacological profile. *Journal of Ethnopharmacology*, Vol.122, No.2, pp. 184-204, ISSN 0378-8741

Trumbeckaite, S.; Benetis, R; Bumblauskiene, D.; Janulis, V.; Toleikis, A.; Viškelis, P. & Jakštas, V. (2011). *Achillea millefolium* L. s.l. herb extract: Antioxidant activity and effect on the rat heart mitochondrial functions. *Food Chemistry*, Vol.127, No.4, pp. 1540-1548, ISSN 0308-8146

Valko, M.; Rhodes, C.J.; Moncol, J.; Izakovic, M. & Mazur, M. (2006). Free radicals, metals and antioxidants in oxidative stress-induced cancer. *Chemico-Biological Interactions*, Vol.160, No.1, pp.1–40, ISSN 0009-2797

Vauzour, D.; Rodriguez-Mateos, A.; Corona, G.; Oruna-Concha, M.J. & Spencer, J.P.E. (2010). Polyphenols and human health: prevention of disease and mechanisms of action. *Nutrients*, Vol.2, No.11, pp. 1106-1131, ISSN 2072-6643

Veberic, R.; Jakopic, J.; Stampar, F. & Schmitzer, V. (2009). European elderberry (*Sambucus nigra* L.) rich in sugars, organic acids, anthocyanins and selected polyphenols. *Food Chemistry*, Vol.114, No.2, pp. 511-515, ISSN 0308-8146

Verma, A.R.; Vijayakumar, M.; Mathela, C.S. & Rao, C.V. (2009). *In vitro* and *in vivo* antioxidant properties of different fractions of *Moringa oleifera* leaves. *Food and Chemical Toxicology*, Vol.47, No.9, pp. 2196-2201, ISSN 0278-6915

Villaño, D.; Fernández-Pachón, M.S.; Moyá, M.L.; Troncoso, A.M. & García-Parrilla, M.C. (2007). Radical scavenging ability of polyphenolic compounds towards DPPH free radical. *Talanta*, Vol.71, No.1, pp. 230-235, ISSN 0039-9140

Virgili, F.; Pagana, G.; Bourne, L.; Rimbach, G.; Natella, F.; Rice-Evans, C. & Packer, L. (2000). Ferulic acid excretion as a marker of consumption of a French maritime pine (*Pinus maritima*) bark extract. *Free Radical Biology and Medicine*, Vol.28, No.8, pp. 1249-1256, ISSN 0891-5849

Vivas, N.; Nonier, M.F.; Pianet, I.; Vivas de Gaulejac, N. & Fouquet, É. (2006). Proanthocyanidins from *Quercus petraea* and *Q. robur* heartwood: quantification and structures. *Comptes Rendus Chimie*, Vol.9, No.1, pp. 120-126, ISSN 1631-0748

Vladimir-Knežević, S.; Blažeković, B.; Bival Štefan, M.; Alegro, A.; Kőszegi, T. & Petrik, J. (2011). Antioxidant activities and polyphenolic contents of three selected *Micromeria* species from Croatia. *Molecules*, Vol.16, No.2, pp. 1454-1470, ISSN 1420-3049

Walle, T.; Ta, N.; Kawamori, T.; Wen, X.; Tsuji, P.A. & Walle, U.K. (2007). Cancer chemopreventive properties of orally bioavailable flavonoids—Methylated versus unmethylated flavones. *Biochemical Pharmacology*, Vol.73, No.9, pp. 1288-1296, ISSN 0006-2952

Wang, H.F.; Provan, G.J. & Helliwell, K. (2003). Determination of hamamelitannin, catechins and gallic acid in witch hazel bark, twig and leaf by HPLC. *Journal of Pharmaceutical and Biomedical Analysis*, Vol.33, No.4, pp. 539-544, ISSN 0731-7085

Weinreb, O.; Mandel, S.; Amit, T. &. Youdim, M.B.H. (2004). Neurological mechanisms of green tea polyphenols in Alzheimer's and Parkinson's diseases. *Journal of Nutritional Biochemistry*, Vol.15, No.9, pp. 506–516, ISSN 0995-2863

Weisz, G.M.; Kammerer, D.R. & Carle, R. (2009). Identification and quantification of phenolic compounds from sunflower (*Helianthus annuus* L.) kernels and shells by HPLC-DAD/ESI-MS. *Food Chemistry*, Vol.1105, No.2, pp. 758-765, ISSN 0308-8146

Weitzel, C. & Petersen, M. (2011). Cloning and characterisation of rosmarinic acid synthase from *Melissa officinalis* L.. *Phytochemistry*, Vol.72, No.7, pp. 572-578, ISSN 0031-9422

Weng, C.J. & Yen, G.C. (2011). Chemopreventive effects of dietary phytochemicals against cancer invasion and metastasis: phenolic acids, monophenol, polyphenol, and their derivatives. *Cancer Treatment Reviews*, In press, ISSN 0305-7372

Willför, S.M.; Smeds, A.I. & Holmbom, B.R. (2006). Chromatographic analysis of lignans. *Journal of Chromatography A*, Vol.1012, No.1-2, pp. 64-77, ISSN 0021-9673

Wolfe, K.L. & Liu, R.H. (2007). Cellular antioxidant activity (CAA) assay for assessing antioxidants, foods, and dietary supplements. *Journal of Agricultural and Food Chemistry*, Vol.55, No.22, pp. 896-8907, ISSN 1520-5118

Zalba, G.; Fortuño, A.; San José, G.; Moreno, M.U.; Beloqui, O. & Díez, J. (2007). Oxidative stress, endothelial dysfunction and cerebrovascular disease. *Cerebrovascular Diseases*, Vol.24, Suppl1, pp. 24-29, ISSN 1421-9786

10

Plant Polyphenols: Extraction, Structural Characterization, Hemisynthesis and Antioxidant Properties

Nour-Eddine Es-Safi

Mohammed V-Agdal University, Ecole Normale Supérieure, Rabat,
Morocco

1. Introduction

Many epidemiological studies showed that the consumption of diets consisting of fruits and vegetables offered protection against some chronic disease (Arts & Hollman, 2005; Chang-Claude et al., 1992; Graf et al., 2005; Phillips et al., 1978). This protection was suggested to be in part due to the intake of some beneficial nutrients including polyphenols which are the most abundant antioxidants in our diets. Indeed, polyphenols are natural products which are recognized as one of the largest and most widespread class of plant constituents occurring throughout the plant kingdom, and are also found in substantial levels in commonly consumed fruits, vegetables and beverages.

Polyphenols have recently aroused considerable interest because of their potential beneficial biochemical and antioxidant effects on human health. Commonly referred to as antioxidants, they may prevent various diseases associated with oxidative stress, such as cancers, cardiovascular diseases, inflammation and others. Most of the experimental results confirmed that polyphenols have several biological activities including radical scavenging, anti-inflammatory, anti-mutagenic, anti-cancer, anti-HIV, anti-allergic, anti-platelet and anti-oxidant activities (Harborne & Williams, 2000).

Consumption of fruits and vegetables has thus been associated with protection against various diseases, including cancers (Steinmetz & Potter, 1996) and cardio-and cerebrovascular diseases (Rimm et al., 1996). This association is often attributed to the antioxidants in the fruits and vegetables such as vitamin C, vitamin E, carotenoids, lycopenes and polyphenols that prevent free radical damage (Steinberg, 1991). Fruits and vegetables consumption may also prevent stroke (Ness & Powles 1997), cancers (Yang & Wang 1993), coronary heart diseases (Tijburg et al. 1997), and osteoporosis (Adlercreutz & Mazur 1997). All these reasons make that polyphenols are receiving increasing interest from consumers and food manufacturers.

Chemically, polyphenols are diverse group of naturally occurring compounds containing multiple phenolic functionalities. They constitute a large and still expanding complex family of molecules, with diverse structures, properties and sizes ranging from monomers to polymers. Polyphenols gather a range of weakly acidic substances possessing aromatic rings bearing hydroxyl substituents and constitute one of the most numerous and widely distributed groups of substances with more than 8000 phenolic structures currently known. Polyphenols can be divided into different classes depending on their basic structure. The main classes of polyphenols are phenolic acids and flavonoids while the less common are stilbenes and lignans. Major subclasses present in food correspond to anthocyanins, flavanols, flavones, flavanones, flavonols and isoflavones.

Several studies have been published about phenolic compounds and their role in the chemistry of fruits (Macheix et al., 1990). In particular, they are responsible for their color intensity, bitterness and their astringent perception. The amount and composition of phenolic compounds in fruit-based foods is dependent on a number of factors including species, varieties, geographical heritage, maturity, growing conditions, production area and yield of fruit as well as on technological processes. The age of fruit derived foods also influences the qualitative and quantitative composition of phenolic compounds in fruit derived foods. The chemical structure of polyphenols will also affect their biological properties such as bioavailability, antioxidant activity, specific interactions with cell receptors and enzymes and other properties.

Food organoleptic properties like color, taste and bitterness are obviously closely connected to the initial phenolic composition. It is also connected to environmental factors such as temperature, light and pH. In addition, the ability of these natural compounds to interact with various molecules is another way to modify these initial properties. Polyphenols are thus also responsible of the alterations usually observed during storage and ageing. While the color of new plant derived product is due to its initial chemical content, the subsequent color changes during storage and ageing involves generally condensation of phenolic compounds. These transformations generally result in browning, discoloration or darkening and this reactivity raises an important economic question. The sensory parameters usually altered during ageing include color and taste.

This chapter constitutes an overview of our findings in the field of polyphenols. Purification and characterization of some flavonoids and phenylethanoids from plants growing in Morocco will be presented. Hemisynthesis and structure determination of derivatized monomeric and dimeric flavanols will be also discussed. Application of spectroscopic methods for the analysis of these natural and derivatized products will be presented. In particular analysis of flavonoids, oligomeric and polymeric procyanidins using electropsray (ESI), matrix-assisted laser desorption ionization (MALDI), and tandem (MS-MS) mass spectrometry will be also reported. Finally the antioxidant properties of these natural/synthesized compounds will be discussed.

2. Results and discussion

2.1 Purification and characterization of some natural phytochemicals

Within a research program aimed at discovering new natural antioxidants, the aerial parts of *Globularia alypum* and *Salvia verbenaca* were extracted with various solvent mixtures, and the reduction of DPPH° was used to evaluate the antioxidant activity of the obtained extracts. The first obtained results showed that the hydromethanolic extracts demonstrated a notable antioxidant activity. The obtained fractions were subjected to SPE column chromatography using a step gradient of MeOH/H$_2$O mixture and each fraction was tested for its antioxidant activity.

Among the obtained fractions, the 50% aqueous methanolic fractions, which exhibited strong activity compared with negative control, were investigated for their phytochemical compositions. Analysis through analytical HPLC showed the presence of several compounds belonging to different families as demonstrated by their UV-visible spectra obtained through the used DAD detector coupled to the HPLC apparatus. Further fractionation by semipreparative HPLC allowed the isolation of sixteen compounds which were tested for their scavenging activity toward DPPH° radical.

The structures of the obtained compounds were elucidated through ESI-MS, CID MS, tandem MS-MS, 1D and 2D homonuclear and heteronuclear NMR analysis (Es-Safi et al., 2005a, 2006b). The phytochemicals isolated from *G. alypum* include syringin **1**, iridoids **2-7**, flavonoids **8-11**, and phenylethanoids **12-15** (Figure 1) while rosmarinic acid **16** was isolated from *S. verbenaca*.

Compound **1** was obtained as an amorphous powder. Its molecular weight 372 Da, determined through ESI-MS analysis ([M+Na]$^+$ and [M-H]$^-$ at *m/z* 395 and 371 Da respectively), was in agreement with the C$_{17}$H$_{24}$O$_9$ formula as confirmed through ^{13}C NMR analysis. The structure of compound **1**, was completely elucidated and was identified as syringin through 1D and 2D NMR analysis. Its spectral data were in agreement with those previously reported in the literature for the same compound (Sugiyama et al., 1993).

Among the isolated compounds, six iridoids **2-7** were isolated. The structure elucidation of the major one **6** was initiated through mass spectroscopy. Its molecular weight was determined as 492 amu by ESI-MS both at negative (*m/z* 491, [M-H]$^-$) and positive (*m/z* 493 [M+H]$^+$, 515 [M+Na]$^+$) ion mode. Among the obtained fragmentation, the loss of a 162 amu was observed suggesting the probable presence of a glucosidic moiety. The structure of compound **6** was further elucidated by NMR analysis. Complete assignments were made using a combination of homonuclear and heteronuclear correlation experiments.

Construction of the iridoid skeleton started with the carbon at 96.5 ppm (C-1), which has an acetal proton at 5.36 ppm (*d, J* = 8.7 Hz, H-1). This acetal proton was coupled to the methine proton at 2.65 ppm (*dd, J* = 8.7 and 9.6 Hz, H-9), which in turn was coupled to the second methine proton located at 2.29 ppm (*dddd, J* = 1.5, 4.5, 7.8 and 9.6 Hz, H-5). H-5 was further coupled to an olefinic proton at 5.04 ppm (*dd, J* = 4.5 and 6.0 Hz, H-4), which in turn was coupled to another olefinic proton at 6.37 ppm (*dd, J* = 1.5 and 6.00 Hz, H-3). In the other direction, the proton H-5 was correlated to the oxymethine proton located at 3.96 ppm (*dd, J* = 1.2 and 7.8 Hz, H-6) which was also correlated, according to the COSY spectrum, with H-7 (3.50 ppm, *bs*). The absence of any other homonuclear coupling observed for H-7 and H-9 indicated a totally substituted C-8 (64.4 ppm). The chemical shift value and coupling constant of C-10 (65.3 ppm, 4.26 and 5.01 ppm, AB system, *J* = 12.6 Hz) also confirmed a C-8 to be a tertiary oxygenated carbon.

The presence of a trans cinnamoyl ester was confirmed by signals due to the five aromatic [7.39 (2H), 7.40 and 7.62 ppm (2H)] and two olefinic protons (6.56 and 7.72 ppm, AB system, *J* = 16.2 Hz) as well as observation of 6 aromatic carbons [130.2 (2C), 130.9 (2C), 132.4 and 136.7 ppm] in addition to the signals located at 119.5, 147.6 and 169.3 ppm corresponding respectively to C(β), C(α) and the carbonyl carbon. Spectral assignment of the glucopyranosyl moiety was easily attributed through 2D COSY experiment, starting from the anomeric proton H-1' which was attributed to the signal located at 4.72 ppm on the basis of its downfield chemical shift. The relative configurations of the stereogenic centres of compound **6** were clarified by 2D NOESY experiment suggesting β configurations for hydrogens at C-5 and C-9 and a β, β, β orientations for the substituents at C-6, C-7 and C-8 (Figure 1). The obtained results for compound **6** were in agreement with the spectral data of globularin previously reported in the literature (Faure et al., 1987).Having in hand the structure of compound **6**, the other known iridoids were easily identified by ESI-MS and NMR spectroscopy by comparison of their spectral data with those of globularin and the spectral data of the literature. Thus compound **4** was identified as globularicisin, compound **5** as globularidin, compounds **2** as globularinin and **3** and **7** as globularimin and globularioside respectively (Figure 1).

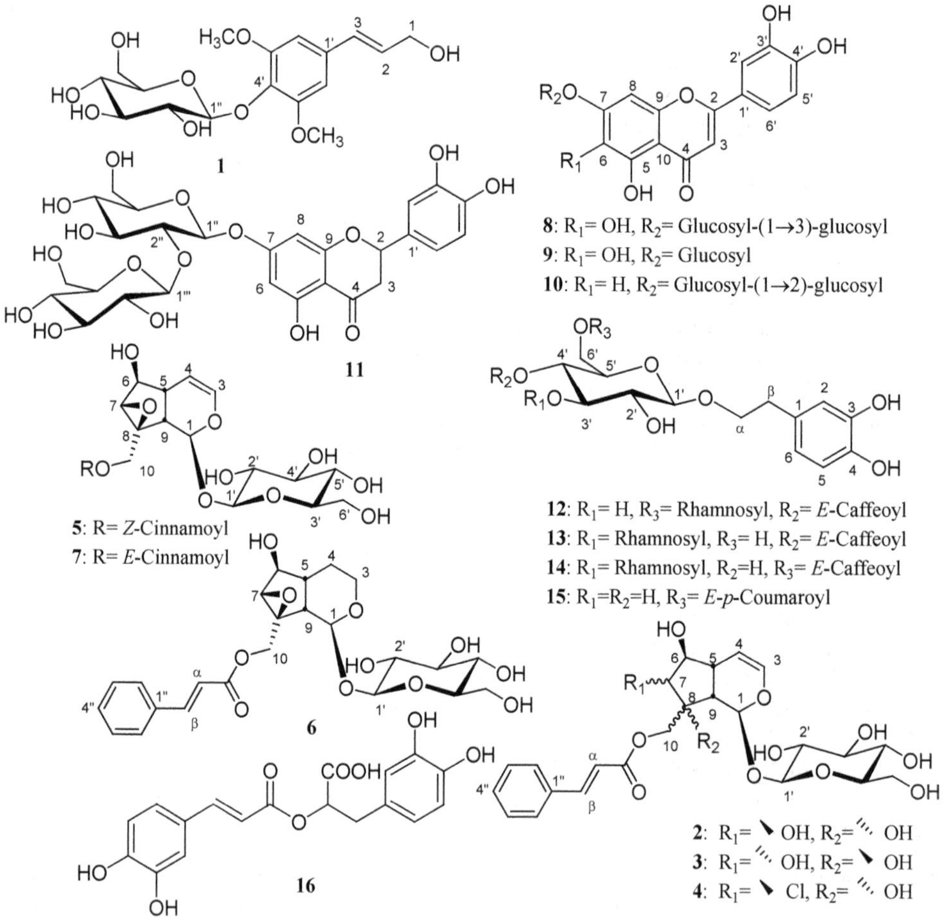

Fig. 1. Structure of the isolated natural compounds.

The ^{1}H NMR signals of compound **9** between 3.50 and 4.00, at 5.06 ppm, and between 6.5 and 7.5 ppm, in connection with a corresponding pattern in the ^{13}C NMR spectrum indicated typical features of a glycosylated flavonoid. Due to the fact that the ^{13}C NMR spectrum showed 21 carbon atoms, the molecular formula $C_{21}H_{20}O_{12}$ obtained through ESI-MS (m/z 463 [M-H]$^-$, 465 [M+H]$^+$) was retained. The positive ESI-MS spectrum also showed an ion signal at m/z 303 which is likely to correspond to a fragment ion, presumably the aglycone. From the mass difference of m/z = 162 between the [M+H]$^+$ peak and the aglycone it was deduced that the sugar moiety was an hexose which was determined as glucopyranosyl unit through NMR analysis.

The ^{13}C NMR spectrum displayed three peak signals in the upfield regions at 146.2, 151.1, and 150.4 ppm corresponding respectively to C-5, C-7 and C-9 in agreement with a 5,6,7-trihydroxylated A-ring of flavones (Horie et al., 1998). Compound **9** had almost identical NMR and MS-MS data for the aglycone 6-hydroxyluteolin as compared with those in **8** (Es-Safi et al., 2005a). The linkage between the sugar H-1″ (5.06 ppm) and the C-7 position (151.1 ppm) of the flavone was established by NOESY experiment showing correlation between the anomeric proton and the residual A ring aromatic proton H-8 (6.99 ppm). Compound **9** was thus identified as 6-hydroxyluteolin 7-O-β-D-glucoside.

The ESI-MS spectra of compound **11** (m/z 609 [M-H]$^-$, 611 [M+H]$^+$) indicated a molecular weight of 610 in agreement with the $C_{27}H_{30}O_{16}$ formula. The observation of a loss of a 324 neutral fragment in the mass spectra of compound **11** confirmed the presence of two hexose moieties. The CID MS-MS spectra of the [M-H]$^-$ ion showed in addition to 609 an intense ion at m/z 285 and 447. The latter was observed with a very low abundance in agreement with a diglucoside structure. The CID MS-MS spectra of the aglycone ion observed at m/z 285 were in agreement with a luteolin unit. This was confirmed through NMR analysis where a singlet at around 6.7 ppm in its ^{1}H NMR spectrum consistent with the H-3 of flavones was observed. This was also supported by the observation of carbon signal at ca 103.5 ppm associated with the C-3 in their ^{13}C NMR spectrum. Compound **11** was concluded to be luteolin-7-O-β-D-sophoroside through NMR analysis which results were in agreement with reported data (Imperato & Nazzaro, 1996).

Compounds **12-15** were obtained as colourless, amorphous compounds. Their UV spectra were very similar showing five absorption bands in the range 230-330 nm. Their IR spectra showed bands for hydroxyl groups and aromatic rings. These data indicated the presence of phenolic compounds with an unsaturated moiety outside the phenol ring. The ESI-MS data provided m/z values of 623 [M-H]$^-$, and 625 [M+H]$^+$ ions giving a molecular weights of 624 consistent with the formula $C_{29}H_{36}O_{15}$ for the three compounds. The CID-MS yielded an apparent peak at m/z = 448. From the mass difference of 146, the presence of a deoxyhexose was deduced.

The ^{1}H NMR spectrum of compound **13** exhibited typical resonances arising from six aromatic protons (2 ABX systems, 6.56-7.05 region), two *trans*-olefinic protons (AB system, 6.27 and 7.59 ppm, J = 15.9 Hz), a benzylic methylene at 2.78 ppm (2H, t, J = 7.2 Hz) and two non-equivalent proton signals at 3.72 and 4.03 ppm (each 1H, m). These data were consistent with the presence of a (E)-caffeic acid unit and 3,4-di0068ydroxyphenethyl alcohol moiety. In addition, two anomeric proton signals at 4.38 (d, J = 7.9 Hz) and 5.17 (d, J = 1.8 Hz) were attributed to the β-D-glucose and α-L-rhamnose units, respectively, indicating the disaccharide structure of **13**.

The presence of a doublet at 1.08 ppm in the ¹H NMR spectrum, the ¹H-¹H COSY interactions, the ¹³C shifts deduced from 2D NMR experiments and the ¹H NMR coupling constants made an α-L-rhamnose-O-β-D-glycoside likely. The acyl group was positioned at the C-4′ position of the glucose unit, on the basis of the strong deshielding of the H-4′ signal (4.91 ppm) of the glucose unit. In the ¹³C NMR spectrum, the C-3′ (82.4 ppm) resonance of the glucose unit showed a remarkable downfield shift, indicating that the rhamnose moiety was attached to the C-3′ position of the glucose. Therefore, based on the NMR data, the structure of **13** was identified as acteoside (Owen et al., 2003).

The proton and carbon resonances of **12** due to the aglycone and sugar moieties were in good agreement with those of **13**, indicating the similar substructures. However the caffeoyl residue was concluded to be attached to glucose C-6 instead of C-4 (normal chemical shift for H4, downfield shifts for H6a,b). Therefore, the structure of **12** was established as isoacteoside (Owen et al., 2003). The NMR data revealed that **14** had most of the structural features of **13** with the exception that the rhamnosyl residue is attached to glucose C-6 instead of C-3 as attested by the downfield shift (4 ppm) of the C-6′ of the glucose moiety. Since the NMR data of **14** was in good agreement with the reported data, its structure was identified as forsythiaside (Shoyama et al., 1986).

Compound **16** which was isolated from *S. verbenaca* was concluded to be rosmarinic acid on the basis of its MS and NMR spectral data. Its ESI-MS spectrum recorded in the negative ion mode presents signal at *m/z* 359 corresponding to the [M-H]⁻ ion in agreement with the proposed structure. The ¹H NMR spectrum presents in particular two doublets (*J*=16 Hz) at 6.2 and 7.5 ppm integrating one proton each and corresponding to the two olefinic protons. The two benzylic protons appeared as two double doublets at 2.9 and 3.1 ppm while the proton in the α position of the carboxyl group appeared as a multiplet at 5.1 ppm. Finally the 6 aromatic protons appeared as multiplets between 6.5 and 7.1 ppm. The ¹³C NMR spectrum showed 18 signals in agreement with the structure of rosmarinic acid. The benzylic carbon atom appeared at 39 ppm and was confirmed through DEPT analysis. The two carbonyl carbon atoms were attributed to the signals located at 175 (COOH) and 169 (CO) ppm. The carbon in the α of the carboxyl group signal was located at 76 ppm. The other observed signals were in agreement with the structure of rosmarinic acid and with previously published results (Mehrabani et al., 2005).

2.2 Hemisynthesis and structure determination of derivatized monomeric and dimeric flavanols

Natural antioxidants have been shown to enhance product stability, quality, and shelf life. Consequently, the development of antioxidants from natural origin has attracted considerable attention and many researchers have focused on the discovery of new natural antioxidants aimed at quenching biologically harmful radicals. However, natural antioxidants are usually difficult to isolate because they are often extracted in complex mixtures. Moreover, they generally occur in few amounts which did not allow achieving the desired biological activity. This prompted us to initiate an investigation program aimed at the hemisynthesis of monomeric and dimeric polyphenols.

The synthesis of some modified monomeric units derived from catechin was initiated with the objectives of exploring the impact of the A ring substitution on their antioxidant properties. For this study, the six 8-substituted derivatives of flavan-3-ols **19-24** in addition to taxifolin **25** (Figure 2) were synthesized and their antioxidative activity investigated.

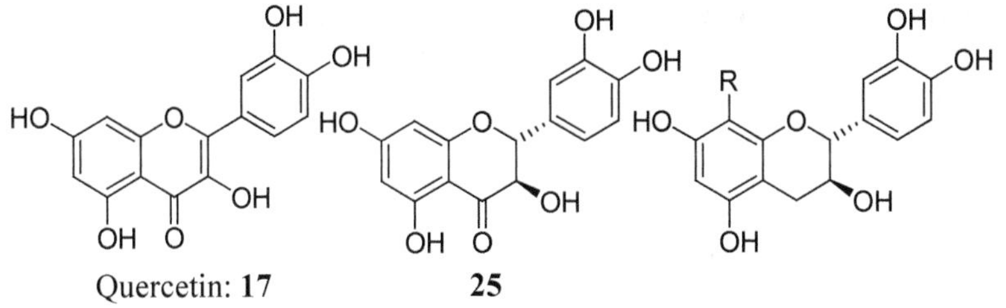

Fig. 2. Structures of the studied modified flavan-3-ol monomers **19-25**.

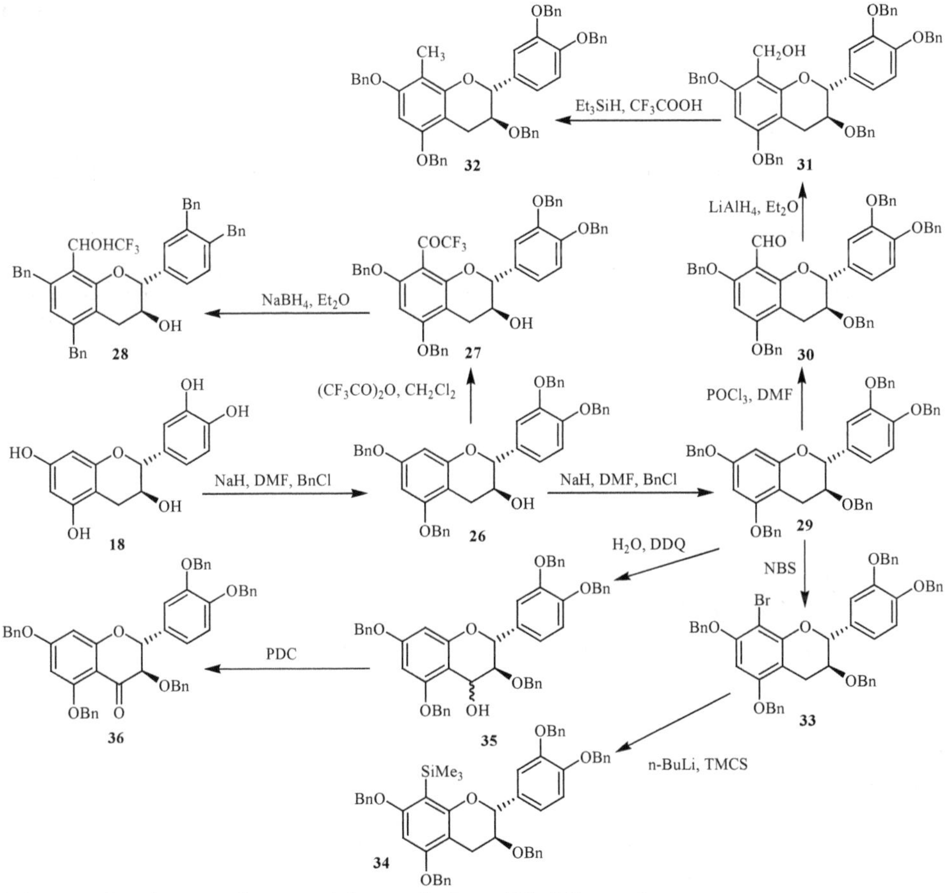

Scheme 1. Synthesis pathways of the studied modified flavanol monomers.

The modified flavan-3-ols monomer derivatives described in this work were synthesized according to the pathways depicted in Scheme 1. Compound **27** was prepared by action of trifluoacetic anhydride on tetrabenzylated catechin **26** following a Friedel-Craft's reaction on the 8 nucleophile position as previously described [Beauhaire et al., 2005; Es-Safi et al.,

2006c]. Further reduction by NaBH$_4$ afforded compound **28**. Compound **30** was prepared starting from the pentabenzylated catechin **29**. After formylation through the classical Vilsmeier reaction, the obtained compound **30** was reduced by LiAlH$_4$ giving the hydroxymethyl derivative **31**. Further reduction of the latter gave the target product **32** with a good yield. The bromided adduct **33** was obtained from **29** by action of NBS. Gram-scale of taxifolin **25** was prepared from (+)-catechin through reactions involving oxidation processes as previously described (Es-Safi & Ducrot, 2006a).

The structures of these modified catechin derivatives were determined through UV, MS and NMR spectroscopy. Structure elucidation of compound **32** will be detailed as example. The ESI-MS spectrum recorded in the positive ion mode showed signals located at m/z 755, 772 and 777 corresponding to [M+H]$^+$, [M+NH$_4$]$^+$ and [M+Na]$^+$ ions respectively and indicating a molecular weight of 754 amu in agreement with the structure of compound **32**. The usual flavan-3-ols characteristic RDA fragmentation was also observed at m/z 423, [M+H-332]$^+$ ion and corresponding to the protonated A moiety (Figure 3).

The remaining outstanding question that needed to be resolved was related to the position of the methyl group on the flavanol A ring. This constitutes the most encountered problem in flavanols structural characterization. Since the two positions 6 and 8 are almost magnetically equivalent, they could not be distinguished on the basis of their chemical shift. In our case, assuming that the substitution occurs at the more nucleophilic positions of the flavanol skeleton, i.e 6 or the 8 as confirmed through ES-MS spectrometry, determination of the residual proton (H6 or H8) could not be achieved based only on its chemical shift but would rather requires the use of 2D NMR analysis.

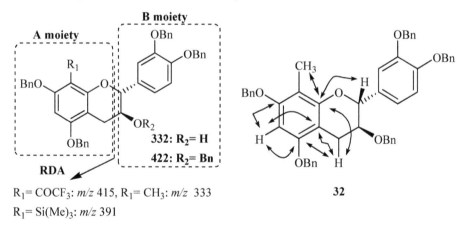

R$_1$= COCF$_3$: m/z 415, R$_1$= CH$_3$: m/z 333
R$_1$= Si(Me)$_3$: m/z 391

Fig. 3. Main fragmentations observed in compounds **27** (R$_1$= COCF$_3$), **32** (R$_1$= CH$_3$) and **34** (R$_1$= Si(Me)$_3$) and main HMBC correlations observed for compound **32**.

The position of the CH$_3$ group on the aromatic A ring was elucidated by long range distance carbon-proton correlations established by 2D NMR HMBC experiments through the following reasoning. The usual pyran ring protons H4 [(2.71 ppm, dd, J= 16.69 and 5.59 Hz) and 3.03 ppm (dd, J= 16.69 and 8.73 Hz)], H3 (6.60 ppm, m) and H2 (7.90 ppm, d, J= 7.99 Hz) were easily assigned by ^{1}H NMR analysis. The three B ring protons were observed between

6.93 and 7.00 ppm. For the aromatic A ring, only one proton signal appearing as a singlet at 6.21 ppm was present indicating a monosubstitution. The presence of the CH_3 group was confirmed through ^1H NMR analysis showing a singulet at 2.06 ppm. The protonated carbon chemical shifts were assigned through NMR HSQC analysis.

The definitive structure elucidation of compound **32** was achieved by HMBC experiment which allowed assignment of all hydrogen and carbon atoms. In addition to their correlations with C2 (79.84 ppm) and C3 (74.97 ppm), H4 protons (2.77 and 3.03 ppm) correlated with 3 carbons located at 102.74, 153.13 and 154.75 ppm. Carbons C4a, C8a and C5 are in a favorable position to give such correlations (Figure 3). The signal observed at 102.74 ppm was attributed to C4a due to its chemical shift position compared to C8a and C5 which are linked to an oxygen atom. The carbon signal located at 153.13 ppm also gave a correlation with H2, which pointed to the C8a carbon and thus the remaining signal observed at 154.75 ppm was attributed to C5. The C8a signal thus attributed did not show any correlation with the residual A ring aromatic protons which is thus H6. This was also confirmed by the presence of a correlation between C5 and the residual aromatic proton and between the methyl protons and the C8a (Figure 3). The position of the methyl group on the A ring 8 position was thus demonstrated.

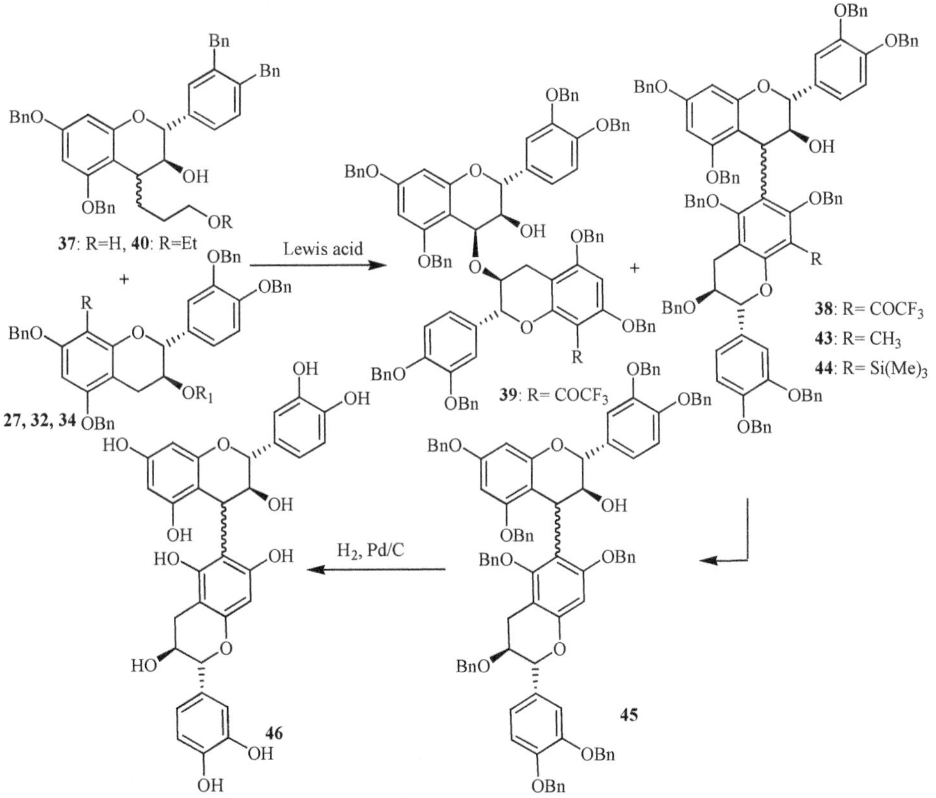

Scheme 2. Lewis acids-catalyzed flavanols coupling reactions.

After having synthesized these modified (+)-catechin derivatives, we tried to synthesize some dimeric flavanols derivatives by coupling flavanols using Lewis acids as catalysts. Indeed lewis acids, like TiCl$_4$, AgBF$_4$, SnCl$_4$, TMSOTf have been employed in literature to synthesize dimeric and oligomeric procyanidins of (+)-catechin and (-)-epicatechin units (Arnaudinaud et al., 2001; Saito et al., 2002; Tückmantel et al, 1999). In these reactions, the role of Lewis acids is to promote the formation of the benzylic carbocation at C4 of a flavanol subunit starting from a C4 hetero substituted flavanol, which thereafter undergoes a Friedel-Craft-like addition on a second flavanol subunit. For this study, the Lewis acid TiCl$_4$ was used as a carbocation promoting agent from the 4-(2-hydroxyethyloxy) flavan-3-ol 37. Coupling reaction between compound 27 and 37 in a 6/1 molar ratio was investigated in CH$_2$Cl$_2$ according to Scheme 2.

The reaction was monitored by CCM and HPLC and showed the disappearance of compound 27 and appearance of new compounds. In order to verify the presence of compounds with the expected dimeric structures the mixture was explored by HPLC coupled to a mass spectrometry detection operating in the positive ion mode. An extracted ion current chromatogram recorded at m/z 1395 and 1412 (Figure 4) and corresponding to a dimeric structure molecular weight showed the presence of a minor and a major compound. The UV spectrum of both compounds exhibited similar maxima (285 and 305 nm) to that of compound 27, indicating that the original flavan structure with the COCF$_3$ group was retained.

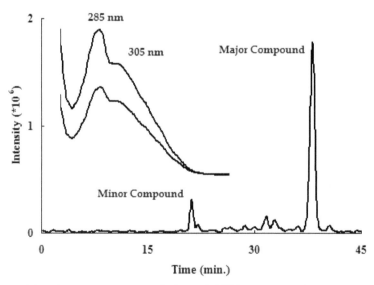

Fig. 4. Extracted ion chromatogram recorded at m/z 1395.

ESI-MS analysis of both compounds showed that the fragmentations observed for minor compound 38 were in agreement with a dimeric structure consisting of tetrabenzylated (+)-catechin 26 coupled to its trifluroacylated derivative 27 through a C4→C6 linkage (Figure 5A). Indeed, MS/MS fragmentation of the minor compound showed only one RDA fragmentation corresponding to the [M+H-332]$^+$ ion.

The mass spectrum obtained of the major compound **39** in the positive ion mode (Figure 5B) showed signals at m/z 1395, 1412, 1417 and 1433 corresponding respectively to $[M+H]^+$, $[M+NH_4]^+$, $[M+Na]^+$ and $[M+K]^+$ indicating a molecular weight of 1394 amu in agreement with a dimeric structure consisting of tetrabenzylated (+)-catechin **26** linked to its trifluoroacylated derivative **27**. However, the remaining problem was the establishment of the position of linkage to compound **27**, as the tetrabenzylated catechin moiety is linked through its 4 position.

In addition to the signals indicated above, the mass spectrum of compound **39** also showed signals at m/z 747 and 649 corresponding to the fission of the bond between the two constitutive units.

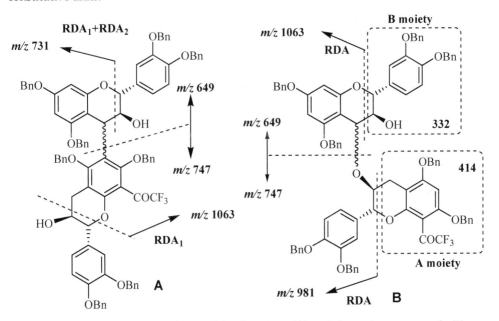

Fig. 5. MS/MS fragmentations observed for the minor (A) and the major compounds (B).

Among the other observed signals two of them were located at m/z 1063 and 981 and were also observed in the spectrum obtained through positive ES CAD MS/MS fragmentation of the signal located at m/z 1395 ($[M+H]^+$ ion). The signal observed at m/z 1063 was attributed to the characteristic RDA fragmentation corresponding to the $[M+H-332]^+$ ion as what was observed for compound **27** through a loss of the B moiety. The second fragmentation observed at m/z 981 correspond in fact to the $[M+H-414]^+$ ion, meaning a loss of the A moiety of compound **27** unit (Figure 5B) and corresponding to another RDA fragmentation. The occurrence of this fission indicated the presence of the A moiety in the structure of compound **39**. In other words, this means that the isolated compound is not a C4→C6 dimer since only one RDA fragmentation corresponding to the $[M+H-332]^+$ ion could be possible in this case as what was observed above for compound **38**. The possible linkage is thus expected to occur *via* the 2 or 3 position of the F ring or possibly the 2′, 5′ or 6′ positions of the ring E.

Through NMR analysis and in conjunction with the absence of a doubly benzylic methylene proton characteristic of a C4→C6 linkage and taking into account the dimeric structure of the compound as supported by MS analysis, the NMR data collectively indicated a dimeric structure with an interflavanyl ether bond connecting the two heterocyclic C and F rings. Taking into account the fact that the linkage did not involve the H2, H3, H4 F ring protons since they were all evidenced through NMR analysis, a (4-O-3) mode of linkage was thus concluded to occur between the two flavan-3-ols units. This was also confirmed by comparison of the chemical shifts of the H4 and H3 resonances of both the C and the E rings with those of their precursors. Finally the structure of compound was univocally confirmed through HMBC analysis where several long range correlations were observed. In particular correlations involving proton and carbon of both C and F rings via the oxygen atom were observed and confirmed thus the ether linkage involved in compound **39**. Full assignment of the protons and carbon chemical shifts was achieved through HMBC analysis (Figure 6) where the main correlations involving H/C of the C and F rings were showed in agreement with the proposed structure.

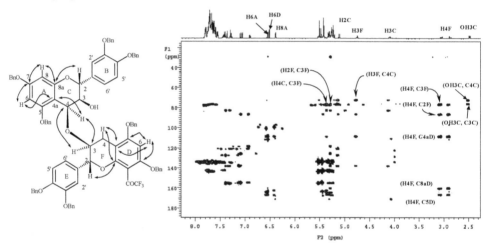

Fig. 6. Main ^{1}H-^{13}C long range correlations observed in compound **39**.

It was concluded that a (4-O-3) linkage was occurred between the two flavan-3-ol units. Moreover, coupling constants for the AMX spin system of the C-ring protons ($J_{3,4}$ = 3.2 Hz) indicated a 3,4 *cis* relative configuration for this ring, that is a 4β linkage between both flavanol units ($J_{3,4}$ = 3.2), which was determined through homonuclear decoupling experiment. The complete stereoselectivity of the reaction remains, however, to be explained and should presumably be due to a participation of the hydroxy group at C3 of **11**. However, its involvement in the stereochemical course of the reaction cannot be, in our case, related to the formation of a protonated epoxide similar to that reported by Bennie et al., 2001 in a work dealing with the dimerization of epioritin-4-ol derivatives.

In addition to TiCl$_4$, TMSOTf was also used to catalyze intermolecular flavanol coupling reactions. When the reaction was conducted between compounds **27** and **40** in the presence of TMSOTf as Lewis acid (Scheme 2), results similar to that obtained with TiCl$_4$ were obtained giving the C4→C6 dimer as minor compound. Intramolecular flavanol coupling reaction was also assayed using the previously reported strategy (Saito et al., 2003). The synthesized compound **41**, which contains both the electrophilic and the nucleophilic parts, was submitted to the flavanol coupling reaction using TMSOTf as Lewis acid (Scheme 3). However, the reaction was difficult to achieve may be due to steric hindrance and the expected C4→C6 **42** was obtained with lower yield.

The almost exclusive, high yielding formation, in these conditions of the novel ether-linked procyanidins as main compound rather than its carbon-carbon C4→C6 coupled analogue reflects the importance of electronic features in the formation of flavan-3-ol dimers. The poor nucleophilicity of the A ring monomeric precursor, caused by the presence of the $COCF_3$ group, permits alternative centers to participate in the interflavanyl bond formation.

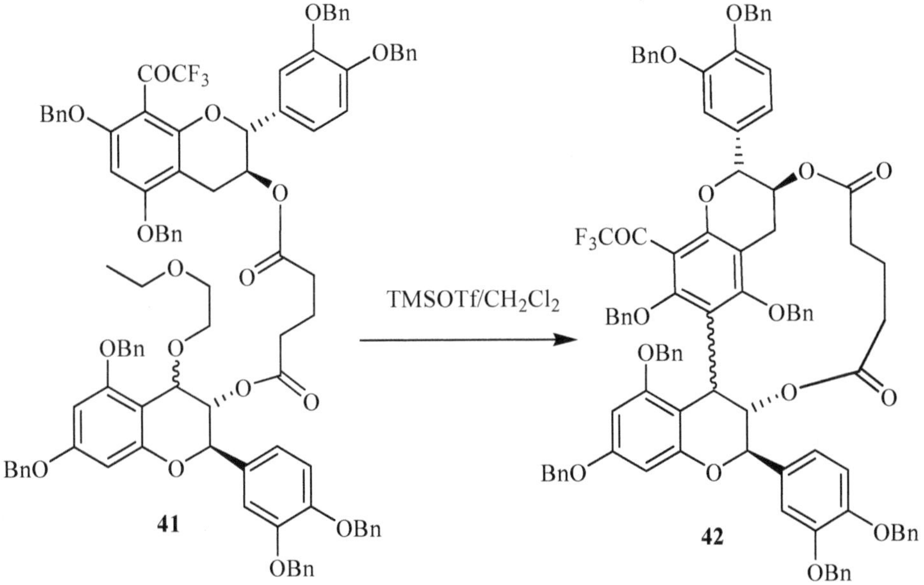

Scheme 3. TMSOTf catalysed intramolecular flavanol coupling.

The obtained results discussed above showed that the interflavanic carbon-carbon linkage formation was largely inhibited during Lewis acid induced flavanols coupling reactions by the presence of an electron-withdrawing group, while this was not the case with an electron-donor group like the methyl substituent. This could constitute thus a setereoselective method for the formation of C4→C6 procyanidin dimers which are usually obtained as minor compounds compared to the C4→C8 ones. In order to apply this technique to the stereoselective preparation of natural dimeric procyanidin of the C4→C6 type, we unsuccefully tried to remove the methyl group from the modified derivatives **43** (Scheme 2). Then we used the trimethylsilyl group which is easily removable by hydrolysis. Indeed, during purification of compound **34** on silicagel chromatography column, we saw that this compound was easily transformed to **29** by loss of the 8 substituent group. This prompts us to use this compound as nucleophile acceptor unit in the Lewis acid coupling reaction. The reaction was monitored through CCM and LC-MS showing the presence of compound with a molecular mass of 1460 amu corresponding to the dimeric compound **44**. After hydrolysis and hydrogenolysis, the corresponding product **46** was separated and analyzed through mass spectroscopy. The obtained results indicated a molecular mass of 578 amu in agreement with the dimeric structure of compounds **46**. Indeed, the mass spectrum of compound **46** showed procyanidin characteristic RDA fragmentation giving an ion fragment by a loss of 152 mass units. We tried to proof the interfalvanic linkage of the obtained compound through 2D NMR technique, but due to degradation of the obtained compound, our attempt was unsuccessful. It may be noted that the lewis acid induced flavanol coupling using compounds **26** and **37** give the C4→C8 adduct **47** as major dimer while the C4→C6 **45** was obtained as minor one (Scheme 4).

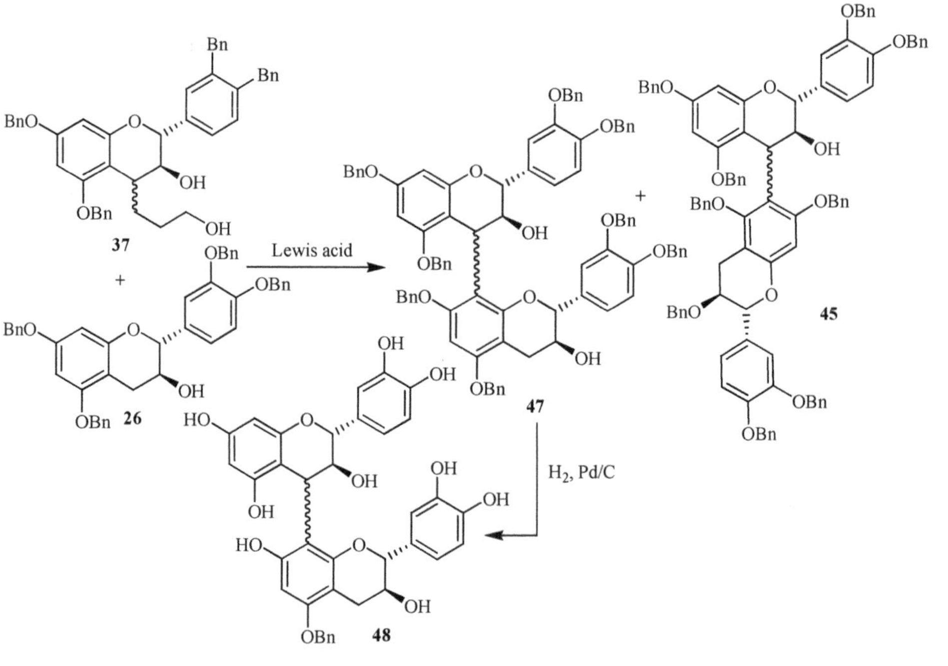

Scheme 4. Formation of dimeric C4→C8 and C4→C6 procyanidins.

After having investigated the Lewis acid induced flavanol coupling reaction involving 4-activated catechin derivatives, we were interested to use other precursors. Experiments were achieved using taxifolin **25**, a natural product often used as starting material in the hemisynthesis of procyanidins (Balas & Vercauteren, 1994). It was prepared as previously described (Es-Safi & Ducrot, 2006a) and was used through two pathways for the preparation of dimeric flavanols (Scheme 5).

In the first pathway, taxifolin was used as precursor of the electrophilic unit by action of NaBH$_4$ giving an 4-hydroxy group which release a 4-carbocation adduct in a mildly acidified medium. The compounds **21** and **24** were used in their free form as nucleophilic units and the reactions were studied through LC-MS techniques (Scheme 5). When the reaction was assayed with compound **24**, new compounds showing a mass signals at m/z 673 and 675 in the negative ion mode were detected. These compounds were interpreted as the dimeric modified procyanidins **49** and **50** formed by action of the carbocation cat+ on the 8-substituted catechin compounds used as nucleophile units. The cat+ unit is issued from the reduction of taxifolin into a flavan-3,4-diol, followed by protonation and dehydration. The action on compound **24** gave thus the dimer **49** while compound **50** was formed after reduction of the carbonyl group by NaBH$_4$ and further action of the cat+ adduct. This was confirmed by detection of compound giving a signal peak at m/z 591 corresponding to the reduced 8-substituted monomer. The same reaction was investigated using the **21** monomer and the corresponding methylated dimer **51** was detected through LC-MS analysis.

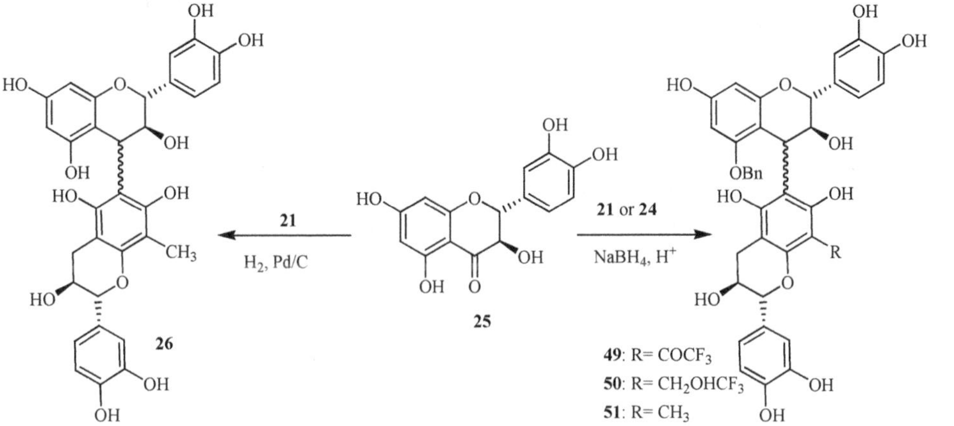

Scheme 5. Flavan-3-ol coupling reactions using taxifolin **25** as starting material.

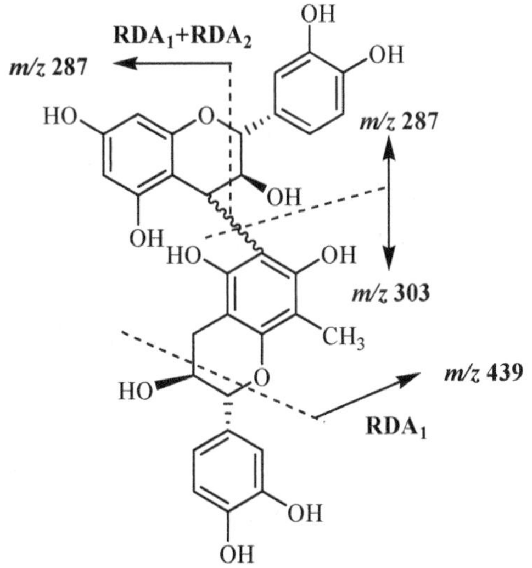

Fig. 7. Mass spectrum and main fragmentations observed in compound 51.

The second pathway using taxifolin was adapted from the recently described methylene linked flavanol dimers synthesis (Boyer & Ducrot, 2005). The application of such reaction to procyanidin synthesis was achieved through hydrogenation of taxifolin **25** in the presence of an excess of the methylated catechin **21** used as nucleophile (Scheme 5). The reaction was explored through LC-MS analysis and the formation of new compounds initially absent in the mixture was observed. Among the obtained products, compound with a molecular mass of 592 amu corresponding to the dimeric procyanidin **51** was observed. The mass spectrum of compound **51** recorded in the negative ion mode showed a molecular ion at m/z 591 and characteristic fragment signals as shown in figure 7.

2.3 Structural elucidation of natural and derivatized polyphenols through spectroscopic methods

The structural elucidation of polyphenols is difficult because of their heterogeneous character. The diversity of polyphenols is given by the structural variability of their basic skeletons with different hydroxylation patterns of the aromatic rings, different configurations at the chiral centers, distinct regio and stereochemistry, ... Due to this complexity and diversity, the characterization of polyphenols remains thus very challenging, and less is known regarding structure-activity relationship.

Various spectroscopic techniques including UV visible, NMR and mass spectroscopy have been used to characterize polyphenols. NMR spectroscopy could be considered as a powerful analytical technique for the determination of polyphenol structures even its poor sensitivity, slow throughput, and difficulties in analysis of mixtures. Technological developments in the field of NMR analysis, such as the LC-NMR analysis, have made of it the most important tool for complete structure elucidation of polyphenols. In addition to NMR, mass spectrometry has also been used for the characterization of polyphenols from various plant sources using various techniques including fast atom bombardment, liquid secondary ion, electrospray, and matrix-assisted laser desorption time of flight.

The examples on the structural elucidation of the compounds described above confirm the usefulness of the different spectroscopic techniques including 1D, 2D NMR and MS analysis. As examples of the usefulness of mass spectroscopy in polyphenols analysis, we gave below two examples. The first one concern the application of MS/MS techniques to the fragmentation study of flavonoids and the second is an application of ESI-MS and MALDI-TOF techniques for the study of a polymeric tannin fraction extracted from pear juice.

Various approaches have been proposed to use mass spectrometric fragmentations for structural characterization of flavonoid aglycones and glycosides (Cuyckens & Claeys, 2004; Es-Safi et al., 2005b; Feketeova et al., 2011; Ma et al., 1997; March & Brodbelt, 2008; Vukics & Guttman, 2010). It has been demonstrated that fragment ions provide important structural information for flavonoids and can be used to establish the distribution of the substituents between the A- and B-rings. A careful study of the fragmentation patterns in CID MS/MS can also be of a particular value in the structural elucidation of glycosides. Even many advances have been achieved in the field of structural identification of flavonoids, it is still a challenge in food chemistry to identify these compounds in foodstuff or those derivatives arising during biotransformation. We present here our results on the MS fragmentation study carried out on natural flavonoids achieved through a combinatory method using positive and negative ESI/MS, CID/MS and tandem MS/MS analysis. The flavonoid glycoside 6-hydroxyluteolin 7-O-glucoside **9** isolated from *Globularia alypum* (Es-Safi et al., 2005a) is given as example.

In order to study the fragmentations of the flavonoid **9**, the CID spectra of the protonated ion [M+H]$^+$ located at m/z 465 were recorded and the obtained result is shown in Figure 8. It showed fragment ions with a relatively high intensity in the higher mass region and corresponding to the glucose moiety fragmentations or loss of small molecules (H$_2$O, CO, CH$_2$O). In addition to the parent ion observed at m/z 465, the spectrum showed an ion signal at m/z 303 which presumably corresponds to the aglycone. The mass difference of m/z 162 Da between the [M+H]$^+$ peak and the aglycone is in agreement with the glucoside structure of compound **9**. The complete obtained MS data and the corresponding fragmentation pathways are gathered in Figure 8.

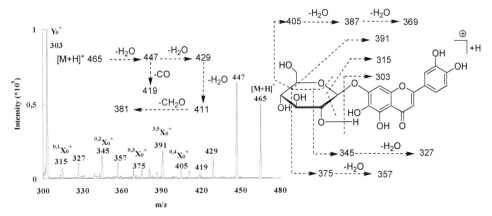

Fig. 8. CID-MS of protonated flavonoid 9 (m/z 465) and the corresponding fragmentations.

In order to characterize the aglycone part of the flavonoid **9**, the Y_0^+ CID spectra are more suited providing data similar to those of free flavonoid aglycones. Low-energy CID spectra of the [M+H]$^+$ ion of 6-hydroxyluteolin (m/z 303) showed various fragment signals. The detected ion species are formed according to the fragmentation pathways shown in Figure 9. The cleavage of the 1 and 3 bonds gave rise to the $^{1,3}A^+$ (m/z 169) and $^{1,3}B^+$ (m/z 135) ions. This pair of product ions clearly provides the substitution pattern in the A (3 OH) and B (2 OH) rings. The obtained ions can also undergo further fragmentations by loss of small molecules giving rise to other ions. By successive losses of 18 (H$_2$O) and 28 (CO) mass units, the ion at m/z 123 which is the base peak could be obtained from that at m/z 169, while that observed at m/z 117 could arise from the ion m/z 135 by loss of a water molecule. An other RDA-type fragmentation corresponding to the cleavage of the 0 and 4 bonds, results in $^{0,4}A^+$ (m/z 125) and $^{0,4}B^+$ (m/z 179) ions that can further fragment by loss of small molecules giving rise to other ions at m/z 161 ($^{0,4}B^+$ - H$_2$O), m/z 151 ($^{0,4}B^+$ - CO) and m/z 123 ($^{0,4}A^+$ - H$_2$). Cleavage of the 0 and 2 bonds leads to the formation of $^{0,2}B^+$ at m/z 137. Cleavage of the 1 and 2 bonds leading to the formation of $^{1,2}B^+$ and $^{1,2}A^+$ +2H ions were also observed giving signals at m/z 123 and 183 respectively. Finally cleavage of the 0 and 3 bonds giving rise to the formation of $^{0,3}B^+$ and $^{0,3}A^+$ ions at m/z 153 were also observed even at low relative intensity.

Mass spectrometry has also been used for the characterization of condensed tannins. In particular electrospray (Cheynier et al., 1997; Hayasaki et al., 2003) and MALDI-TOF (Behrens et al., 2003; Kruger et al., 2000) were used to characterize the degree of polymerization and structure of proanthocyanidins. The lyophilized proanthocyanidin fraction of a pear juice was investigated through mass spectroscopy. After extraction, the purified condensed tannin fraction was first initiated by ESI-MS and MALDI-TOF techniques and the obtained results are discussed below.

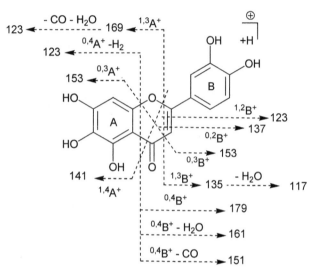

Fig. 9. CID MS-MS data and proposed fragmentation cleavage of the $[M+H]^+$ ion of compound 9 aglycone.

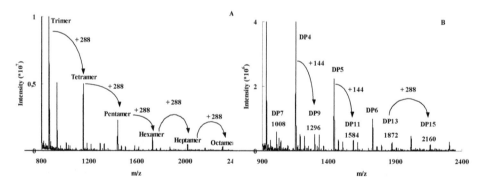

Fig. 10. ESI-MS spectra showing monocharged (A) and doubly charged (B) procyanidin ions.

ESI-MS analysis was performed in the negative ion mode as proanthocyanidin molecules are thereby better detected than in the positive ion mode due to the acidity of the phenolic protons. They are also more negatively charged as the chain length increases. An example of the obtained results is shown in figure 10.

Among the observed peak signals, figure 10A showed molecular ion species consistent with procyanidin oligomers containing singly linked units. A first series of abundant ions separated by 288 Da were observed from m/z 865 to 2306 Da corresponding to the molecular masses of procyanidins with DP3 to DP8. Indeed these signals could be interpreted as [M-H]$^-$ ion peaks of trimeric (m/z 865 Da), tetrameric (m/z 1153 Da), pentameric (m/z 1441Da), hexameric (m/z 1729 Da), heptameric (m/z 2017 Da), and octameric (m/z 2305 Da) procyanidins respectively. In addition to the signals indicated above, other less intense signals were also observed in the higher m/z region values. These peaks could correspond to nonameric (m/z 2593 Da), decameric (m/z 2881 Da), and undecameric (m/z 3169 Da) proanthocyanidins or to doubly charged ions [M-2H]$^{2-}$ of DP6, DP8, DP10, DP12, DP14, DP16, DP18, DP20, and DP22 species.

Mass spectra also proved evidence for a series of compounds that are 144 mass units higher than those described above. Compounds of this series were separated by 288 mass units with the most intense signals at m/z 1008, 1296, 1584, 1872, and 2160 Da (Figure 10B). These signals were attributed to doubly charged ions due to their narrower signal width compared to the singly charged species. Existence of the doubly charged ions was proven by the presence of additional signals that can be unambiguously attributed to the doubly charged ions [M-2H]$^{2-}$ of odd polymerization degree, starting from DP7. Such multiply charged species are reported to be more frequently observed in ES-MS and became more intense as the molecular weight increases, probably as a result of longer chain length which allows a better charge separation, thus minimizing the electrostatic repulsive forces. The ion peaks at m/z 1008, 1296, 1584, 1872, and 2160 Da were attributed to the doubly charged species of heptameric, nonameric, undecameric, tridecameric, and pentadecameric procyanidins respectively. No clear multiply charged species beyond the doubly charged ones were detected, presumably because of the lower concentration of larger tannin molecules. However, the apparent decrease of polymer concentration as the molecular weight increases may also be due to an increased dispersion of signal among variously charged ions, including large ones that cannot be detected.

This study shows the importance of ESI-MS analysis in determining the molecular weight of condensed tanins revealing the presence of various oligomeric proanthocyanidins detected as singly and doubly charged ions. However, the limited range imposed by the quadrupole analyzer as well as the easy generation of multiple ions for the larger molecules, inducing peak dispersion and frequent overlapping, result in an increased difficulty of interpretation and quantification of the signals due to higher DP procyanidins.

In order to overcome the problem related to the detection of higher molecular weight proanthocyanidins with a good precision, MALDI-TOf analysis was used. Since its introduction this technique has revealed itself as powerful method for the characterization of synthetic and natural polymers and has been recently introduced for the analysis of condensed tannins in food science (Kruger et al., 2000).

The obtained MALDI-TOF mass spectra of the studied polymeric mixture, recorded as sodium adducts in the positive reflectron ion mode and showing a series of repeating procyanidin polymers. The polymeric character is reflected by the periodical occurrence of peak series representing different chain lengths. The obtained results indicated that pear juice condensed tannins are characterized by mass spectra with a series of peaks with distances of 288 Da corresponding to a mass difference of one catechin/epicatechin between each polymer. Therefore prolongation of condensed tannins is due to the addition of catechin/epicatechin monomers.

Higher molecular weight ions but with significantly less signal intensity were also observed and were attributed to procyanidin consisting of 20 to 25 flavanol units. These observations fully corroborated the interpretation accorded to the ESI-MS data and demonstrated that both techniques were comparable in usefulness for the analysis of low to moderate size proanthocyanidin polymers.

For the condensed tannins indicated above, each peak was always followed by mass signals in a distance of 152 Da corresponding to the addition of one galloyl group at the heterocyclic ring C. Thus peak signals corresponding to monogalloylated derivatives of various procyanidin oligomers were easily attributed. No procyanidin containing more than one galloyl group was detected. Therefore, MALDI-TOF mass spectrometry indicates the simultaneous occurrence of pure procyanidin polymers and monogalloylated polymers. This showed that only monogalloylation occurs in pear juice procyanidin oligomers. To our knowledge, this is the frst mass spectrometric evidence confirming the existence of of galloylated procyanidin oligomers in pear fruits.

2.4 Antioxidant properties of natural and synthesized compounds

Free radicals are known to be a major factor in biological damages, and DPPH° has been used to evaluate the free radical-scavenging activity of natural antioxidants (Yokozawa et al., 1998). DPPH°, which is a molecule containing a stable free radical with a purple color, changes into a stable compound with a yellow color by reacting with an antioxidant which can donate an electron to DPPH°. In such case, the purple color typical of the free DPPH° radical decays, a change which can be followed spectrophotometrically at 517 nm. This simple test can provide information on the ability of a compound to donate an electron, the number of electrons a given molecule can donate and on the mechanism of antioxidant action. In cases where the structure of the electron donor is not known (e.g. a plant extract), this method can afford data on the reduction potential of unknown materials. The DPPH° test is a very convenient method for screening small antioxidant molecules because the reaction can be observed visually using common TLC and also its intensity can be analysed by simple spectrophotometric assays (Sanchez-Moreno et al., 1998). The DPPH° radical is scavenged by antioxidants through the donation of hydrogen to form the stable reduced DPPH molecule.

Because of the ease and convenience of this reaction, this technique was thus used for exploring the antioxidant activity of the natural and synthesized compounds described above. The natural isolated compounds described in the first part of this chapter were tested for their antioxidant scavenging effects on DPPH radical and their activity was compared to the synthetic antioxidant BHT and quercetin used as positive control. The free radical scavenging activity is usually expressed as percentage of DPPH° inhibition but also by the antioxidant concentration required for a 50 % DPPH° reduction (IC_{50}). IC_{50} value is considered to be a good measure of the antioxidant efficiency of pure compounds and extracts.

The obtained results are summarized in figure 11. It showed that 6-hydroxyluteolin derivatives **8** (6.6 µM) and **9** (7.1 µM) were the most potent radical scavenging compounds. The little differences found in the radical scavenging activities among these compounds is may be due to the presence of an additional glucose moiety in compound **8**. Among the flavonoid derivatives, eriodictyol- and luteolin-diglucosides **11** and **10** also showed strong activity compared to the positive control (7.8 and 12.2 µM). Figure 11 also showed that the four phenylethanoids **12-15** possessed the ability to act as a hydrogen donors with an IC_{50} around 12-15 µM due to their ortho-dihydroxy structures. The results showed that acteoside, isoacteoside and forsythiaside exhibited higher activity than the positive control BHT, but there was no significant difference between them (IC_{50} around 12 µM). Within the phenylethanoid family compound **15** (15.5 µM) was slightly less active than the three others. The obtained results are in agreement with previous reports, where phenyl propanoid glycosides are described as potent antioxidant agents (Aligiannis et al., 2003; Wang et al., 1996), as well as flavonoids (Bors et al., 1990) due to their catechol groups. On the other hand, figure 11 showed that the iridoid derivatives **2-7** exhibited moderate to weak DPPH-scavenging activities compared to the tested flavonoids and phenylethanoids.

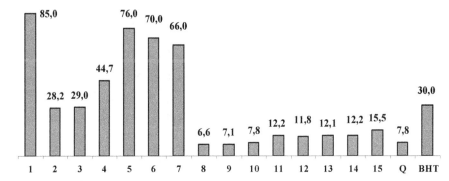

Fig. 11. IC_{50} (µM) of the natural compounds **1-15** compared to that of quercetin (Q) and BHT.

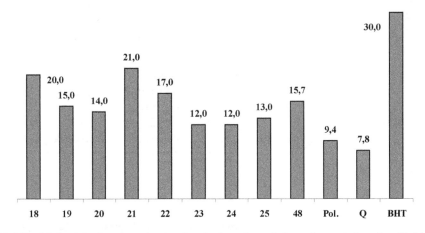

Fig. 12. IC_{50} (µM) of the hemisynthesized polyphenols and the polymeric fraction (Pol.) compared to that of quercetin (Q) and BHT.

The results concerning the antioxidant activity of the synthesized modified (+)-catechin using the DPPH° method are summarized in Figure 12 which showed that the new flavan-3-ol derivatives are potent free radical scavenging agents in the DPPH° free radical assay. It can be noticed that some of the tested compounds were more efficient than (+)-catechin **18** and BHT. Compound **25** is clearly the most efficient of the new tested molecules. Among all the tested compounds, only compound **21** with a methyl group as substituent was less active than (+)-catechin.

The proanthocyanidins pear juice fraction investigated above through ESi-MS and MALDI-TOF analysis was tested in an *in vitro* free radical scavenging assay as well as the monomeric catechin and its dimer B3 and their antioxidant power were compared to BHT and quercetin used as positive control. The obtained results are summarized in Figure 12. It showed that the polymeric procyanidin was the most potent radical scavenging fraction followed by the dimer B3 and catechin. The polymeric procyanidin fraction and the dimer B3 are as effective as quercetin and significantly better than BHT.

3. Conclusion

This chapter showed the importance of phenolic compounds as one of the largest and most widespread class of plant constituents occurring throughout the plant kingdom. The use of a combination of chromatographic and spectroscopic methods, allowed the purification and structural elucidation of several compounds and their capacity to scavenge the stable DPPH° free radical was evaluated.

The use of various synthesis pathways allowed the hemisynthesis of derivatized monomeric and dimeric flavanols. The obtained results showed that the introduction of a substituent onto position 8 of (+)-catechin yielded compounds with improved antiradical efficacy in solution. The usefulness of mass spectrometry in the analysis of polyphenols was demonstrated on a flavonoid glycoside and a polymeric condensed tannin fraction. Detailed informations were obtained through tandem mass spectrometry (MS/MS) in combination with collision-induced dissociation (CID) and various oligomeric procyanidins with increasing polymerization degree were thus detected. The antioxidant activity of the studied polymeric fraction was also investigated.

In summary, this chapter showed that the field of polyphenols remains an open research area of a good interest. Given their importance in food industry, it is interesting to know which factors can influence their use and in which manner this could be achieved. It is noteworthy to mention that the possible use of the studied phytochemicals could not be envisaged without taking into account the toxicological aspect and current legislative rules, in addition to the influence of these compounds on the organoleptic properties of food like taste, color, odor, and stability.

4. References

Adlercreutz, H. & Mazur, W. (1997) Phyto-oestrogen and Western disease. *Annales of Medicine*, Vol. 29, pp. 95–120.

Aligiannis, N.; Mitaku, S., Tsitsa-Tsardis, E., Harvala, C., Tsaknis, I., Lalas, S. & Haroutounian, S. (2003). Methanolic extract of Verbascum macrurum as a source of natural preservatives against oxidative rancidity. *Journal of Agricultural and Food Chemistry*, Vol. 51, pp. 7308–7312.

Arnaudinaud, V.; Nay, B., Verge, S., Nuhrich, A., Deffieux, G., Merillon, J. –M., Monti, J. -P. & Vercauteren, J. (2001). Total synthesis of isotopically labelled flavonoids. Part 5: Gram-scale production of ^{13}C-labelled (–)-procyanidin B3. *Tetrahedron Letters*, Vol. 42, pp. 5669-5671.

Arts, I. C. W. & Hollman, P. C. H. (2005). Polyphenols and disease risk in epidemiologic studies. *American Journal of Clinival Nutrition*, Vol. 81, pp. 317–325.

Balas, L. & Vercauteren, J. Extensive high-resolution reverse 2D NMR analysis for the structural elucidation of procyanidin oligomers. (1994). *Magnetic Resonance in Chemistry*, Vol. 32, pp. 386-393.

Beauhaire, J.; Es-Safi, N.-E., Boyer, F. D., Kerhoas, L., Le Guernevé, C. & Ducrot, P.H. (2005). Synthesis of modified proanthocyanidins: Introduction of acyl substituents at C-8 of catechin.Selective synthesis of a C-4→O→C-3 Ether-linked Procyanidin-like Dimer. *Bioorganic and Medicinal Chemistry Letters*, Vol. 15, pp. 559-562.

Behrens, A.; Maie, N., Knicker, H. & Kögel-Knabner, I. (2003). MALDI-TOF mass spectrometry and PSD fragmentation as means for the analysis of condensed tannins in polant leaves and needles. *Phytochemistry*, Vol. 62, pp. 1159-1170.

Bennie, L.; Coetzee, J., Malan, E., Woolfrey, J. R. & Ferreira, D. (2001). Oligomeric flavanoids. Part 34: Doubly-linked proteracacinidin analogues from Acacia caffra and Acacia galpinii. *Tetrahedron*, Vol. 57, pp. 661-667.

Bors, W.; Heller, W., Michel, C. & Saran, M. (1990). Flavonoids as antioxidants: determination of radical-scavenging efficiencies. In *Methods in Enzymology*, Packer, L., pp. 343–355, Academic Press, San Diego, CA, .

Boyer, F. D. & Ducrot, P.H. (2005). Hydrogenation of substituted aromatic aldehydes: nucleophilic trapping of the reaction intermediate, application to the efficient synthesis of methylene linked flavanol dimers. *Tetrahedron Letters*, Vol. 46, pp. 5177-5180.

Chang-Claude, J.; Frentzel-Beyne, R. & Eilber, U. (1992). Mortality pattern of German vegetarians after 11 years of follow up. *Epidemiology*, Vol. 3, pp. 195–401.

Cheynier, V.; Doco, T., Fulcrand, H., Guyot, S., Le Roux, E., Souquet, J. M., Rigaud, J. & Moutounet, M. (1997). ESI-MS analysis of polyphenolic oligomers and polymers. *Analusis*, Vol. 25, pp. M32- M37.

Cuyckens, F. & Claeys, M. (2004). Mass spectrometry in the structural analysis of flavonoids. *Journal of Mass Spectrometry*, Vol. 39, pp. 1–15.

Es-Safi, N. & Ducrot, P. H. (2006a). Oxidation of flavan-3-ol, gram-scale synthesis of taxifolin. *Letters in Organic Chemistry*, Vol. 3, pp. 231-234.

Es-Safi, N.; Kerhoas, L., Ducrot, P. H. (2005b). Application of positive and negative ESI-MS, CID/MS and tandem MS/MS to a study of fragmentation of 6-hydroxyluteolin 7-O-glucoside and 7-O-glucosyl-(1→3)-glucoside. *Rapid Communications in Mass Spectrometry*, Vol. 19, pp. 2734-2742.

Es-Safi, N.; Khlifi, S., Kerhoas, L., Kollmann, A., El Abbouyi, A. & Ducrot, P. H. (2005a). Antioxidant constituents of the aerial parts of *Globularia alypum* growing in Morocco. *Journal of Natural Products*, Vol. 68, pp. 1293–1296.

Es-Safi, N.; Khlifi, S., Kollmann, A., Kerhoas, L., El Abbouyi, A. & Ducrot, P. H. (2006b). Iridoid glucosides from the aerial parts of *Globularia alypum* L. (Globulariaceae). *Chemical and Pharmaceutical Bulletin*, Vol. 54, pp. 85-88.

Es-Safi, N.; Le Guernevé, C., Kerhoas, L. & Ducrot, P. H. (2006c). Influence of an 8-trifluoroacetyl group on flavanol couplings. *Tetrahedron*, Vol. 62, pp. 2705-2714.

Faure, R., Babadjamian, A., Balansard, G., Elias, R. & Maillard, C. (1987). Concerted use of two-dimensional NMR spectroscopy in the complete assignment of the ^{13}C and ^{1}H NMR spectra of globularin. *Magnetic Resonance in Chemistry*, Vol. 25, pp. 327-330.

Feketeová, L.; Barlow, C. K., Benton, T. M., Rochfortd, S. J. & O'Haira, R. A. J. (2011). The formation and fragmentation of flavonoid radical anions. *International Journal of Mass Spectrometry*, Vol. 301, pp. 174–183

Graf, B. A.; Milbury, P. E. & Blumberg, J. B. (2005). Flavonols, flavonones, flavanones and human health: Epidemological evidence. *Journal of Medicinal Food.*, Vol. 8, pp. 281–290.

Harborne, J. B., Williams, C. A. (2000). Advances in flavonoid research since 1992. *Phytochemistry*, Vol. 55, pp. 481- 504.

Hayasaka, Y.; Waters, E. J., Cheynier, V., Herderich, M. J. & Vidal, S. (2003). Characterization of proanthocyanidins in grape seeds using electrospray spectrometry. *Rapid Communications in Mass Spectrometry*, Vol. 17, pp. 9-16.

Horie, T.; Ohtsura, Y., Shibata, K., Yamashita, K., Tsukayama, M. & Kawamura, Y. (1998). ^{13}C NMR spectral assignment of the A-ring of polyoxygenated flavones. *Phytochemistry*, Vol. 47, pp. 865-874.

Imperato, F. & Nazzaro, R. (1996). Luteolin 7-O-sophoroside from *Pteris cretica*. *Phytochemistry*, Vol. 41, pp. 337-338.

Kruger, C. G.; Dopke, N. C., Treichel, P. M., Folts, J. & Reed, J. D. (2000). Matrix-assisted laser desorption/ionization time-of-flight mass spectrometry of polygalloyl polyflavan-3-ols in grape seed extract. *Journal of Agricultural and Food Chemistry*, Vol. 48, pp. 1663-16667.

Ma, Y. L.; Li, Q. M., Van den Heuvel, H. & Claeys M. (1997). Characterization of flavone and flavonol aglycones by collision-induced dissociation tandem mass spectrometry. *Rapid Communications in Mass Spectrometry*, Vol. 11, pp. 1357–1364.

Macheix, J. J.; Fleuriet, A. & Billot, J. (1990). *Fruit phenolics*. CRC Press, Boca Raton, FL.

March, R. & Brodbelt, J. (2008). Analysis of flavonoids: tandem mass spectrometry, computational methods, and NMR. *Journal of Mass Spectrometry*, Vol. 43, pp. 1581–1617.

Mehrabani, M.; Ghassemi, N., Sajjadi, E., Ghannadi, A., Shams-Ardakani, M. (2005). Main phenolic compound of petals of Echium amoenum fisch. and c.a. mey., a famous medicinal plant of Iran. *DARU Journal of Pharmaceutical Sciences*, Vol. 13, pp. 65-69

Ness, A. R. & Powles, J. W. (1997). Fruit and vegetables, and cardiovascular disease: a review. *International Journal of Epidemiology*, Vol. 26, pp. 1-13.

Owen, R.W.; Haubner, R., Mier, W., Giacosa, A., Hull, W.E., Spiegelhalder, B. & Bartsch, H. (2003). Isolation, structure elucidation and antioxidant potential of the major phenolic and flavonoid compounds in brined olive drupes. *Food and Chemical Toxicology*, Vol. 41, pp. 703-717.

Phillips, R.; Lemon, F., Beeson, L. & Kuzma, J. (1978). Coronary heart disease mortality among Seventh-Day Adventists with differing dietary habits: A preliminary report. *American Journal of Clinical Nutrition*, Vol. 31, pp. S191–S198.

Rimm, E. B.; Ascherio, A., Giovannucci, E., Spiegelman, D., Stampfer, M. J. & Willett, W. C. (1996). Vegetable, fruit and cereal fiber intake and risk of coronary heart disease among men. *Journal of the American Medical Association*, Vol. 275, pp. 447-451.

Saito, A.; Nakajima, N., Tanaka, A. & Ubukata, M. (2002). Synthetic studies of proanthocyanidins. Part 2: Stereoselective gram-scale synthesis of procyanidin-B3. *Tetrahedron*, Vol. 39, pp. 7829-7837.

Saito, A.; Nakajimab, N., Tanakac, A. & Ubukata, M. (2003). Synthetic studies of proanthocyanidins. Part 3: Stereoselective 3,4-*cis* catechin and catechin condensation by TMSOTf-catalyzed intramolecular coupling method. *Tetrahedron Letters*, Vol. 44, pp. 5449-5452

Sanchez-Moreno, C.; Larrauri, J. A. & Sauro-Calixto, F. A. (1998). Procedure to measure the antiradical efficiency of polyphenols. *Journal of the Science of Food Agriculture*, Vol. 76, pp. 270-276.

Shoyama, Y.; Matsumoto, M., Koga, S. & Nishioka, I. (1986). Four caffeoyl glycosides from callus tissue of Rehmannia glutinosa. *Phytochemistry*, Vol. 25, pp. 1633-1636.

Steinberg, D. (1991). Antioxidants and atherosclerosis: a current assessment. *Circulation*, Vol. 84, pp. 1420-1425.

Steinmetz, K. A. & Potter, J. D. (1996). Vegetables, fruit and cancer prevention: a review. *Journal of the American Diet Association*, Vol. 96, pp. 1027-1039.

Sugiyama, M.; Nagayama, E. & Kikuchi, M. (1993). Lignan and phenylpropanoid glycosides from Osmanthus asiaticus. *Phytochemistry*, Vol. 33, pp. 1215-1219.

Tijburg, L. B. M.; Mattern, T., Folts, J. D., Weisgerber, U. M. & Katan, M. B. (1997). Tea flavonoids and cardiovascular diseases: A review. *Critical Reviews in Food Science and Nutrition*, Vol. 37, pp. 693-704.

Tückmantel, W.; Kozikowski, A. P. & Romanczyk, L. J. Jr. (1999). Studies in polyphenol chemistry and bioactivity. 1. Preparation of building blocks from (+)-catechin. Procyanidin formation. Synthesis of the cancer cell growth inhibitor, 3-O-galloyl-(2R,3R)-epicatechin-4β,8-[3-O-galloyl-(2R,3R)-epicatechin]. *Journal of the American Chemical Society*, Vol. 121, pp. 12073-12081.

Vukics, V. & Guttman, A. (2010), Structural characterization of flavonoid glycosides by multi-stage mass spectrometry. *Mass Spectrometry Reviews*, Vol. 29 pp. 1–16.

Wang, P.; Kang, J., Zheng, R., Yang, Z., Lu, J., Gao, J. & Jia, Z. (1996). Scavenging effects of phenylpropanoid glycosides from Pedicularis on superoxide anion and hydroxyl radicals by the spin trapping method. *Biochemical Pharmacology*, Vol. 51, pp. 687–691.

Yang, C.S. & Wang, Z.Y. (1993). Tea and cancer, a review. *Journal of the Natinal Cancer Institute*, Vol. 85, pp. 1038-1049.

Yokozawa, T.; Chen, C. P., Dong, E., Tanaka, T., Nonaka, G. I. & Nishioka, I. (1998). Study
    on the inhibitory effect of tannins and flavonoids against the 1,1-diphenyl-2-
    picrylhydrazyl radical. *Biochemical Pharmacology*, Vol. 56, pp. 213-222.

11

Potato Peel as a Source of Important Phytochemical Antioxidant Nutraceuticals and Their Role in Human Health – A Review

A. Al-Weshahy and V.A. Rao*

*Department of Nutritional Sciences, Faculty of Medicine,
University of Toronto, Toronto, Ontario,
Canada*

1. Introduction

Food processing as one of the most important industries over the globe, however, by-products of such industrial activity that are mainly organic material must be handling in appropriate manner to avoid any environmental violence. Sanitation and disposal problem of food processing by-products is priority hence many approaches were suggested including recycling of such ingredients and utilize in several food and / or non-food applications (1). By-products of food processing is an inexpensive, affordable, and valuable starting material for the extraction of value added products such as dietary fiber, natural antioxidants, biopolymers, and natural food additives(2-4). However, the central dogma is still the stability, and economic feasibility of the processing development (5,6).

Potato (*Solanum tuberosum* L.) is one of the major world crops with world annual production of 180 million tones on 2009 according to the Food and Agriculture Organization (FAO) (7). Potato vegetation is dated back to South America around 500 B.C (8) and over centuries, it becomes a cornerstone in human nutrition in which nutritional quality was well established and documented and considers a source for many nutrients as shown in (table 1).

Of over 30 MT of annual production, tenth goes to industry to produce variable products including French fries and potato chips while the rest consumes freshly (7). By-products from potato processing, as like as any other food processing industry, are principally organic materials thus management and disposal are crucial toward a clean industry.

Potato peel (PP) has been studied as feed for pigs (9).However, potato peel is not suitable, without further treatments, as feed for non-ruminants because it is too fibrous to be digested (10). On the other hand, potato peel has been successfully used in feeding of multi-gastric animals. Milk fat from cows fed with PP was reported to be 3.3 g/kg higher than that of control (11).

* Corresponding Author

Water (g)	79.3	Calcium (mg)	12	Vitamin A, RAE (mcg)	0	Monounsaturated fatty acids, total (g)	0
Energy (kcal)	77	Copper (mg)	0.11	Vitamin C (mg)	19.7	16:1 (g)	0
Protein (g)	2.02	Iron (mg)	0.78	Vitamin B-6 (mg)	0.3	18:1 (g)	0
Fat, total (g)	0.09	Magnesium (mg)	23	Choline, total (mg)	12.1	20:1 (g)	0
Carbohydrate (g)	17.5	Phosphorus (mg)	57	Vitamin B-12 (mcg)	0	22:1 (g)	0
Sugars, total (g)	0.78	Potassium (mg)	421	Vitamin B-12, added (mcg)	0	Polyunsaturated fatty acids, total (g)	0.04
Fiber, total dietary (g)	2.2	Selenium (mcg)	0.3	Vitamin E, alpha tocopherol (mg)	0.01	18:2 (g)	0.03
Alcohol (g)	0	Sodium (mg)	6	Vitamin E, added (mg)	0	18:3 (g)	0.01
Cholesterol (mg)	0	Zinc (mg)	0.29	Vitamin D (D2 + D3) (mcg)	0	18:4 (g)	0
Saturated fatty acids, total (g)	0.03	Carotene, beta (mcg)	1	Folate, DFE (mcg)	16	20:4 (g)	0
4:0 (g)	0	Carotene, alpha (mcg)	0	Folate, food (mcg)	16	20:5 n-3 (g)	0
6:0 (g)	0	Cryptoxanthin, beta (mcg)	0	Folate, total (mcg)	16	22:5 n-3 (g)	0
8:0 (g)	0	Lutein + zeaxanthin (mcg)	8	Folic acid (mcg)	0	22:6 n-3 (g)	0
10:0 (g)	0	Lycopene (mcg)	0	Vitamin K (mcg)	1.9		
12:0 (g)	0	Caffeine (mg)	0	Niacin (mg)	1.05		
14:0 (g)	0	Theobromine (mg)	0	Retinol (mcg)	0		
16:0 (g)	0.02			Riboflavin (mg)	0.03		
18:0 (g)	0			Thiamin (mg)	0.08		

Values calculated per 100 gm fresh weight
Source: USDA Food and Nutrient Database for Dietary Studies (FNDDS)

Table 1. Chemical composition and nutritional value of potato.

The present review summarizes most attempts of potato peels utilization in food and non-food applications that include the extraction and verification of bioactive ingredients and nutritional quality of potato peels and their applications.

Although PP is being used for feeding livestock, by-products from potato processing industry still outpace such limited utilization. Another aspect was its utilization as a source for natural antimicrobial compounds (12).

2. Potato peels as a source of dietary fibers in food applications

Dietary fiber is well known as a bulking agent, increasing the intestinal mobility and hydration of the feces (13). Several authors have reviewed the importance of consumption of moderate amounts of dietary fibers for human health (14).

Scientifically speaking, dietary fiber is a broad term that includes several carbohydrates; cellulose, hemicelluloses, lignins, pectins, gums etc. (15). (16) reported that PP fibers are primarily insoluble, and can bind bile acids in-vitro. It is believed that binding of bile acids is one of the mechanisms whereby certain sources of dietary fibers lower plasma cholesterol. (17) studied the hypocholesterolemic effect of dietary fiber from PP and found that after four weeks of feeding on potato peels, rats showed 40 % reduction in plasma cholesterol content and 30% of hepatic fat cholesterol levels were reduced as compared with animals fed only with cellulose supplemented diet. Defects of dietary fiber on lipid-profile influence several health related issues. High concentrations of low-density lipoprotein (LDL) cholesterol, other dyslipidemia (high

concentration of triglycerides and low concentration of high-density lipoprotein [HDL] cholesterol), leads to blood platelets aggregation (18), risk factors for cardiovascular diseases (CVD) (19), and hypertension (20). Moreover, high intake of dietary fibers has a positive influence on blood glucose profile and it is related health complications, in healthy and diabetic individuals of both types. By altering the gastric emptying time, dietary fibers are able to affect the absorption of other simple sugars.

The effect of dietary fibers on blood glucose and insulin response has been demonstrated by many other authors as well (21,22).

Different sources of dietary fibers have been used to replace wheat flour in the preparation of bakery products. Potato peel was introduced as a promising source of dietary fiber. Since approximately 50% of potato peels (w/w) is dietary fibers (23). (24) studied the physical and chemical characteristics of PP and reported PP as being superior to wheat bran in its content of total dietary fiber, water holding capacity, and low quantities of starchy components. Wheat flour was also substituted with PP in the production of white bread, but it increased crumb darkening and reduced the loaf volume (24).

(25) found that PP caused a musty odor in breads, but the extrusion of potato peel before its utilization can diminish this aroma from the final product. (26) mentioned the effect of using PP in biscuit processing. The resulted biscuits produced using 5 and 10 % (w/w) of PP replaced wheat flour were smaller in terms of their stack weight and sensory score (color and appearance) in proportion to the levels used. In addition, supplementary biscuits were harder to bite than control biscuits.

(27) found that muffins with 25 % PP were darker, lower in height and more resistant to compression. Similarly, cookies with 10 and 15 % PP (w/w) were darker, harder, and smaller in diameter than control cookies. From a different prospect, (23) suggested the possible effect of potato peel as a good source of dietary fiber to be acting as anticarcinogenic material. Dietary fibers are known as protective materials against mutagenesis and carcinogenesis via several well established mechanisms that include binding of carcinogenic and mutagenic substances, reduce intestines-transit time, increase water absorption and fecal bulk, and lower fecal pH through the fermentation by intestinal

microflora (28). The probable role of extruded vs. unextruded potato peel, in comparison with wheat bran and cellulose as other sources of dietary fiber, in binding of the carcinogenic benzopyrene in designed in-vitro digestion model were investigated(16).

Un-extruded steam peels bound more benzopyrene than did peels extruded at temperature of 110 °C and feed moisture of 30%. Moreover, binding of benzopyrene by abrasion potato peels was lower than that by steam potato peels. In addition, abrasion peels contain approximately 25% dietary fiber and 50% starch, which may have maintained benzopyrene in suspension and / or higher amount of polyphenols remaining in abrasion peel, in contrast with steam peel, which may also have role in lowering of levels of benzopyrene by interaction and binding (16).

The method of peeling was found to be a key factor influencing the chemical composition of peels and its suitability for further utilization. (29) compared the influence of peeling method on composition of PP. Abrasion, method of peeling used by potato chip manufacturers, results in more starch and less dietary fiber than the steam peeling method used in the production of dehydrated potatoes. Potato peels with either abrasion or steam peeling methods were extruded; at barrel temperatures of either 110 °C or 150 °C and fed moistures of either 30 or 35%. Extrusion was associated with an increase in total dietary fiber and lignin contents and a decrease in starch content in steam peels. Lignin content was found to decrease but total dietary fiber content was unaffected in extruded abrasion peels. Soluble nonstarch polysaccharides increased in both types of peeling because of extrusion.

The higher quantity of glucose recovered from the insoluble fiber fraction of extruded steam peels was reported to be the possible reason in the formation of resistant starch. On the other hand, manual peeling of potato produced peels with approximately 63%, on a dry weight basis of alcohol-insoluble fibers, which was separated into pectic substances, hemicellulose, cellulose, and lignin. These fractions consisted of 3.4% pectin, 2.2% cellulose, 14.7% protein, 66.8% starch, and 7.7% ash. The sugars in the alcohol-soluble fraction consisted of 1.4% total soluble sugars and 0.9% reducing sugars (30).

3. Potato peels contribution in biotechnology

Several agro-industrial byproducts such as wheat bran, rice bran, molasses bran, barley bran, maize meal, soybean meal, potato peel and coconut oil cake have been screened as low-cost solid substrates for microbial production of enzymes to be use either in food applications or in other industrial sectors. Potato peel was reported to be an excellent substrate for the production of thermostable alpha-amylase, a starch hydrolyzing enzyme extensively used in different food industries, under solid-state controlled growth conditions (31) and was successfully used in some applications (32). Moreover, (33) and (34) used potato peel as a low-cost agro-industrial medium in production of both alpha-amylase and alkaline protease enzymes, respectively, to be used as detergents.

The antibacterial activity of the potato peel was found to be species dependent and the water extract of potato peel was effective only at high concentration against gram negative and one gram positive bacteria (35). (12) also investigated the extract of potato peel as antimicrobial agent against different types of bacteria and fungi. The results indicated the antibacterial and antifungal activities of potato peel to be species independent and when compared to one of antibiotics, streptocycline, potato peel had significant effect against *Pseudomonas aeruginosa* and *Clavibacter michigenensis*. In addition to its antimicrobial properties, potato peel can also function as a metal binder, probably due to its contents of polyphenolic compounds.

Potato peel also was able to support the economical growth and production of several extracellular hydrolytic enzymes, using *Bacillus subtilis* (30). (36) achieved the highest productivity, in terms of amount and activity, using Bacillus amylolequifaciens grown on solid media of potato peels, compare to peel samples of several fruits and vegetables, to produce β-mannanase (Figure 1). The growing interest in mannanase production for Industrial applications is due to its importance in the bioconversion of agro-industrial residues, which randomly hydrolyzes the axial chain of hetero-mannans, the major softwood hemicellulose (37).

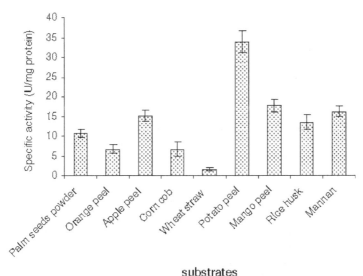

substrates

Fig. 1. Specific activity of mannanase produced by *B. amyloliquefaciens* gown on different lignocellulosic materials. Source {Mabrouk, 2008 #87932}

Mannanases have been tested in several industrial processes, such as extraction of vegetable oils from leguminous seeds, viscosity reduction of extracts during the manufacturing of instant coffee and oligosaccharides as well as it is importance in textile and paper industries. (38,39).

4. Potato peels in food applications

Potato peel also has acquired attention as a natural antioxidant in food system due to its high content of polyphenols, which was reported to be 10 times higher than their levels in the flesh (40) accounting for approximately 50 % of all polyphenols in potato tuber (41). Therefore, the effective utilization of potato peel as an antioxidant in food has been investigated extensively. Synthetic antioxidants, especially butylated hydroxytoluene (BHT) and butylated hydroxyanisole (BHA) are commonly used to prevent the oxidation process (42).

Concerns have been raised regarding the use of these synthetic antioxidants as being toxic and carcinogenic (43). Synthetic antioxidants may cause liver swelling and disturb the normal levels of liver enzymes (44). There is a strong need for alternative and effective antioxidants, from natural sources, to prevent deterioration of foods.

One of the first attempts to re-utilize PP was using it as a natural antioxidant in food systems. The oxidative deterioration of fats and oils is responsible for rancid odors and flavors, with a consequent decrease in nutritional quality and safety caused by the formation of secondary, potentially toxic, compounds. Thus, addition of antioxidants is an important step in processing to preserve flavor and color deterioration and to avoid nutrient loss. Due to the concerns of synthetic antioxidants in humans' foods, potato peel and extracts was proposed as a possible potential antioxidant in food systems (45). The same authors also measured the composition of fatty acids and polyphenolic content in peel of different potato varieties they also measured the antioxidant capacity of the petroleum-ether extracts in comparison with commercial antioxidants, tertiary butylhydroquinone (TBHQ), butylated hydroxyanisol, and butylated hydroxytoluene. Based on the results of their work, they suggested potato peel extract as a possible effective natural antioxidant retarding the oxidation process in vegetable oils; in particular colored skin-potato varieties which have been shown to contain the highest antioxidant activity reflecting high content of polyphenols (anthocyanins) that are responsible for their appearance (45).

(46) measured both amounts and type of phenolic compounds in freeze-dried, aqueous extract of potato peel. Chlorogenic (50.31%), gallic (41.67%), protocatechuic (7.815%), and caffeic (0.21%) acids were the major phenolic compounds detected in this study. They also measured the stability of sunflower oil heated at 63 oC when spiked with individual phenolic compounds that were detected in extract and with potato peel-water extract, respectively. When compared with control, sunflower oil in presence of aqueous potato peel extract was superior to BHT but not ascorbic acid derivative in preventing rancidity-related deteriorations in heated oil. On the other hand, (47) qualitatively and quantitatively, assessed polyphenols in either methanolic extract at 4 oC or water extract at 25 and 100 oC, respectively, of potato peel. Methanol extract of PP was shown to contain highest amounts of total polyphenolic compounds than water extract. (46). (47) reported that the main polyphenol detected in potato peel extract was chlorogenic acid. In terms of its safety as natural antioxidants in foods, potato peel freeze-dried extract was found not to be mutagenic when tested with *Salmonella typhimurium- Escherichia coli* microsome assay (35).

Moreover, the extract of potato peel had both bactericidal and bacteriostatic effects but only at a high concentration. Thus, potato peel was suggested as a possible safe, natural antioxidant to preserve foods.

More recently, potato peels, as well as some other agro-industrial by products, were examined for their content of total polyphenols and related antioxidant capacities (48). When extracted with mixture of 0.1 % of HCL in methanol: acetone: water (60:30:10, v/v/v), potato peel was found to contain approximately 177mg of total polyphenols /100 gm of fresh weight of peel.

In addition, (48) measured the total antioxidant capacity of potato peel extracts by measuring their antiradical scavenging activities and reducing power. A strong positive correlation was observed between total polyphenolic compounds in potato peel extracts and their antioxidant potency.

Lipid oxidation is a major cause of muscle food deterioration, affecting color, flavor, texture, and nutritional value ((49) and ((50). This oxidative deterioration of muscle involves the oxidation of the unsaturated fatty acids, catalyzed by hemoproteins as well as non-heme iron. (51) used freeze-dried extract of potato peel at two different levels of 500 and 1000 ppm as a natural antioxidant in ground beef patties to measure the efficacy of PP extract against the commercial antioxidant, control.

Freeze-dried extract of potato peel showed maximum antioxidant capacity at pH range of 5-6 while lost this activity at neutral and alkaline pH. In addition, antioxidant capacity, as measured with β-carotene linolate method, was significantly decreased when freeze-dried extract was boiled for more than 30 minutes and at temperature higher than 80 ºC. (51) also studied the effect of heat, time, and pH on stability of potato peel extract. Further development in terms of amount being use and optimum storage conditions of food product was suggested.

(52) explored if the potato peel extract possess antioxidant potentiality in retarding lipid oxidation in lamb meat preserved with radiation. Radiation processing is one of the most effective technologies that can extend shelf life and eliminate pathogenic bacteria in raw meat and meat products. However, meat on irradiation may undergo pronounced oxidative changes that influence the sensory quality of meat (53). When added to lamb meat in ratio of 0.04%, before irradiation process, potato peel extract was able to retard lipid oxidation in a similar manner as butylated hydroxytoluene (BHT). More recently, potato peel extract were studied as a natural antioxidant to prevent deteriorations of food lipids (54). Using six different solvents and two other food processing by-products.

Compared to sesame cake and sugar beet pulp, potato peel was superior in its content of polyphenolic compounds also showed the strongest antioxidant capacity using three different confirming assays (54).

(55) and his colleagues also evaluated the effectiveness of potato peel extract, as natural antioxidant during 60 days storage of refined soy-bean oil at 25 and 45 ºC. Free fatty acids, peroxide values, and iodine values were the criteria to assess the antioxidant activity of potato peels extract. Different organic solvents, including ethanol, methanol, acetone, hexane, petroleum-ether, and diethyl ether, were used to prepare extracts of potato peels.

The maximum efficiency of extraction was achieved by petroleum ether meanwhile diethyl ether, methanol, hexane, ethanol, and acetone, respectively, had had lower amounts of polyphenolic compounds in the extract. Potato peel extracted with petroleum ether exhibited strongest antioxidant activity in soybean oil during storage, equal almost to the antioxidant activity of synthetic antioxidants (BHA and BHT). However, the level of potato peel extract needed was 8–12 times higher than that of the synthetic antioxidants to control the development of rancidity during storage of cooking oils at high temperature. They suggested that potato peel extract in oils, fats and other food products can safely be used as natural antioxidant to suppress lipid oxidation (55).

Polyphenols in plants are present in either free form or bound to cell wall polysaccharides. Not all polyphenols are, therefore, readily extracted resulting in their underestimation by many researches.

(56) and (57) mention the incompleteness of data related to polyphenols in potato peel. They discussed the presence of other polyphenols in potato peel that were ignored by previous works. Principally they were interested to figure out the amount of ferulic acid-sugar esters in potato peels since many established works showed its ability to suppress the LDL-cholesterol oxidation in human plasma (58).

In their work (59) and his colleagues studied the thermal stability of ferulic acid which affects adhesion and texture of plant foods. (57) measured both free and bound forms of polyphenols in potato peel and their related free radical scavenging activities. Their results showed the superiority of bound- form of polyphenols, ferulic acid, in potato peels to quench free radicals, as measured by free radical scavenging activity technique, and strongly recommended it as a strong natural antioxidant.

5. Potentiality of potato peels antioxidants in biological systems

In light of above investigations, the potentiality of potato peel or potato peel extracts to act as antioxidant in biological systems have draw great scientific attention. The antioxidant potency of freeze-dried aqueous extract of potato peel was investigated, employing various established antioxidant measurement techniques in vitro; lipid peroxidation in rat liver homogenate,1,1-diphenyl-2-picrylhydrazyl (DPPH), as well as superoxide/hydroxyl radical scavenging, reducing power, and iron ion chelation (60).

The freeze-dried aqueous extract of potato peel powder showed strong inhibitory activity toward lipid peroxidation in rats' liver homogenate induced by the $FeCl_2$-H_2O_2 system. Furthermore, the water extract of PP exhibited a strong concentration-dependent inhibition of deoxyribose (DNA) oxidation.

The antioxidant activity measurements of potato peel extract did emphasis its strong reducing power activity, superoxide scavenging ability as well as its ion chelating potency. The in vitro results suggest the possibility that potato peel waste could be effectively employed as an ingredient in health or functional food, to alleviate oxidative stress (60).

In patients with diabetes mellitus, either type I or type II, it is well known that the production of ROS and lipid peroxides (LPO) increase (61). It has been suggested that oxidative stress (OS) is responsible for the pathophysiology of diabetes (62). The OS was reported to be related to hyperglycemia (63).

Hyperglycemia causes nonenzymatic glycation of protein through the Maillard reaction and alters energy metabolism, which results in an elevation of ROS levels and further development of diabetic complications (64). Potato peel was found to influence both glycemic index and antioxidant status in streptozotocin (STZ)-induced diabetic male Wistar rats (65). In that study, diabetic rats fed potato peel-powder-supplemented diet for 4 weeks showed significant decrease in blood glucose levels. In addition, Incorporation of PP powder into the diet reduced significantly the hypertrophy of both liver and kidney in STZ-diabetic rats and normalized the activities of serum alanine-aminotransferase (ALT) and aspartate-aminotransferase (AST).

Serum enzymes such as aspartate aminotransferase and alanine aminotransferase are employed in the evaluation of hepatic disorders and the increase in their levels reflects acute liver damage and inflammatory hepatocellular disorders (66). In addition, (65) measured both hepatic and renal-lipids oxidation, glutathione as well as activities of various antioxidant enzymes in liver and kidney of STZ-diabetic rats. It is suggested that PP powder in the diet may also be able to attenuate the eye lens damage associated with the diabetic conditions.

The strong antioxidant properties of potato peel extract (PP), which have been attributed to high content of polyphenolic compounds, was tested as a protective agent against erythrocytes-oxidative induced-damage in vitro (67) and by the measurement of morphological alterations and the structural alterations in the cell membrane. The total polyphenolic content in aqueous PP in this experiment was found to be 3.93 mg/g, dry weight based.

The major phenolic acids present were: gallic acid, caffeic acid, chlorogenic acid and protocatechuic acid. An experimental pro-oxidant system was used to induce lipid peroxidation in rat red blood cells (RBCs) and human RBC membranes. PP was found to inhibit lipid peroxidation with similar effectiveness in both the systems (about 80–85% inhibition by PP at 2.5 mg/ml).

While PP *per se* did not cause any morphological alteration in the erythrocytes, under the experimental conditions used, PP significantly inhibited the H_2O_2-induced morphological alterations in rat RBCs as revealed by scanning electron microscopy. (67) also suggested PP extract as a significant protector of human erythrocyte membrane proteins from oxidative damage probably by acting as a strong antioxidant. By virtue of its unique vascular and metabolic features, the liver is exposed to absorbed drugs and xenobiotics in concentrated form.

Detoxification reactions (phase I and phase II) metabolize xenobiotics aiming to increase substrate hydrophilicity for excretion. Drug-metabolizing enzymes detoxify many xenobiotics but bioactivate or increase the toxicity of others (68). In case of bioactivation, the liver is the first organ exposed to the damaging effects of the newly formed toxic substance.

Therefore, protective mechanisms relevant to the liver are of particular interest. Because free radicals and reactive oxygen species play a central role in liver diseases pathology and progression, dietary antioxidants have been proposed as therapeutic agents counteracting liver damage (69). (70) predicted a possible protective role of the potato peel extrcat against induced liver injury in rats.

Prior to the treatment with tetrachlorocarbon (CCL_4), the animals received doses of 100 mg, freeze-dried aqueous potato peel extract, / kg of body weight for seven consecutive days. The animals receiving an acute dose of carbon tetrachloride (CCL_4) to induce liver injury followed this. Liver enzymes as well as biomarkers of oxidative stress either in liver or in blood serum were measured. The administration of PP to rats orally at 100 mg/kg body weight/day reduced the risk of hepatic damage induced as a result of CCl_4 administration, as observed by evaluating of serum lactate dehydrogenase (LDH), aspartate aminotransferase (AST), and alanine aminotransferase (ALT) levels in CCl_4-treated rats. Also, the deteriorations of malondialdehyde (MDA); which is one of the end products of lipid peroxidation in the liver tissue, and depletion of hepatic glutathione (GSH) level; which is an important indicator of oxidative stress (71), were significantly higher in CCl_4-treated rats in comparison with animals that were pretreated with potato peel extract.

Super oxidase dismutase (SOD), catalse (CAT), and glutathione peroxidase (GPX) constitute a mutually supportive team of antioxidant defense against reactive oxygen species. SOD is the first line of antioxidant defense and it hastens the dismutation of superoxide radical to H_2O_2, while CAT/GPX converts H_2O_2 to water (72).

According to this scenario, a significant increase in SOD activity as a defense against the presence of free radicals can, generate overwhelmingly large amounts of H_2O_2. This in turn would disable the organism to handle the excessive H_2O_2, which would again result in oxidative stress.

Thus, increase in SOD accompanied by a decrease in CAT/GPX activity indicates a state of oxidative stress due to free radical generation (73). (70) elucidated the significant positive correlation between dosing of potato peel extract and SOD levels in rats treated with CCl_4. Additionally, histopathological studies showed that CCl_4 induced a remarkable degeneration in hepatocytes and focal necrosis. However, in general, lesions were markedly diminished in rats that were pre-administered with potato peel extract prior CCl_4 administration.

Study	Results	Reference
Solubility of PP fibres and its ability to bind bile salts	Are primarily insoluble, and can bind bile acids in-vitro. It is believed that binding of bile acids is one of the mechanisms whereby certain sources of dietary fibers lower plasma cholesterol	{Camire, 1993 #88855}
The hypocholesterolemic effect of dietary fiber from PP	40 % reduction in plasma cholesterol content and 30% of hepatic fat cholesterol levels were reduced in rats fed on potato peels compared to normal diet	{Lazarov, 1996 #88875}
Physical and chemical characteristics of PP and substitution of PP wheat flour in the production of white bread	Being superior to wheat bran in its content of total dietary fiber, water holding capacity, and low quantities of starchy components. Potato peels increased crumb darkening and reduced the loaf volume	{Toma, 1979 #88853}
The probable role of extruded vs. unextruded potato peel, in comparison with wheat bran and cellulose as other sources of dietary fiber, in binding of the carcinogenic benzopyrene in designed in-vitro digestion model	1. Un-extruded steam peels bounds more benzopyrene than did peels extruded at temperature of 110 ºC and feed moisture of 30%. 2. Binding of benzopyrene by abrasion potato peels was lower than that by steam potato peels. 3. Abrasion peels contain approximately 25% dietary fiber and 50% starch, which may have maintained benzopyrene in suspension and / or higher amount of polyphenols remaining in abrasion peel, in contrast with steam peel, which may also have role in lowering of levels of benzopyrene by interaction and binding	{Camire, 1993 #88855}.

Raw and extruded PP fibres in the production of bread	PP caused a musty odor in breads, but the extrusion of potato peel before its utilization can diminish this aroma from the final product.	{Orr, 1982 #88797}
The effect of using PP in biscuit processing.	The resulted biscuits produced using 5 and 10 % (w/w) of PP replaced wheat flour were smaller in terms of their stack weight and sensory score (color and appearance) in proportion to the levels used. In addition, supplementary biscuits were harder to bite than control biscuits.	{Abdel-Magied, 1991 #88876}
Potato peels in the production of muffins and cookies	Muffins with 25 % PP were darker, lower in height and more resistant to compression. Similarly, cookies with 10 and 15 % PP (w/w) were darker, harder, and smaller in diameter than control cookies.	{Arora, 1994 #86730}
The influence of peeling method on chemical composition of PP.	1. Abrasion method used by potato chip manufacturers, results in more starch and less dietary fiber than the steam peeling method used in the production of dehydrated potatoes. 2. Extrusion was associated with an increase in total dietary fiber and lignin contents and a decrease in starch content in steam peels. 3. Lignin content was found to decrease but total dietary fiber content was unaffected in extruded abrasion peels. 4.Soluble nonstarch polysaccharides increased in both types of peeling because of extrusion.	{Camire, 1997 #88802}
Manual peeling of potato peels	Approximately 63%, on a dry weight basis of alcohol-insoluble fibers was separated into pectic substances, hemicellulose, cellulose, and lignin. These fractions consisted of 3.4% pectin, 2.2% cellulose, 14.7% protein, 66.8% starch, and 7.7% ash. The sugars in the alcohol-soluble fraction consisted of 1.4% total soluble sugars and 0.9% reducing sugars	{Mahmood, 1998 #88884}.

Potato peel used as a low-cost agro-industrial medium in production of both alpha-amylase and alkaline protease enzymes and several extracellular hydrolytic enzymes	High yield and high activity of the produced enzymes	{Mukherjee, 2008 #88896}, {Mukherjee, 2009 #88895}, {Fadel, 1999 #88873} and {Fadel, 2002 #88874} {Mahmood, 1998 #88884}. {Mabrouk, 2008 #88880} {McCleary, 1988 #88881} {Gubitz, 1996 #88882; Ademark, 1998 #88883}.
The extract of potato peel as antimicrobial.	Antibacterial and antifungal activities of potato peel to be species independent	{Prasad, 2007 #88515
Potato peel extracts was proposed as a possible potential antioxidant in food systems	Extract was superior to BHT but not ascorbic acid derivative in preventing rancidity-related deteriorations in heated oil	{Onyeneho, 1993 #88898} {Rodriguez De Sotillo, 1994 #80192} ({Rhee, 1996 #88903} ({Yin, 1997 #88904}., {Makrisa, 2007 #88902} {Mansour, 2000 #80194} {Formanek, 2003 #88897}. {Kanatt, 2005 #89686} {Mohdaly, 2010 #88957}. {Mohdaly, 2010 #88957}. {Rehman, 2004 #86733} {Rehman, 2004 #86733}.
Amounts and type of phenolic compounds in freeze-dried, aqueous extract of potato peel.	1. Chlorogenic (50.31%), gallic (41.67%), protocatechuic (7.815%), and caffeic (0.21%) acids were the major phenolic compounds detected in this study. 2. Qualitatively and quantitatively, assessed polyphenols in either methanolic extract at 4 °C or water extract at 25 and 100 °C, respectively, of potato peel. Methanol extract of PP was shown to contain highest amounts of total polyphenolic compounds than water extract. reported that the main polyphenol detected in potato peel extract was chlorogenic acid.	{Rodriguez De Sotillo, 1994 #80192} {Ishii, 1997 #88910}. {Nara, 2006 #45746} {Rodriguez De Sotillo, 1994 #80191}

Safety of potato peels extract when used as natural antioxidants in foods,	Potato peel freeze-dried extract was found not to be mutagenic when tested with *Salmonella typhimurium- Escherichia coli* microsome assay	{Rodriguez De Sotillo, 1998 #80193}.
The potentiality of potato peel or potato peel extracts to act as antioxidant in biological systems	1. Inhibitory activity toward lipid peroxidation in rats' liver homogenate induced by the $FeCl_2$–H_2O_2 system. the water extract of PP exhibited a strong concentration-dependent inhibition of deoxyribose (DNA) oxidation. 2. Potato peel was found to influence both glycemic index and antioxidant status in streptozotocin (STZ)-induced diabetic male Wistar rats reduced significantly the hypertrophy of both liver and kidney and normalized the activities of serum alanine-aminotransferase (ALT) and aspartate-aminotransferase (AST). 3. PP extract as a significant protector of human erythrocyte membrane proteins from oxidative damage probably by acting as a strong antioxidant.	{Singh, 2004 #79 {Singh, 2005 #88890}. 926}. {Singh, 2005 #88890}
Protective role of the potato peel extract against induced liver injury using CCL_4 in rats.	1. The administration of PP to rats orally at 100 mg/kg body weight/day reduced the risk of hepatic damage induced as a result of CCl_4 administration, as observed by evaluating of serum lactate dehydrogenase (LDH), aspartate aminotransferase (AST), and alanine aminotransferase (ALT) levels in CCl_4-treated rats. 2. Significant positive correlation between dosing of potato peel extract and SOD levels in rats treated with CCl_4 3. histopathological studies showed that CCl_4 induced a remarkable degeneration in hepatocytes and focal necrosis. However, in general, lesions were markedly diminished in rats that were pre-administered with potato peel extract prior CCl_4 administration.	{Singh, 2008 #87208}

Table 2. Summary of potato peels (PP) attempts of reutilization.

6. References

[1] Schieber A, Stintzing FC, Carle R. By-products of plant food processing as a source of functional compounds-recent developments. Trends in Food Science and Technology 2001;12(11):401-413.

[2] Chiellini E, Cinelli P, Chiellini F, Imam SH. Environmentally degradable bio-based polymeric blends and composites. Macromolecular Bioscience 2004;4:218-231.

[3] Bildstein MO, García J, Faraldi M, Colvine S. Value-added for the european tomato processing industry. Acta Horticulturae 2009;823:195-198.

[4] Di Mauro A, Arena E, Fallico B, Passerini A, Maccarone E. Recovery of anthocyanins from pulp wash of pigmented oranges by concentration on resins Journal of Agricultural and Food Chemistry 2002;50(21):5968-5974.

[5] Bhushan S, Kalia K, Sharma M, Singh K, Ahuja PS. Processing of apple pomace for bioactive molecules. Critical Reviews in Biotechnology 2008;28:285-296.

[6] Chiu SW, Chan SM. Production of pigments by *Monascus purpureus* using sugar-cane bagasse in roller bottle cultures. World Journal of Microbiology and Biotechnology 1992;8(1):68-70.

[7] FAOSTAT. Volume 2009; 2009.

[8] Bradshaw JE, Ramsay G, Jaspreet S, Lovedeep K. Potato Origin and Production. Advances in Potato Chemistry and Technology. San Diego, U.S.A.: Academic Press; 2009. p 1-26.

[9] Natu RB, Mazza G, Jadhav SJ. Waste utilization. In: Salunkhe DK, Kadam SS, Jadhav SJ, editors. Potato: production, processing, and products: CRC Press, Boca Raton, U.S.A.; 1991. p 175-199.

[10] Birch GG, Blakebrough N, Parker KJ. Enzymes and Food Processing. London: Applied Science Publishers Ltd; 1981. 296 p. p.

[11] Jurjanz S, Colin-Schoellen O, Gardeur JN, Laurent F. Alteration of milk fat by variation in the source and amount of starch in a total mixed diet fed to dairy cows. Journal of Dairy Science 1998;81(11):2924-2933.

[12] Prasad AGD, Pushpa HN. Antimicrobial activity of potato peel waste. Asian Journal of Microbiology, Biotechnology and Environmental Sciences 2007;9(3):559-561.

[13] Forsythe WA, Chenoweth WL, Bennink MR. The effect of various dietary fibres on serum cholesterol and laxation in the rat. Journal of Nutrition 1976;106:26-32.

[14] Ballesteros MN, Cabrera RM, Saucedo MS, Yepiz-Plascencia GM, Ortega MI, Valencia ME. Dietary fiber and lifestyle influence serum lipids in free living adult men. Journal of the American College of Nutrition 2001;20(6):649-655.

[15] Gallaher D, Schneeman BO. Dietary fibre. In: Bowman AB, Russell MR, editors. Present knowledge in nutrition. Washington, DC, USA: ILSI; 2001. p 805.

[16] Camire ME, Zhao J, Violette DA. In vitro binding of bile acids by extruded potato peels. Journal of Agricultural and Food Chemistry 1993;41(12):2391-2394.

[17] Lazarov K, Werman MJ. Hypocholesterlaemic effect of potato peels as a dietary fiber source. Journal of Medical Sciences Research 1996;24:581-582.

[18] Bagger M, Andersen O, Nielsen JB, Ryttig KR. Dietary fibres reduce blood pressure, serum total cholesterol and platelet aggregation in rats. British Journal of Nutrition 1996;75(3):483-493.

[19] Erkkila AT, Lichtenstein AH. Fiber and cardiovascular disease risk: how strong is the evidence? Journal of Cardiovascular Nursing 2006;21(1):3-8.

[20] Alonso A, Beunza JJ, Bes-Rastrollo M, Pajares RM, Martinez-Gonzalez MA. Vegetable protein and fiber from cereal are inversely associated with the risk of hypertension in a Spanish cohort. Archives of Medical Research 2006;37(6):778-786.

[21] Onyechi UA, Judd PA, Ellis PR. African plant foods rich in non-starch polysaccharides reduce postprandial blood glucose and insulin concentrations in healthy human subjects. British Journal of Nutrition 1998 80(5):419-428.

[22] Chandalia M, Garg A, Lutjohann D, von Bergmann k, Grundy SM, Brinkley LJ. Beneficial effect of high dietary fiber intake in patients with type 2 diabetes mellitus. The New England Journal of Medicine 2000;342:1392-1398.

[23] Camire ME, Zhao J, Dougherty MP, Bushway RJ. In vitro binding of benzo[a]pyrene by extruded potato peels. Journal of Agricultural and Food Chemistry 1995;43:970-973.

[24] Toma RB, Orr PH, D'appolonia B, Dintzis FR, Tabekhia MM. Physical and chemical properties of potato peel as a source of dietary fiber in bread. Journal of Food Science 1979;44:1403-1407.

[25] Orr PH, Toma RB, Munson ST, D'Appolonia B. Sensory evaluation of breads containing various levels of potato peel. American Potato Journal 1982;59(12):605-612.

[26] Abdel-Magied MM. Effect of dietary fiber of potato peel on the rheological and organoleptic characteristics of biscuits. Egyptian Journal of Food Science 1991;19:293-300.

[27] Arora A, Camire ME. Performance of potato peels in muffins and cookies. Food Research International 1994;27:15-22.

[28] Harris PJ, Ferguson LR. Dietary fibre: Its composition and role in protection against colorectal cancer. Mutation Research 1993;290:97-110.

[29] Camire ME, Violette D, Dougherty MP, McLaughlin MA. Potato peel dietary fiber composition: effects of peeling and extrusion cooking processes. Journal of Agricultural and Food Chemistry 1997;45(4):1404-1408.

[30] Mahmood AU, Greenman J, Scragg AH. Orange and potato peel extracts : Analysis and use as Bacillus substrates for the production of extracellular enzymes in continuous culture. Enzyme and Microbial Technology 1998;22(2):130-137.

[31] Fadel M. Utilization of potato chips industry by products for the production of thermostable bacterial alpha amylase using solid state fermentation system: 1. Effect of incubation period, temperature, moisture level and inoculum size. Egyptian Journal of Microbiology 1999;34:433-445.

[32] Fadel M. Utilization of potato chips industry by products for production of thermostable bacterial alpha-amylase using solid state fermentation system. 2. Effect of moistening agent, supplementary substrates nitrogen source, and application of the solid fermented substrate for some starches digestion. Egyptian Journal of Microbiology 2002;34(4):533-546.

[33] Mukherjee KA, Adhikari H, Rai KS. Production of alkaline protease by a thermophilic Bacillus subtilis under solid-state fermentation (SSF) condition using Imperata cylindrica grass and potato peel as low-cost medium: Characterization and application of enzyme in detergent formulation. Biochemical Engineering Journal 2008;39:353-361.

[34] Mukherjee KA, Borahb M, Rai KS. To study the influence of different components of fermentable substrates on induction of extracellular α-amylase synthesis by *Bacillus subtilis* DM-03 in solid-state fermentation and exploration of feasibility for inclusion of α-amylase in laundry detergent formulations. Biochemical Engineering Journal 2009;43:149-156.

[35] Rodriguez De Sotillo D, Hadley M, Wolf-Hall C. Potato peel extract a nonmutagenic antioxidant with potential antimicrobial activity. Journal of Food Science 1998;63(5):907-910.

[36] Mabrouk EMM, El Ahwany MDA. Production of β-mannanase by Bacillus amylolequifaciens 10A1 cultured on potato peels. African Journal of Biotechnology. 2008;7(8):1123-1128.

[37] McCleary BV. β-Mananasa. Methods in Enzymology 1988;160:596-610.

[38] Gubitz GM, Hayn M, Urbanz G, Steiner W. Purification and properties of an acid β-mannanase from *Sclerotium rolfsii*. Journal of Biotechnology 1996;45:165-172.

[39] Ademark P, Varga A, Medve J, Harjunpa AV, Drakenberg T, Tjerneld F. Softwood hemicellulose-degrading enzymes from *Aspergillus niger*: Purification and properties of a β-mannanase. Journal of Biotechnology 1998;63:199-210.

[40] Malmberg A, Theander O. Free and conjugated phenolic acids and aldehydes in potato tubers. Swedish Journal of Agricultural Research 1984;14:119-125.

[41] Friedman M. Chemistry, biochemistry, and dietary role of potato polyphenols. Journal of Agricultural and Food Chemistry 1997;45(5):1523-1540.

[42] Sobedio JL, Kaitaramita J, Grandgiral A, Malkkl Y. Quality assessment of industrial pre-fried French fries. American Oil Chemical Society 1991;68:299-302.

[43] Ito N, Hiroze M, Fukushima G, Tauda H, Shira T, Tatematsu M. Studies on antioxidant; their carcinogenic and modifying effects on chemical carcinogensis. Food Chemistry Toxicology 1986;24:1071-1081.

[44] Madhavi DL, Deshpande SS, Salunkhe DK. Butylated hydroxyanisole (BHA; tert-butyl-4-hydroxyanisole) and Butylated hydroxytoluene (BHT; 2,6-di-tert-butyl-p-cresol). In: Madhavi DL, Deshpande SS, Salunkhe DK, editors. Food antioxidants: Technological, toxicological, and health perspectives. New York, U.S.A.: Marcel Dekker; 1996. p 1-215.

[45] Onyeneho NS, Hettiarachchy SN. Antioxidant activity, fatty acids and phenolic acids compositions of potato peels. Journal of the Science of Food and Agriculture 1993;62:345-350.

[46] Rodriguez De Sotillo D, Hadley M, Holm ET. Potato peel waste: Stability and antioxidant activity of a freeze-dried extract. Journal of Food Science 1994;59(5):1031-1033.

[47] Rodriguez De Sotillo D, Hadley M, Holm ET. Phenolics in aqueous potato peel extract: Extraction, identification and degradation. Journal of Food Science 1994;59(3):649-651.

[48] Makrisa PM, Boskou G, Andrikopoulos KN. Polyphenolic content and in vitro antioxidant characteristics of wine industry and other agri-food solid waste extracts. Journal of Food Composition and Analysis 2007;20:125-132.

[49] Rhee KS, Anderson LM, Sams AR. Lipid oxidation potential of beef, chicken and pork. Journal of Food Science 1996;61:8-12.

[50] Yin MC, Cheng WS. Oxymyoglobin and lipid oxidation in phosphatidylcholine liposomes retarded by α-tocopherol and β- carotene. Journal of Food Science 1997;62:1095-1097.

[51] Mansour EH, Khalil AH. Evaluation of antioxidant activity of some plant extracts and their application to ground beef patties. Food Chemistry 2000;69(2):135-141.

[52] Kanatt SR, Chander R, Radhakrishna P, Sharma A. Potato peel extract: a natural antioxidant for retarding lipid peroxidation in radiation processed lamb meat. Journal of Agricultural and Food Chemistry 2005;53(5):1499-1504.

[53] Formanek Z, Lynch A, Galvin K, Farkas J, Kerry JP. Combined effects of irradiation and the use of natural antioxidants on the shelf-life stability of overwrapped minced beef. Meat Science 2003;63:433-440.

[54] Mohdaly AA, Sarhan MA, Smetanska I, Mahmoud A. Antioxidant properties of various solvent extracts of potato peel, sugar beet pulp and sesame cake. Journal of the Science of Food and Agriculture 2010;90(2):218-226.

[55] Rehman Z, Habib F, Shah WH. Utilization of potato peels extract as a natural antioxidant in soy bean oil. Food Chemistry 2004;85:215-220.

[56] Fry SC. Cross-linking of matrix polymers in the growing cell walls of angiosperms. Annual Review of Plant Physiology 1986;37:165-186.

[57] Nara K, Miyoshi T, Honma T, Koga H. Antioxidative activity of bound-form phenolics in potato peel. Bioscience, Biotechnology, and Biochemistry 2006;70(6):1489-1491.

[58] Ohta T, Semboku N, Kuchii A, Egashira Y, Sanada H. Antioxidant activity of corn bran cell-wall fragments in the LDL oxidation system. Journal of Agricultural and Food Chemistry 1997;45(5):1644-1648.

[59] Ishii T. Structure and functions of feruloylated polysaccharides. Plant Science 1997;127(2):111-127.

[60] Singh N, Rajini PS. Free radical scavenging activity of an aqueous extract of potato peel. Food Chemistry 2004;85(4):611-616.

[61] Kuyvenhoven JP, Meinders AE. Oxidative stress and diabetes mellitus. Pathogenesis of long-term complications. European Journal of Internal Medicine 1999;10:9-19.

[62] Dandona P, Thusu K, Cook S, Synder B, Makaowski J, Armstrong D, Nicotera T. Oxidative damage to DNA in diabetes mellitus. Lancet 1996;347:444-445.

[63] Baynes JW, Thorpe SR. Role of oxidative stress in diabetic complications: A new perspective on an old paradigm. Diabetes 1999;48:1-9.

[64] Shimoi K, Okitsu A, Green MHL, Lowe JE, Ohta T, Kaji K, Terato H, Ide H, Kinae N. Oxidative DNA damage induced by high glucose and its suppression in human umbilical vein endothelial cells. Mutation Research 2001;480–481:371–378.

[65] Singh N, Kamath V, Rajini PS. Attenuation of hyperglycemia and associated biochemical parameters in STZ-induced diabetic rats by dietary supplementation of potato peel powder. Clinica Chimica Acta 2005;353(1-2):165-175.

[66] El BK, Hashimoto Y, Muzandu K, Ikenaka Y, Ibrahim ZS, Kazusaka A, Fujita S, Ishizuka M. Protective effect of *Pleurotus cornucopiae* mushroom extract on carbon tetrachloride-induced hepatotoxicity. Japanese Journal of Veterinary Research 2009;57(2):109-118.

[67] Singh N, Rajini PS. Antioxidant-mediated protective effect of potato peel extract in erythrocytes against oxidative damage. Chemico-Biological Interactions 2008;173(2):97-104.

[68] Jaeschke H, Gores GJ, Cederbaum AI, Hinson JA, Pessayre D, Lemasters JJ. Mechanisms of hepatotoxicity. Toxicological Sciences 2002;65(2):166-176.

[69] Higuchi H, Gores GJ. Mechanisms of liver injury: An overview. Current Molecular Medicine 2003;3(6):483-490.

[70] Singh N, Kamath V, Narasimhamurthy K, Rajini PS. Protective effect of potato peel extract against carbon tetrachloride-induced liver injury in rats. Environmental Toxicology and Pharmacology 2008;26(2):241-246.

[71] Souza MF, Rao VSN, Silveira ER. Inhibition of lipid peroxidation by ternatin, a tetramethoxyflavone from *Egletes viscosa* L. Phytomedicine 1997;4(1):27-31.

[72] Halliwell B, Gutteridge JM. Role of free radicals and catalytic metal ions in human disease: An overview. Methods in Enzymology 1990;186:1-85.

[73] Tasaduq SA, Singh K, Sethi S, Sharma SC, Bedi KL, Singh J, Jaggi BS. Hepatocurative and antioxidant profile of HP-1, a polyherbal phytomedicine Human and Experimental Toxicology 2003;22(12):639-645.

12

Polyamines of Plant Origin – An Important Dietary Consideration for Human Health

Denise C. Hunter and David J. Burritt
Food & Wellness Group, The New Zealand Institute
for Plant & Food Research Limited, Auckland,
The Department of Botany, The University of Otago, Dunedin,
New Zealand

1. Introduction

Ubiquitous in nature, polyamines are a group of aliphatic amines, cationic at neutral pH, that are essential for cell growth and viability. Because of their positive charge, polyamines are able to bind by electrostatic linkages to many cellular macromolecules, including DNA, RNA, and proteins (Kusano et al. 2008). Polyamines are involved in the regulation of a diverse range of vital cellular processes in both eukaryotic and prokaryotic cells, including cell proliferation, signal transduction and membrane stabilization (Wang et al. 2003; Kusano et al. 2008). They are also involved in the regulation of gene expression and translation (Igarashi & Kashiwagi, 2000; Kusano et al., 2008), and control programmed cell death in some organisms (Seiler & Raul, 2005). The diamine putrescine and the triamine spermidine are found in nearly all organisms and are the most abundant polyamines in prokaryotic cells, such as bacteria, while the tetraamine spermine is mainly found in eukaryotic cells. In plants the most common polyamines are putrescine, spermidine and spermine (Tiburcio et al., 1993; Grimes et al. 1986), which are present as free amines, conjugated to small molecules such as hydroxycinnamic acid, or bound to larger macromolecules such as proteins or nucleic acids. Less common polyamines found in plants are cadaverine, and the spermidine- and spermine-related compounds, homospermidine, norspermidine, homospermine, norspermine and thermospermine (Martin-Tanguy, 2001). The structures of the common and less common polyamines found in plants are shown in Table 1. Polyamines are involved in many aspects of plant development (Martin-Tanguy, 2001; Li & Burritt, 2003; Hunter & Burritt, 2005; Baron & Stasolla, 2008) and are important molecules associated with both abiotic and biotic stress tolerance (Burritt, 2008). Because of their roles in a diverse array of fundamental processes, polyamines are found within all the compartments that make up the plant cell, including mitochondria, chloroplasts and the nucleus (Martin-Tanguy, 2001).

In recent years there has been considerable interest in the influence of ingested polyamines from plant-based foods on human health (Lima et al., 2011). In a recent study comparing several vegetable crops cultivated using organic or conventional procedures, Lima et al. (2011) reported that organic vegetables contained higher concentrations of polyamines than those produced by conventional cultivation, and suggested that this could be due to plants cultivated organically being subjected to stress from pests and/or diseases. Hence an understanding of the factors regulating polyamine metabolism in plants could be of great value when considering the importance of polyamines of plant origin on human health. Polyamines are important to human health, particularly because they are involved in an array of specific roles that are essential to cell growth and proliferation (Kalač & Krausová, 2005). Therefore, polyamines may be considered especially important in the young. However, it is well established that the capacity for polyamine synthesis decreases with age (Larqué, 2007). Considering the array of specific roles that polyamines fulfil, a decrease in polyamines could contribute to the ageing process. Therefore, this chapter examines the content of polyamines in plants and plant-based foods, the role of polyamines in human health throughout the ageing process, and the benefit that might be achieved with consumption of high polyamine plant-based foods by older people.

Name	Structure
Diamines	
1,3-Diaminopropane	$NH_2(CH_2)_3NH_2$
Putrescine	$NH_2(CH_2)_4NH_2$
Cadaverine	$NH_2(CH_2)_5NH_2$
Triamines	
Spermidine	$NH_2(CH_2)_3\ NH(CH_2)_4NH_2$
Homospermidine	$NH_2(CH_2)_4\ NH(CH_2)_4NH_2$
Norspermidine	$NH_2(CH_2)_3\ NH(CH_2)_3NH_2$
Tetraamines	
Spermine	$NH_2(CH_2)_3NH(CH_2)_4\ NH(CH_2)_3NH_2$
Homospermine	$NH_2(CH_2)_3NH(CH_2)_4\ NH(CH_2)_4NH_2$
Norspermine	$NH_2(CH_2)_3NH(CH_2)_3\ NH(CH_2)_3NH_2$
Thermospermine	$NH_2(CH_2)_3NH(CH_2)_3\ NH(CH_2)_4NH_2$

Table 1. Common and uncommon diamines and polyamines found in plants

2. Polyamines and plants

2.1 Polyamine biosynthesis and catabolism

In animals and most plants, with the notable exception of *Arabidopsis thaliana*, putrescine can be synthesized directly by decarboxylation of ornithine via the enzyme ornithine decarboxylase (ODC; EC 4.1.1.17) (Figure 1). However, unlike in animal cells, where the existence of the enzyme arginine decarboxylase (ADC; EC 4.1.1.19) is debatable, plants can synthesise putrescine from arginine, via ADC, agmatine iminohydrolase (EC 3.5.3.12) and N-carbamoylputrescine amidohydrolase (EC 3.5.1.53) (Alcázar et al. 2006; Slocum, 1991). Interestingly, plants also contain the enzyme arginase that allows the inter-conversion of ornithine and arginine, although in most plants the concentration of arginine is generally much higher than that of ornithine suggesting that the formation of arginine is generally favoured. In plants that contain both ADC and ODC the two pathways for putrescine biosynthesis appear to be physically separated within the cell, with ADC mostly found associated with the thylakoid membranes of chloroplasts and in the nucleus (Borrell et al., 1995; Bortolotti et al., 2004), and ODC localized in the cytosol (Borrell et al., 1995). Irrespective of the pathway of biosynthesis, the pool of cellular putrescine can be used for the synthesis of spermidine, spermine and other polyamines. Addition of an aminopropyl group from decarboxylated S-adenosyl-methionine (dcSAM), synthesized by the enzyme S-adenosyl-methionine decarboxylase (SAMDC; EC 4.1.1.50), to putrescine via the action of spermidine synthase (SPDS; EC 2.5.1.16), produces spermidine, while the addition of a second aminopropyl group to spermidine via the action of spermine synthase (SPMS; EC 2.5.1.22) produces spermine (Alcázar et al. 2006; Slocum, 1991). While the tetraamine found at the highest concentration in most flowering plants is spermine, recent studies have shown that in non-flowering plants, thermospermine may be synthesized in preference to spermine. In this reaction, catalyzed by thermospermine synthase (tSPMS; EC 2.5.1.79), the aminopropyl group is added to the opposite end of the spermidine molecule to that used by SPMS. While most of the pool of cellular putrescine is used to synthesize other polyamines, in some plant species putrescine can be used to initiate the synthesis of alkaloids, via the activity of putrescine N-methyltransferase, or to generate H_2O_2 in a reaction catalyzed by diamine oxidase (DAO; EC 1.4.3.22), a copper-containing enzyme (Figure 1). This reaction plays an important role in plant pathogen interactions (Martin-Tanguy, 2001). In addition to DAO, the flavin-containing polyamine oxidases (PAOs) found in plants can also generate H_2O_2. Unlike DAOs, which display a high affinity for putrescine, PAOs oxidize the secondary amine groups of spermidine and spermine (Medda et al., 1995). Both DAO and PAO are cell wall-associated enzymes (Slocum, 1991).

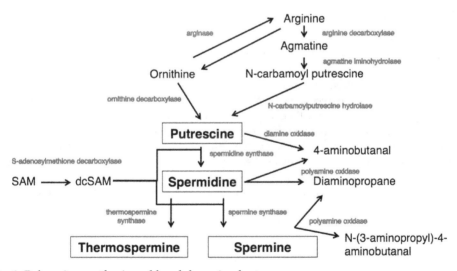

Fig. 1. Polyamine synthesis and breakdown in plants

2.2 Polyamine conjugation

While the bulk of cellular polyamines found in plants usually exist as free forms, polyamines can also be conjugated to small molecules like phenolic acids and various macromolecules such as DNA, RNA and proteins. Conjugation to phenolic acids is common in plants with polyamines often covalently bonded to phenolic acids, such as hydroxycinnamic acids by the formation of an amide linkage (Martin-Tanguy, 2001). The formation of this linkage is catalyzed by a group of enzymes known as transferases and uses activated carboxyl groups provided by esters of coenzyme A (CoA) (Negrel, 1989). Conjugates occur as basic or as neutral forms (Martin-Tanguy, 1985); with the former, a single amine group of an aliphatic amine is linked to cinnamic acid with the resulting conjugate being basic, while if each terminal amine group is bound to a cinnamic acid, a neutral conjugate is formed (Martin-Tanguy, 1985). Polyamines conjugated to hydroxycinnamic acids are also referred to as hydroxycinnamic acid amides (HCAAs). HCAAs are found in many families of higher plants (Martin-Tanguy, 1985). The most common hydroxycinnamoyl substituants of spermidine include the coumaroyl, caffeoyl, feruloyl, hydroxyferuloyl, and sinapoyl acyl groups (Bienz et al., 2005). Mono-, di-, and trisubstituted hydroxycinnamoyl spermidine conjugates have also been reported (Bienz et al., 2005). Other HCAAs found in crop plants include diferuloylputrescine, diferuloylspermidine, and feruloyltyramine in *Oryza sativa* (rice) (Bonneau et al., 1994), hydroxycinnamoyl agmatine in *Hordeum vulgare* (barley) (Smith & Best, 1978), and 4-coumaroyltryptamine and feruloyltryptamine in *Zea mays* (maize) (Collins, 1989). Polyamines can also be post-translationally linked to proteins via covalent bonds. These reactions are catalyzed by transglutaminases (TGases; EC 2.3.2.13), a group of enzymes able to modify proteins post-translationally (Lorand & Graham, 2003). TGases are found in both intra- and extra-cellular locations in plants (Folk, 1980) and can modify protein substrates by "cationisation" or by forming inter- or intra-molecular bridges, using polyamines of different lengths (Serafini-Fracassini et al., 2009).

2.3 The functions of polyamines in plants

Polyamines appear to have numerous physiological functions in plants. They are associated with plant growth and development, playing roles in embryogenesis, root and shoot formation, floral initiation and fruit development (Evans & Malmberg, 1989; Galston & Kaur-Sawhney, 1990). In recent years there has been an increasing interest in the roles polyamines play as molecules that help to protect plants against environmental stresses. Research has clearly demonstrated that cellular polyamines show significant fluctuations in both composition and concentrations in response to environmental conditions (Bouchereau et al., 1999; Smith et al., 2001; Groppa & Benavides; 2008, Burritt, 2008). While it is clear that polyamines play an important role in protecting plant cells from adverse environmental conditions, their precise mode of action remains largely a matter of speculation. However, stress-driven fluctuations in polyamine metabolism could significantly influence the concentrations of bioavailable polyamines in plant-based foods.

3. Polyamines as cytoprotective molecules

3.1 Polyamines as antioxidants

Reactive oxygen species (ROS) are produced within cells as a consequence of normal metabolic processes. When cells are under stress, the production of ROS often increases (Halliwell & Gutteridge, 1999). When ROS are produced at high enough concentrations to overcome the antioxidant defences that normally keep an organism's ROS concentrations in check, oxidation of DNA, proteins and membrane fatty acids occurs, the latter resulting in lipid peroxidation and a loss of membrane function (Halliwell & Gutteridge, 1999). Such damage is commonly referred to as oxidative stress and is considered a very sensitive biomarker of many important environmental stressors (Lesser, 2006; Burritt & MacKenzie 2003; Burritt, 2008). Numerous studies have shown that cells with reduced concentrations of polyamines are more sensitive to oxidative damage (Chattopadhyay et al., 2002; Rider et al., 2007; Burritt, 2008), which suggests that polyamines may play a role in protecting the cells of a wide range of organisms from oxidative damage caused by elevated ROS concentrations. Hence one of the potential modes of action by which polyamines could protect cells is to act as antioxidants. While several studies have tested the ability of polyamines to act as antioxidants, whether they can be classified as cellular antioxidants is still a matter of debate (Chattopadhayay et al., 2002; Kakkar & Sawhney, 2002; Groppa & Benavides, 2008). Bors et al. (1989) proposed that polyamines could act as antioxidants as their anion- and cation-binding properties involve radical scavenging and they have been shown to inhibit both lipid peroxidation and metal-catalyzed induction of oxidative stress (Kitada et al., 1979; Tadolini, 1988). However, other studies have shown that polyamines lack antioxidant activity and could even act as pro-oxidants (Groppa & Benavides, 2008).

3.2 Polyamines and DNA protection

Several studies have shown that both natural and synthetic polyamines can enhance the stability of DNA, and protect DNA from damage caused by oxidative stress and ionizing radiation, and from endonuclease digestion (Nayvelt et al., 2010). Two protective mechanisms have been proposed by which polyamines could protect DNA. It has been suggested that polyamines can directly scavenge ROS, in particular hydroxyl radicals that readily target DNA, and/or promote DNA packaging into nanoparticles (Nayvelt et al., 2010). Because of their positive charge, polyamines can interact electrostatically with DNA that has a negative charge, and spectroscopic evidence has shown that polyamine analogues can bind to guanine bases and the backbone phosphate groups of DNA, while spermidine and spermine bind to both the major and minor grooves of DNA, as well as to the phosphate groups. When 89-90% of the charges associated with DNA have been neutralised by the binding of polyamines, DNA compaction is induced, limiting the accessibility of hydroxyl radicals to target sites within the DNA and hence protecting against oxidative damage (Vijayanathan et al., 2002).

4. Polyamines and human health

4.1 Polyamines and healthy ageing

As in plants, polyamines (putrescine, spermidine and spermine) are also ubiquitous amongst mammalian cells, including human cells. Their diversity of roles in cellular metabolism and growth requires them to be available in large amounts in rapidly growing tissues (Bardócz et al., 1993), but they are also active in the control of various biological processes, such as mediating the action of hormones and growth factors (Bardócz et al., 1995), modifying the immune response, blocking calcium ion channels and regulating apoptosis (Larqué et al., 2007). Polyamines are, therefore, essential to maintaining health at all life stages. It was originally thought that polyamines were synthesised *in situ* within cells when they were required (Bardócz et al., 1996). However, it is now recognised that there are three sources of polyamines in humans: intracellular *de novo* synthesis of polyamines, dietary polyamines, and polyamines produced as metabolites from gut microbiota. As humans age, the capacity for *in situ* polyamine biosynthesis reduces, because the activity of one of the key polyamine biosynthetic enzymes, ODC, decreases (Larqué et al., 2007; Das & Kanungo, 1982). Therefore, the importance of dietary polyamines may become elevated with age. Unfortunately, there are a limited number of studies examining the importance of polyamines in human health and ageing, and therefore the influence of polyamines on health is mostly extrapolated from *in vitro* and small animal studies.

As a result of unprecedented public health advances and successes in many parts of the world, the proportion of people aged 60 and over is growing faster than any other age group (Henry, 2002). Ageing is a multi-faceted process, and is the result of the combination of genetic and environmental factors, but a healthy diet and lifestyle are key components to healthy ageing. Undernutrition is most prevalent in developing countries, but it is also present in some elderly people of developed countries (Calder & Kew, 2002). The benefits of good nutrition can only be realised if the integrity and function of the gastrointestinal tract is maintained with age, making gut health an important health target in the elderly. Nutritional status is an important factor for maintaining optimal immune function, and one process that is central to ageing is immunosenescence. Age-associated changes affecting the immune system contribute to increased morbidity and mortality in the elderly as a result of higher incidence of infections, and possibly autoimmune diseases and cancer (Kalula & Ross, 2008; Pawelec, 1999). Immunosenescence not only results in an increase in infections, but is considered a contributor to systemic low-level inflammation (Fulop et al., 2010), termed 'inflammageing', an underlying cause of many common chronic diseases and frailty in elderly. It appears, therefore, that nutrition is a key aspect in achieving healthy ageing, and given the function of polyamines outlined above, it is reasonable to assume that polyamines play a part in maintaining health as people age.

4.2 Polyamines derived from dietary sources

In 1995, Bardócz and colleagues estimated that the average total polyamine daily intake by an adult in Britain was 388 µmol, represented by 220 µmol of putrescine, 99 µmol of spermidine and 69 µmol of spermine (Bardócz et al., 1995). However, until recently there were a limited number of reports detailing the polyamine content of food, but with the increased availability of high-through put analysis techniques, specifically high performance liquid chromatography, information on the polyamine content in food is accumulating. As detailed in section 1, polyamines exist in free, conjugated and bound forms, but unfortunately reports examining the polyamine content in foods do not tend to examine the form in which polyamines are present within the foods. What also is not clear at this stage is whether the form of polyamine present in foodstuffs influences the bioavailability and/or bioactivity of diet-derived polyamines.

A wide variation in the concentration of polyamines in different foods is reported. Meat, fish and meat products tend to be high in putrescine and spermine, and low in spermidine, which is in contrast to plant-derived foods, which tend to be high in putrescine and spermidine (Kalač & Krausová, 2005). Fermentation of food enhances the polyamine content of some products. For example, the putrescine content of cooked cabbage was reported to be 5.6 mg kg[-1] (Eliassen et al., 2002, as cited by Kalač & Krausová, 2005), and that of sauerkraut was 146 mg kg[-1] (Kalač et al., 1999, as cited by Kalač & Krausová, 2005). The polyamine content in cheese is reportedly high, particularly in mature cheddar, but is relatively low in yoghurt (Eliassen et al., 2002). Interestingly, cooking appears to have little effect on the composition and concentration of polyamines in most foods tested (e.g. carrot and potato), but does influence content in others (Eliassen et al., 2002). For example, mean putrescine content decreases slightly in broccoli after cooking, but spermidine decreases quite considerably (Eliassen et al., 2002). A decrease in polyamine content tends to occur as fruits and vegetables ripen (Valero, 2010; La Vizzari et al., 2007; Simon-Sarkadi et al., 1994, as cited by Kalač & Krausová, 2005), indicating that ripeness and length of time from harvesting to consumption may also influence the polyamine content of plant-derived foods.

An early study reporting the polyamine content of specific foods reported that green vegetables were high in spermidine, whereas other vegetables, fruits and fish were high in putrescine, and red meat and poultry were high in spermine (Bardócz et al., 1995). More detailed studies of the polyamine content of food have since been completed, and have revealed that corn, peas and potatoes are particularly rich vegetable sources of putrescine and spermidine; peas are also rich in spermine compared with the other foods of plant origin tested (with the exception of cashews); oranges are the richest fruit source of polyamines, particularly putrescine; and pears are a relatively rich source of putrescine and spermidine (Farriol et al., 2004, as cited in Larqué et al., 2007). In a recent study, Binh et al. (2010a) reported the polyamine content of Asian foods. The highest putrescine concentrations were found in maize, citrus fruits, peas, soybeans, and other beans; soybeans, other beans, and vegetables were the richest sources of spermidine; and edible offal, molluscs, meats, soybeans and other beans were rich sources of spermine (Binh et al., 2010a). Furthermore, an examination of the polyamine content of 227 foods, with a focus on Japanese foods, was reported by Nishimura et al. (2006). High polyamine plant-based foods included rice bran, wheat germ, green pepper, Japanese pumpkin, soybean, fermented soybeans (natto), pistachio nut, shimeji and dried agaricus (mushrooms), nukazuke (fermented cucumber), orange, Philippine mango, and green leaf tea.

Metabolites from intestinal microbiota are also considered an important source of polyamines (Bardócz et al., 1996). For example, *Bacteroides* spp. and *Fusobacterium* spp. produce polyamines when cultured *in vitro* in the absence of polyamines (Noack et al., 1998), and the administration of probiotics, e.g. *Bifidobacterium lactis* LKM512, has been shown to enhance faecal polyamine concentration (Matsumoto & Benno, 2004). The fibre and polyphenol compounds within plant foods are also capable of modulating growth and proliferation of gut microflora species (Parkar et al., 2008; Noack et al., 2000; Noack et al., 1998). Furthermore, purified fibre derived from plant material (pectin) stimulated proliferation of microflora species that promote polyamine production, thereby enhancing polyamine in the caecal contents (Noack et al., 2000). Interestingly, there was a decline of polyamines from caecum to faeces in all treatments and controls, suggesting that the polyamines synthesized by intestinal microbes are absorbed in the caecum and colon. Whether different plant foods or plant-derived ingredients stimulate the proliferation of different gut microflora, both *in vitro* and *in vivo*, continues to be investigated, and it would also be interesting to examine their effect on polyamine synthesis, to determine the extent to which plant foods might also indirectly contribute to the total body polyamine pool.

The polyamine content of a large range of different foods has recently been reported by Binh et al. (2010a, 2010b) and polyamine intake was correlated with gross domestic product (GDP) and longevity. In a study of 49 European and other Western countries, differences in dietary intake were detected according to GDP (Binh et al., 2010b). The dietary profile of those countries with a higher GDP (>20,000 current international dollars) included higher amounts of animal products, seafood, and fruits, which was associated with increased supply of spermine and putrescine per total calorie intake. The dietary profile of countries with a lower GDP (<20,000 current international dollars) included higher amounts of whole milk, and crops, resulting in slightly higher supply of spermidine compared with the profile of higher GDP countries, although not significantly so. Overall, there was a significantly higher supply of total polyamines in higher GDP countries, and it was suggested that increased polyamine intake may have some role in the difference in the prevalence of diseases associated with socioeconomic disparity (Binh et al. 2010b). Although the daily amount of polyamine availability from foods in Asian countries was considerably lower than that reported in European countries, GDP of Asian countries was also positively correlated with polyamine content per energy (Binh et al. 2010a). Furthermore, increased life expectancy was also associated with greater polyamine content per energy in Asian countries. However, it was recognised that there may be other confounding factors contributing to increased life expectancy.

Importantly, there is good evidence that dietary polyamines contribute directly to the total body polyamine pool. An early classical experiment using a rat model demonstrated that radio-labelled putrescine, spermidine, and spermine were taken up by the small intestine in a dose-dependent manner (Bardócz et al., 1995). However, the uptake and fate of the polyamines varied. One hour after the rats were given ^{14}C-labelled putrescine by intubation, only 29-39% of the label was recovered as polyamines, of which 11-15% was present as putrescine. In contrast, 79% and 72-74% of labelled spermidine and spermine, respectively, were recovered in the same form as given, and, if conversion to other polyamines was also included in the calculations, up to 96% and 82% of the radio-labelled spermidine and spermine were recovered, respectively. Bardócz et al. (1995) suggested therefore, that diet could provide polyamines for absorption and contribution to the total polyamine pool through the systemic circulation, thereby reaching every tissue of the body. Similarly, putrescine uptake and metabolism from the small intestinal lumen of healthy volunteers was demonstrated following perfusion with increasing concentrations of putrescine (Milovic et al., 1997, as cited in Milovic, 2001). Some 60-80% of the putrescine disappeared from the lumen linearly with time, although putrescine *per se* was not recovered in the blood. There was, however, a transitory increase in acetylated putrescine, and a steady increase in spermidine and spermine concentrations, suggesting the polyamines were absorbed from the intestinal lumen in humans and putrescine underwent extensive metabolism before reaching the systemic circulation (Milovic, 2001), although spermidine and spermine uptake was not examined in this study.

Long-term supplementation of diets with polyamines or polyamine rich foods has been shown to increase polyamine concentrations in the blood in animal models and humans. For example, mice fed experimental chow containing high concentrations of polyamines for 26 weeks had significantly higher concentrations of blood spermine and spermidine than mice fed chow containing low or normal concentrations of polyamines (Soda et al., 2009a). Soda et al. (2009a) noted that there was considerable blood spermine and spermidine variability between mice, which was exaggerated in mice fed the high polyamine diet. These findings are supported with human data. Healthy human male volunteers were asked to either exclude soybean products and fermented foods from their diet, or include 50-100 g of natto, a fermented soybean product, in their diet for 2 months (Soda et al., 2009b). Following long-term daily consumption of natto, blood spermine concentrations significantly increased, but concentrations remained unchanged in those from the control (no natto) group. The blood spermidine concentrations did not change for either group. Interestingly, although not statistically significant (p=0.06), age had a positive correlation (r=0.62) with changes in blood spermine concentration. The findings from this study demonstrate that long-term intake of a polyamine-rich diet can increase blood polyamine concentrations, and the effect of dietary polyamines might be greater in older people.

4.3 Effect of age on polyamine concentrations

Polyamines are present in all tissues, although their concentration and the ratio between polyamines vary between different tissues. For example, in rats aged 3 months the highest concentration of spermidine was detected in the thymus, and large amounts were also detected in the liver, spleen, lungs and different parts of the gastro-intestinal tract (Jänne et al., 1964). These tissues, as well as the kidneys, also contained relatively large amounts of spermine. In a more recent study, similar trends were reported for the polyamine content of mice, although the pancreas was found to contain the highest concentration of spermidine, and in this study the concentration of putrescine was also considered (Nishimura et al., 2006). The putrescine concentration of a range of tissues was typically low, below approximately 2 nmol/mg protein in all tissues of mice aged 3 weeks, compared with spermidine and spermine, which ranged from approximately 1.0 nmol/mg protein in muscle, heart and skin tissues, up to approximately 25 nmol of spermidine/mg protein in the pancreas and 5 nmol of spermine/mg protein in the thymus (Nishimura et al., 2006). These data tend to support the suggestion that putrescine undergoes extensive metabolism upon uptake, although the content of the relative polyamines in the mouse chow was not described.

The effect of age on polyamine concentrations in tissues was also examined by Jänne et al. (1964) and Nishimura et al. (2006). Overall, the concentration of polyamines (spermidine and spermine) decreased with increasing age (0-9 months) in all tissues examined from rats (Jänne et al., 1964). However, the decrease in spermidine was most marked during the first month of life, decreasing relatively slowly after one month, and the concentrations of spermine increased slightly during the first month in the liver, thymus, spleen and kidneys, and remained unchanged or decreased slightly after one month, and from birth in other tissues. Similar trends were observed in ageing mice (3 to 26 weeks), with a significant decrease of spermidine in the thymus, spleen, ovary, liver, stomach, lung, kidney, heart and muscle, as well as skin from the ear and abdomen (Nishimura et al., 2006). In contrast, however, the polyamine concentrations in the pancreas, brain and uterus were maintained in the ageing mice. It was suggested that stimulation of protein synthesis and modulation of the ion channels are the most important functions of polyamines, and these functions are necessary activities in these organs/tissues, therefore mechanisms exist in these tissues to maintain polyamine concentrations through ageing (Nishimura et al., 2006). Furthermore, Nishimura et al. (2006) recommended that since the decrease in spermidine was most marked, either foods containing putrescine, spermidine and spermine or foods particularly rich in spermidine should be consumed. As indicated above, green vegetables, corn, peas, beans and potatoes are particularly rich sources of spermidine, possibly suggesting that a predominantly plant-based diet would provide the polyamines of most benefit as humans' age.

4.4 Role of dietary polyamines in maintaining health during ageing

There is a consensus among the literature that polyamine concentrations within the body decrease with age, although this may be tissue specific. The effect that this has on health is still being understood; however, enhancing polyamine intake appears to have a positive effect on health as ageing progresses. For example, in a study where mice were fed a low, normal or high polyamine diet from 8 weeks of age, whole blood spermidine concentrations were significantly higher after 26 weeks of feeding with the high polyamine experimental chow, and mice fed the high polyamine chow lived significantly longer than mice fed the low or normal polyamine chow (Soda et al., 2009a). Furthermore, pathological changes associated with ageing were inhibited in mice consuming the high polyamine chow, specifically lower incidence of glomerulosclerosis and higher protein expression of SMP-30, a protein expressed in multiple organs and tissues that protects from oxidative stress during ageing.

The dietary intake of polyamines has been cautioned in the past because the increased requirement for polyamines by rapidly dividing cells and tissues, such as tumour cells, is well recognised. Interfering with the supply of polyamines with ODC inhibitors, polyamine structural analogues and derivatives, and deprivation of exogenous polyamines, are potential therapeutic targets for tumour growth (Kalač & Krausová, 2005). However, the study described above (Soda et al., 2009a) suggests that in the absence of a tumour, a high polyamine diet is beneficial to maintaining health through ageing. Further support for this is afforded with the use of transgenic mouse models. For example, a transgenic mouse line over-expressing human ODC gene was used to examine whether constitutively over-expressed ODC pre-disposes the animals to enhanced tumorigenesis (Alhonen et al., 1995). At 2 years of age, the tissue ODC activity in the transgenic animals was 20- to 50-fold that in their syngenic littermates, but the occurrences of spontaneous tumours between the two groups of animals was comparable.

Notwithstanding the requirement for polyamines in tumorigenic tissue, evidence suggests that enhanced endogenous polyamine concentrations promote health during ageing via a number of mechanisms. A recent study by Eisenberg et al. (2009) examined the influence of spermidine on a number of ageing models, and demonstrated extended lifespan with exogenous application of spermidine. Using a yeast cell model of chronologically ageing cells, exogenous supply of spermidine increased lifespan by up to four times that of untreated cells, and using a yeast model of replicative ageing (representing the lifespan of dividing cells in higher eukaryotes), spermidine caused a significant increase in the replicative lifespan of old cells. Furthermore, spermidine-treated cells were resistant to stress from heat shock or hydrogen peroxide treatment, which supports the theory that improved longevity often correlates with increased stress resistance (Eisenberg et al., 2009). Enhancement of lifespan in human cells was then demonstrated, using long-term culture of peripheral blood mononuclear cells (PBMCs), treated with or without exogenous spermidine in the culture medium, and measuring cell survival by flow cytometry. After 12 days, only 15% of the control cells had survived, whereas 50% of spermidine (20 nM)-treated cells survived (Eisenberg, et al. 2009). Staining indicated that enhanced cell survival by spermidine was not as a result of inhibition of apoptosis, but rather an inhibition of necrosis.

As discussed by Eisenberg et al. (2009), necrosis culminates in the leakage of intracellular compounds resulting in local inflammation, a suspected cause of 'inflammageing'. Following on from this, the effect of exogenous spermidine on oxidative stress was examined, given that, in the free radical theory, ageing is attributed to the accumulation of oxidative stress. Indeed, mice fed spermidine (3 mM added to drinking water) for 200 days had an increase in free thiol groups compared with control mice, suggesting a lower degree of oxidative stress and protein damage (Eisenberg et al., 2009). Furthermore, autophagy, the major lysosomal degradation pathway for recycling damaged and potentially harmful cellular material, is thought to be essential for healthy ageing and longevity and Eisenberg et al. (2009) also examined the involvement of spermidine in autophagy. Spermidine enhanced autophagy, as determined both directly and indirectly, in a number of cell types including cultured human cells, and it was suggested that spermidine-induced autophagy increased lifespan in the variety of model organisms used. Given that polyamines appear to increase lifespan, their involvement in preventing or delaying the onset of the major underlying pathologies that contribute to ageing is also worthy of consideration.

4.4.1 Gut health

Whilst the growth of many organs ceases with adolescence, the integrity of the mucosa of the gastrointestinal (GI) tract is maintained by continuous cell renewal (Majumdar, 2003). Deviation in these replicative processes may result in the loss of structural and functional integrity of the gut; therefore maintenance of normal growth and general properties of the adult GI tract is a key aspect to healthy ageing. Polyamines have been implicated in the maintenance of gut integrity. The strongest evidence of the involvement of polyamines in the development, maturation and maintenance of gut integrity comes from studies using young animals. For example, suckling rats were either fed a polyamine-deficient diet, a polyamine-deficient diet plus antibiotics, a polyamine-deficient diet plus polyamine supplementation at normal concentrations, or normal standard laboratory chow for six months (Löser et al., 1999). Although after six months there were no differences in body weight gain, food consumption or general behaviour, consumption of a polyamine-deficient diet with or without antibiotics resulted in significant decreases in organ weight, protein content, and DNA content in the small intestinal and colonic mucosa. Interestingly, there was no significant difference in the intracellular polyamine metabolism between any of the treatment groups, indicating that intracellular *de novo* synthesis of polyamines was not activated to compensate for a deficiency in exogenous polyamines (Löser et al., 1999). Conversely, oral administration of polyamines to neonatal mice resulted in precocious maturation of the gut, as evidenced by increased villus and crypt length, changes of the activities of brush-border membrane hydrolases (Dorhout et al., 1997, as cited by Seiler and Raul, 2007), as well as precocious development of the intestinal immune system after spermine administration (ter Steege et al., 1997, as cited by Seiler and Raul, 2007). Importantly, the action of polyamines in gut development has been demonstrated using a human model, albeit *in vitro*. Caco-2 cells, derived from a colorectal adenocarcinoma, are commonly used for studies of the gastric mucosa, because they spontaneously express characteristics of enterocyte differentiation upon confluence, including the formation of tight junctions. Depletion of the putrescine and spermidine pools with the specific inhibitor α-difluoromethylornithine (DFMO), prevented the growth of microvilli and differentiation of Caco-2 cells (Herold et al., 1993, and Duranton et al., 1998, as cited by Seiler and Raul, 2007). Whilst polyamines are clearly required for gut development and maturation in the young, these studies also suggest implications of polyamines for gut integrity with ageing, because the continual renewal process in the gut is characterized by active proliferation of stem cells localized near the base of the crypts, progression of these cells up the crypt-villus axis with cessation of proliferation and subsequent differentiation and apoptosis (Zou et al., 2008).

Maintenance of gut integrity, such as through formation of tight junctions and production of mucus, is essential to good health because this helps to prevent a leaky gut, limiting the incidence of infection from pathogenic bacteria and food intolerance. An insult to the intestinal mucosa is repaired via two mechanisms: restitution and replacement. Restitution is a rapid process whereby existing viable cells from adjacent areas migrate to the lesion and cover denuded spots, and is therefore suitable for superficial mucosal damage (Seiler and Raul, 2007). Replacement of damaged cells occurs via cell division, and is a slower process than restitution. As reviewed by Seiler and Raul (2007), polyamines are involved in many aspects of these processes, including the production of cytoskeletal components, cell adhesion factors, and crypt reproduction. In addition to these functions, a novel function of polyamines within the gut was postulated by Bardócz et al. (1998). Radiolabelled putrescine was administered to fasted rats and 70% of the putrescine was converted to succinate, more than double the rate of rats fed *ad libitum*. Bardócz et al. (1998) suggested, therefore, that dietary polyamines may serve as a source of instantly metabolisable energy and further support the metabolic needs of the gut tissue.

The involvement of polyamines in the maintenance of gut integrity would suggest that polyamines are essential for the process of healthy ageing, as opposed to pathological ageing. Evidence that this is the case in humans is limited, given the difficulty in obtaining suitable tissue samples. Nevertheless, faecal polyamine concentrations provide supporting evidence of higher polyamine concentrations within the gut in young and healthy adults compared with the elderly. For example, the concentration of spermidine in the faeces of the elderly was found to be significantly less than that in healthy young adults, and this was linked with changes to gut microbiota (Mäkivuokko et al., 2010). Further evidence suggests that hospitalised elderly subjects have significantly lower intestinal polyamine concentrations than healthy adults, and polyamine concentration was significantly influenced by the faecal microflora pattern present between the two groups (Matsumoto & Benno, 2007). It is possible that the difference in faecal microflora is indicative of different dietary habits, or the difference in faecal microflora results in variation between other microflora metabolites with health benefits, such as short chain fatty acids, but it is also possible that differences in polyamine uptake from diet and microflora directly influence health status through ageing. An interesting aspect that has not yet been examined, to our knowledge, is whether synergistic interactions between microflora metabolites, namely polyamines and short chain fatty acids, promote gut integrity and/or immune function (as detailed below).

4.4.2 Immune function and inflammation

The decrease in polyamine concentrations with age has clearly been demonstrated in numerous tissues and blood. Given that the majority of circulating polyamines are contained in the erythrocytes and leukocytes (Cohen et al., 1976), and polyamines play a pivotal role in numerous cellular functions, it is natural to consider whether decreasing polyamine concentrations with ageing plays a role in immunosenescence and 'inflammaging'.

With age, increased expression of several adhesion molecules occurs, playing a crucial role in cell adhesion and mediating cell-cell interactions, resulting in augmented capability of cell adhesion and activation of immune cells, thereby mediating inflammation (Soda et al., 2005). Lymphocyte function-associated antigen-1 (LFA-1) is an adhesion molecule, and modulating its function can control cellular immunity and inflammation. Soda et al. (2005) demonstrated that exogenous application of spermine to cultured PBMCs suppressed LFA-1 expression, which was accompanied with a decrease in adhesion capacity of PBMCs to human umbilical vein endothelial cells. Similar, but weaker effects were also observed with the application of spermidine. These results suggest that elevated polyamine concentrations, in this case spermidine and spermine only, inhibit a very early and important event that is involved in invoking inflammation.

Further support for the positive effects that polyamines have on modulation of inflammation is given through examination of their effects on the production of inflammatory cytokines. For example, exogenously supplied spermine inhibited the synthesis of a number of pro-inflammatory cytokines from PBMCs stimulated with lipopolysaccharide, including tumour necrosis factor (TNF), interleukin (IL)-1, IL-6, macrophage inflammatory protein (MIP)-1α and MIP-1β (Zhang et al., 1997). Whilst inhibition of MIP-1α and MIP-1β, and IL-6 approached 100%, complete inhibition of TNF and IL-1β by spermine was not achieved. Coupled with an earlier report that administration of spermine failed to inhibit the production of transforming growth factor β, a potent anti-inflammatory cytokine (Tsunawaki et al., 1988), and the fact that TNF and IL-1β are involved in important antimicrobial and antiviral immune responses, spermine appears implicated in maintaining an appropriate inflammatory status. Importantly, these findings translate into a dampening down of the inflammatory response *in vivo*. For example, co-administration of spermine with carrageenan protected mice against the development of acute inflammation of the foot pad, using the carrageenan-induced paw edema model (Zhang et al., 1997). A mouse model for inflammation-mediated intestinal damage also showed that spermine exerted a protective effect, inhibiting the expression of inducible nitric oxide synthase and nitrotyrosine, and decreasing serum concentrations of pro-inflammatory mediators, including nitrate, nitrite and interferon-γ, whilst enhancing the concentration of IL-10, an anti-inflammatory cytokine (ter Steege et al., 1999). Taken together, these findings suggest that although endogenous polyamine production decreases with age, enhancement of exogenous sources of polyamines might be useful in mitigating the loss of gut function and integrity, and regulation of inflammatory processes that occurs with ageing. The specific effects that exogenous sources of polyamines have on human health with ageing still largely remains to be investigated, but through understanding the effect of polyamines on processes of immune function and chronic inflammation, and the effect this has on non-communicable diseases that become more prevalent with ageing, the roles of polyamines in these diseases may be suggested. For example, Soda (2010) suggested that by considering the inhibition of cell adhesion through suppression of LFA-1 by dietary polyamines, and increased availability of arginine for nitric oxide synthesis (which is important for vascular physiology and function) in the presence of dietary polyamines, polyamines may inhibit cardiovascular disease.

4.4.3 Other potential health benefits of polyamines

The causes of pathological ageing and frailty are complex and multidimensional, based on the interplay of genetics, biological, physical, psychological, social and environmental factors (Fulop et al., 2010). Given the ubiquity of polyamines within the body, and their centrality in maintaining normal cell function, it might be expected that polyamines are integral to many processes in ageing. The use of transgenic animals has given some insight into what these might be (Alhonen et al., 2009).

Social factors play an important part in maintaining good health and physical functionality with age. Central to social interaction is the ability to communicate, and age-related hearing loss may prevent or reduce social interaction. Clinical studies have shown that DFMO, a specific inhibitor of putrescine synthesis, can cause hearing loss in some patients (Meyskins & Gerner, 1999). A transgenic mouse model has been developed that is completely deficient in spermine synthase, has reduced concentrations of spermine and increased spermidine in all cells examined, and is profoundly hearing impaired (Wang et al., 2009). The hearing loss was attributed to a large reduction in endocochlear potential, and it was reversed by breeding the deficient strain with a strain that ubiquitously expresses spermine synthase. The application of DFMO in the mice deficient in spermine synthase resulted in profound weight loss and death within a few days, from a severe loss of balance that prevented normal feeding and drinking (Wang et al., 2009). It was suggested that polyamines are important in auditory physiology because of their role as regulators of potassium channels, thereby influencing endocochlear potential. Although the importance of polyamines in maintaining hearing and balance has been highlighted, what is not clear is whether it is the absence of spermine or an altered spermidine:spermine ratio that causes the hearing loss. Given this study, it is possible that a greater body pool of polyamines could help to prevent hearing loss with ageing, although this study considered the effect of endogenous polyamine production and it is not known whether uptake of dietary polyamines would influence hearing. Furthermore, oxidative damage has also been implicated in age-related hearing loss (Someya & Prolla, 2010), which provides another potential mechanism by which polyamines may assist in the prevention of hearing loss. It should be noted that the involvement of polyamines in age-related hearing loss is, at this stage, largely speculative, and considering the difficulty in determining polyamine concentrations within the ear, at least in humans, it is not an issue that will be quickly resolved. Epidemiological studies correlating dietary habits and intake with the onset of age-related hearing loss may give some insights into the impact of diet on hearing loss.

Considering that the pancreas contains the highest concentration of spermidine (Nishimura et al., 2006), it might be expected that spermidine, or polyamines in general, play an important role in maintaining the function of the pancreas. A transgenic rat model has been used to demonstrate that a depletion of pancreatic spermidine and spermine, through over-expression of the catabolic polyamine enzyme spermidine/spermine N^1-acetyltransferase (SSAT), leads to onset of acute pancreatitis (Alhonen et al., 2000), and this could be prevented with the application of 1-methylspermidine, a metabolically stable analogue of spermidine (Räsänen et al., 2002). It should be kept in mind that Nishimura et al. (2009) demonstrated a steady-state of polyamines were present in the pancreas even with ageing, but given that the total body pool of polyamines generally decreases with age, diet-derived polyamines could still be an important source to maintain pancreatic polyamine concentrations. Liver injury as a result of xenobiotic insult causes cell death, and requires quiescent hepatocytes to proliferate and restore liver mass and hepatic function, but the capacity to achieve this diminishes with age (Sanz et al., 1999). The main age-related changes in the process of recovery from liver injury are a delayed response in the development of cell killing and regeneration, and decreased regenerative ability (Sanz et al., 1999). Using the transgenic rat model over-expressing SSAT, it was shown that a profound decrease in hepatic spermidine and spermine pools caused a failure to initiate liver regeneration (Räsänen et al., 2002). Furthermore, supplementation with 1-methylspermidine restored early liver regeneration. These results might suggest that, despite the capacity for endogenous polyamine production reducing with age, a diet high in polyamines, particularly spermidine, could support a higher total body polyamine pool and promote liver regeneration and function into old age.

5. Conclusions

Because of their ubiquity in human tissue and involvement in a wide range of vital cellular processes, the importance of polyamines to maintenance of human health is well recognised. Despite this, however, the specific mechanisms by which polyamines influence human health, particularly with increasing age, are less well understood. It is likely that the implication of polyamines in the growth of tumours has meant that research into the health benefits of polyamines has been largely overlooked. The evidence provided within this chapter indicates that polyamines are important molecules for maintaining good health into old age, and the total body polyamine pool may be influenced by diet. Polyamines are also ubiquitous in plant tissues, and they have similarly important functions in plants and animals, particularly as cytoprotective molecules. The production of polyamines in plants can be manipulated through cultivation practices and environmental stressors, and the polyamine content of plant-derived foods may also be influenced by postharvest practices and conditions. Plant-derived foods tend to be a rich source of putrescine and spermidine; however, research is lacking an examination of the form in which polyamines are present in plant-derived foods (free, conjugated or bound) and whether this influences the bioavailability and bioactivity of polyamines in humans. Nevertheless, plant-derived foods represent an important source of dietary polyamines. The evidence presented here, that maintaining endogenous polyamine concentrations with increasing age and in the absence of tumour tissue has a positive influence on sustaining good health, has largely been derived from the use of animal models. This is because demonstrating unequivocal cause and effect of polyamines in health or disease prevention requires determination of polyamine content within the tissues under consideration, and human tissue samples are usually not readily available. An alternative approach to this, as has been taken with other phytonutrients such as polyphenols and carotenoids, is the completion of epidemiological studies that could examine estimates of typical polyamine consumption from diet records, and correlate it with health status and disease prevalence in the elderly. Further strength could be provided by these studies, if blood samples were obtained and blood polyamine concentrations determined. Nevertheless, there is good evidence to suggest that polyamines assist with healthy ageing. However, more research is required before recommendations on optimal and safe polyamine intake can be made.

6. References

Alcázar, R.; Marco, F.; Cuevas, J.C.; Patron, M.; Ferrando, A.; Carrasco, P.; Tiburcio, A.F.; Altabella, T. (2006). Involvement of polyamines in plant response to abiotic stress. *Biotechnology Letters*, Vol.28, 1867-1876.

Alhonen, L.; Halmekytö, M.; Kosma, V.-M.; Wahlfors, J.; Kauppinen, R.; Jänne, J. (1995). Life-long over-expression of ornithine decarboxylase (ODC) gene in transgenic mice does not lead to generally enhanced tumorigenesis or neuronal degradation. *International Journal of Cancer*, Vol.63, 402-404.

Alhonen, L.; Parkkinen, J.J.; Keinänen, T.A.; Sinervirta, R.; Herzig, K.H.; Jänne, J. (2000). Activation of polyamine catabolism in transgenic rats induces acute pancreatitis. *Proceedings of the National Academy of Sciences of the United States of America*, Vol.97, 8290-8295.

Alhonen, L.; Uimari, A.; Pietilä, M.; Hyvönen, M.T.; Pirinen, E.; Keinänen, T.A. (2009). Transgenic animals modelling polyamine metabolism-related diseases. *Essays in Biochemistry*, Vol.46, 125-144.

Bardócz, S.; Dugid, T.G.; Brown, D.S.; Grant, G.; Pusztai, A.; White, A.; Ralph, A. (1995). The importance of dietary polyamines in cell regeneration and growth. *British Journal of Nutrition*, Vol.73, 819-828.

Bardócz, S.; Grant, G.; Brown, S.B.; Pusztai, A. (1998). Putrescine as a source of instant energy in the small intestine of the rat. *Gut*, Vol.42, 24-28.

Bardócz, S.; Grant, G.; Brown, S.B.; Ralph, A.; Pusztai, A. (1993). Polyamines in food – implications for growth and health. *Journal of Nutritional Biochemistry*, Vol.4, 66-71.

Bardócz, S.; White, A.; Grant, G.; Brown, D.S.; Dugid, T.J.; Pusztai, A. (1996). Uptake and bioavailability of dietary polyamines. *Biochemical Society Transactions*, Vol.24, 226S.

Baron, K.; Stasolla, C. (2008). The role of polyamines during in vivo and in vitro development. *In Vitro Cellular & Developmental Biology-plant*, Vol.44, 384-395.

Bienz, S.; Bisegger, P.; Guggisberg, A.; Hesse, M. (2005). Polyamine alkaloids. *Natural Product Reports* Vol.22, 647–658.

Binh, P.N.T.; Soda, K.; Maruyama, C.; Kawakami, M. (2010a). Relationship between food polyamines and gross domestic product in association with longevity in Asian countries. *Health*, Vol.2, 1390-1396.

Binh, P.N.T.; Soda, K.; Kawakami, M. (2010b). Gross domestic product and dietary pattern among 49 western countries with a focus on polyamine intake. *Health*, Vol.2, 1327-1334.

Bonneau, L.; Carre, M.; Martin-Tanguy, J. (1994). Polyamines and related enzymes in rice seeds differing in germination potential. *Plant Growth Regulation*, Vol.15, 75-82.

Borrell, A.; Culianezmacia, F.A.; Altabella, T.; Besford, R.T.; Flores, D.; Tiburcio, A.F. (1995). Arginine decarboxylase is localized in chloroplasts. *Plant Physiology*, Vol.109, 771-776.

Bors, W.; Langebartels, C.; Michel, C.; Sandermann, J.H. (1989). Polyamines as radical scavengers and protectants against ozone damage. *Phytochemistry*, Vol.28, 1589-1595.

Bortolotti, C.; Cordeiro, A.; Alcazar, R.; Borrell, A.; Culianez-Macia, F.A.; Tiburcio, A.F.; Altabella, T. (2004). Localization of arginine decarboxylase in tobacco plants. *Physiologia Plantarum*, Vol.120, 84-92.

Bouchereau, A., Aziz, A., Larher, F., Martin-Tanguy, J. (1999). Polyamines and environmental challenges: recent development. *Plant Science*, Vol.140, 103–125.

Burritt, D.J. (2008). The polycyclic aromatic hydrocarbon phenanthrene causes oxidative stress and alters polyamine metabolism in the aquatic liverwort *Riccia fluitans* L. *Plant Cell & Environment*, Vol.31, 1416–1431.

Burritt, D.J.; MacKenzie, S. (2003). Antioxidant metabolism during the acclimation of *Begonia x erythrophylla* to high-light. *Annals of Botany*, Vol.91, 783-794.

Calder, P.C.; Kew, S. (2002). The immune system: a target for functional foods. *British Journal of Nutrition*, Vol. 88, S165-S176.

Chattopadhayay, M.K.; Tiwari, B.S.; Chattopadhayay, G.; Bose, A.; Sengupta, D.N.; Ghosh, B. (2002). Protective role of exogenous polyamines on salinity-stressed rice (Oryza sativa) plants. *Physiologia Plantarum*, Vol.116, 192–199.

Cohen, L.F.; Lundgren, D.W.; Farrel, P.M. (1976). Distribution of spermidine and spermine in blood from cystic fibrosis and control subjects. *Blood*, Vol.48, 469-475.

Collins, F.W. (1989). Oat phenolics: Avenanthramides, novel substituted N-cinnamoyl-anthranilate alkaloids from oat groats and hulls. *Journal of Agricultural and Food Chemistry*, Vol.37, 60–66.

Das, R.; Kanungo, M.S. (1982). Activity and modulation of ornithine decarboxylase and concentration of polyamines in various tissues of rats as a function of age. *Experimental Gerontology*, Vol.17, 95-103.

Eisenberg, T.; Knauer, H.; Schauer, A.; Büttner, S.; Ruckenstuhl, C.; Carmona-Gutierrez, D.; Ring, J.; Schroeder, S.; Magnes, C.; Antonacci, L.; Fussi, H.; Deszcz, L.; Hartl, R.; Schraml, E.; Criollo, A.; Megalou, E.; Weiskopf, D.; Laun, P.; Heeren, G.; Breitenbach, M.; Grubeck-Loebenstein, B.; Herker, E.; Fahrenkrog, B.; Fröhlich, K.-U.; Sinner, F.; Tavernarakis, N.; Minois, N.; Kroemer, G.; Madeo, F. (2009). Induction of autophagy by spermidine promotes longevity. *Nature Cell Biology*, Vol.11, 1305-1314.

Eliassen, K.A.; Reistad, R.; Risøen, U.; Rønning, H.F. (2002). Dietary polyamines. *Food Chemistry*, Vol.78, 273-280.

Evans, P.T.; Malmberg, R.L. (1989). Do polyamines have roles in plant development? *Annual Review of Plant Physiology and Molecular Biology*, Vol.40, 235–269.

Folk, J.E. (1980). Transglutaminases. *Annual Review of Biochemistry*, Vol.49, 517-531.

Fulop, T.; Larbi, A.; Witkowski, J.M.; McElhaney, J.; Loeb, M.; Mitnitski, A.; Pawelec, G. (2010). Aging, frailty and age-related diseases. *Biogerontology*, Vol.11, 547-563.

Galston, A.W.; Kaur-Sawhney, R.K. (1990). Polyamines in plant physiology. *Plant Physiology*, Vol.94, 406–410.

Groppa M. D.; Benavides M. P. (2008). Polyamines and abiotic stress: Recent advances. *Amino Acids* Vol.34, 35-45.

Halliwell, B.; Gutteridge, J.M.C. (1999). Free Radicals in Medicine and Biology, Edition 3. Oxford: Oxford University Press.

Henry, M. (2002). Healthy ageing is vital for development. World Health Organisation Media Centre, 24/07/2011, available from http://www.who.int/mediacentre/news/releases/release24/en/

Hunter, D.C.; Burritt, D.J. (2005). Light quality influences the polyamine content of lettuce (*Lactuca sativa* L.) cotyledon explants during shoot production *in vitro*. *Plant Growth Regulation*, Vol.45, 53–61.

Igarashi, K.; Kashiwagi, K. (2000). Mysterious modulators of cellular functions. *Biochemical & Biophysical Research Communications*, Vol.271, 559-564.

Jänne, J.; Raina, A.; Siimes, M. (1964). Spermidine and spermine in rat tissues at different ages. *Acta Physiologica Scandinavia*, Vol.62, 352-358.

Kakkar, R.K; Sawhney, V.K. 2002. Polyamine research in plants – a changing perspective. *Physiologia Plantarum*, Vol.116, 281-292.

Kalač, P.; Krausová, P. (2005). A review of dietary polyamines: Formation, implications for growth and health and occurrence in foods. *Food Chemistry*, Vol.90, 219-230.

Kalula, S.Z.; Ross, K. (2008). Immunosenescence – inevitable or preventable? *Current Allergy & Clinical Immunology*, Vol.21, No.3, 126-130.

Kitada, M.; Igarashi, K.; Hirose, S.; Kitagawa, H. (1979). Inhibition by polyamines of lipid peroxide formation in rat liver microsomes. *Biochemical & Biophysical Research Communications*, Vol.87, 388–394.

Kusano, T.; Berberich, T.; Tateda, C.; Takahashi, Y. (2008). Polyamines: essential factors for growth and survival. *Planta*, Vol.228, 367-381.

Larqué, E.; Sabater-Molina, A.; Zamora, S. (2007). Biological significance of dietary polyamines. *Nutrition*, Vol.23, 87-95.

La Vizzari, T.; Veciana-Nogués, M.T.; Weingart, O.; Bover-Cid, S.; Mariné-Font, A.; Vidal-Carou, M.C. (2007). Occurrence of biogenic amines and polyamines in spinach and changes during storage under refrigeration. *Journal of Agricultural and Food Chemistry*, Vol.55, 9514-9519.

Lesser, M.P (2006). Oxidative stress in marine environments: biochemistry and physiological ecology. *Annual Review of Physiology*, Vol.68, 253-278.

Li, Z.L.; Burritt, D.J. (2003). Changes in endogenous polyamines during the formation of somatic embryos from isogenic lines of *Dactylis glomerata* L. with different regenerative capacities. *Plant Growth Regulation*, Vol.40, 65–74.

Lima, G.P.P.; Vianello, F. (2011). Review on the main differences between organic and conventional plant-based foods. *International Journal of Food Science & Technology*, Vol.46, 1-13.

Lorand, L.; Graham, R.M. (2003). Transglutaminases: Crosslinking enzymes with pleiotropic functions. *Nature Reviews Molecular Cell Biology*, Vol.4, 140-156.

Löser, C.; Eisel, A.; Harms, D.; Fölsch, U.R. (1999). Dietary polyamines are essential luminal growth factors for small intestinal and colonic mucosal growth and development. *Gut*, Vol.44, 12-16.

Majumdar, A.P.N. (2003). Regulation of gastrointestinal mucosal growth during aging. Journal of Physiology and Pharmacology, Vol.54, Suppl 4, 143-154.

Mäkivuokko, H.; Tiihonen, K.; Tynkkynen, S.; Paulin, L.; Rautonen, N. (2010). The effect of age and non-steroidal anti-inflammatory drugs on human intestinal microbiota composition. *British Journal of Nutrition*, Vol. 103, 227-234.

Martin-Tanguy, J. (1985). The occurrence and possible function of hydroxycinnamoyl acid amides in plants. *Plant Growth Regulation*, Vol.3, 381–399.

Martin-Tanguy J (2001). Metabolism and function of polyamines in plants: recent development (new approaches). *Plant Growth Regulation*, Vol.34, 135-148.

Matsumoto, M.; Benno, Y. (2004). Anti-inflammatory and antimutagenic activity of polyamines produced by *Bifidobacterium lactis* LKM512. *Current Topics in Nutraceutical Research*, Vol.2, 219-226.

Medda, R.; Padiglia, A.; Floris, G. (1995). Plant Copper-amine Oxidases. *Phytochemistry*, Vol.39, 1-9.

Meyskins, F.L. Jnr; Gerner, E.W. (1999). Development of difluoromethylornithine (DFMO) as a chemoprevention agent. *Clinical Cancer Research*, Vol.5, 945-951.

Milovic, V. (2001). Polyamines in the gut lumen: bioavailability and biodistribution. *European Journal of Gastroenterology & Hepatology*, Vol.13, 1021-1025.

Nayvelt, I.; Hyvonen, M.T.; Alhonen, L.; Pandya, I.; Thomas, T.; Khomutov, A.R.; Vepsalainen, J.; Patel, R.; Keinanen, T.A.; Thomas, T.J. (2010). DNA condensation by chiral alpha-methylated polyamine analogues and protection of cellular DNA from oxidative damage. *Biomacromolecules*, Vol.11, 97-105.

Negrel, J. (1989). The biosynthesis of cinnamoylputrescines in callus tissue cultures of *Nicotiana tabacum*. *Phytochemistry*, Vol.28, 477–481.

Nishimura, K.; Kashiwagi, S.K.; Igarashi, K. (2006). Decrease in polyamines with aging and their ingestion from food and drink. *Journal of Biochemistry*, Vol.139, 81-90.

Noack, J.; Dongowski, G.; Hartmann, L.; Blaut, M. (2000). The human gut bacteria *Bacteroides thetaiotaomicron* and *Fusobacterium varium* produce putrescine and spermidine in cecum of pectin-fed gnotobiotic rats. Journal of Nutrition 130, 1225-1231.

Noack, J.; Kleessen, B.; Proll, J.; Dongowski, G.; Blaut, M. (1998). Dietary guar gum and pectin stimulate intestinal microbial polyamine synthesis in rats. *Journal of Nutrition*, Vol.128, 1385-1391.

Parkar, S.G.; Stevenson, D.E., Skinner, M.A. (2008). The potential influence of fruit polyphenols on colonic microflora and human gut health. *International Journal of Food Microbiology*, Vol,124, 295-298.

Pawelec, G. (1999). Immunosenescence: impact in the young as well as the old? *Mechanisms of Ageing and Development*, Vol.108, 1-7.

Räsänen, T.L.; Alhonen, L.; Sinervirta, R.; Keinänen, T.; Herzig, K.H.; Suppola, S.; Khomutov, A.R.; Vepsäläinen, J.; Jänne, J. (2002). A polyamine analogue prevents acute pancreatitis and restores early liver regeneration in transgenic rats with activated polyamine catabolism. *The Journal of Biological Chemistry*, Vol.277, 39867-39872.

Rider, J.E.; Hacker, A.; Mackintosh, C.A.; Pegg, A.E.; Woster, P.M.; Casero, R.A. (2007). Spermine and spermidine mediate protection against oxidative damage caused by hydrogen peroxide. *Amino Acids*, Vol.33, 231-240.

Sanz, N.; Díez-Fernández, C.; Alvarez, A.M.; Fernández-Simón, L.; Cascales, M. (1999). Age-related changes on parameters of experimentally-induced liver injury and regeneration. *Toxicology and Applied Pharmacology*, Vol.154, 40-49.

Seiler, N.; Raul, F. (2005). Polyamines and apoptosis. *Journal of Cellular & Molecular Medicine*, Vol.3, 623-642.

Seiler, N.; Raul, F. (2007). Polyamines and the intestinal tract. *Critical Reviews in Clinical Laboratory Sciences*, Vol.44, No.4, 365-411.

Serafini-Fracassini, D.; Della Mea, M.; Tasco, G.; Casadio, R.; Del Duca, S. (2009). Plant and animal transglutaminases: do similar functions imply similar structures? *Amino Acids*, Vol.36, 643-657.

Slocum, R.D. (1991). Polyamine biosynthesis in plants. In: Slocum, R.D.; Flores, H.E. (eds) Biochemistry and Physiology of Polyamines in Plants. CRC Press Boca Raton Ann Arbor London Publishers, pp23-40.

Smith, J., Burritt, D., Bannister, P. (2001). Ultraviolet-B radiation leads to a reduction in free polyamines in *Phaseolus vulgaris* L. *Plant Growth Regulation*, Vol.35, 289-294.

Smith, T.A.; Best, G.R. (1978). Distribution of the hordatines in barley. *Phytochemistry*, Vol.17, 1093–1098.

Soda, K. (2010). Polyamine intake, dietary pattern, and cardiovascular disease. *Medical Hypotheses*, Vol. 75, 299-301.

Soda, K.; Dobashi, Y.; Kano, Y.; Tsujinaka, S.; Konishi, F. (2009a). Polyamine-rich food decreases age-associated pathology and mortality in aged mice. *Experimental Gerontology*, Vol.44, 727-732.

Soda, K.; Kano, Y.; Nakamura, T.; Kasono, K.; Kawakami, M.; Konishi, F. (2005). Spermine, a natural polyamine, suppresses LFA-1 expression on human lymphocyte. *The Journal of Immunology*, Vol.175, 237-245.

Soda, K.; Kano, Y.; Sakuragi, M.; Takao, K.; Lefor, A.; Konishi, F. (2009b). Long-term oral polyamine intake increases blood polyamine concentrations. *Journal of Nutritional Science and Vitaminology*, Vol.55, 361-366.

Someya, S.; Prolla, T.A. (2010). Mitochondrial oxidative damage and apoptosis in age-related hearing loss. *Mechanisms of Ageing and Development*, Vol.131, 480-486.

Tadolini, B. (1988) Polyamine inhibition of lipid peroxidation. *Biochemical Journal*, Vol.249, 33-36.

ter Steege, J.C.A.; Forget, P.Ph., Buurman, W.A. (1999). Oral spermine administration inhibits nitric oxide-mediated intestinal damage and levels of systemic inflammatory mediators in a mouse endotoxin model. *Shock*, Vol.11, 115-119.

Tiburcio, A.F.; Campos, J.L.; Figueras, X.; Besford, R.T. (1993) Recent advances in the understanding of polyamine functions during plant development. *Plant Growth Regulation*, Vol.12, 331-340.

Tsunawaki, S.; Sporn, M.; Ding, A.; Nathan, M.P. (1988). Deactivation of macrophages by transforming growth factor-beta. *Nature (London)*, Vol.334, 260-262.

Valero, D. (2010). The role of polyamines on fruit ripening and quality during storage: what is new. *Acta Horticulturae*, Vol.884, 199-206.

Vijayanathan, V.; Thomas, T.; Thomas, T.J. (2002). DNA nanoparticles and development of DNA delivery vehicles for gene therapy. *Biochemistry*, Vol.41, 14085-14094.

Wang, C.J.; Delcros, J.G.; Cannon, L.; Konate, F.; Carias, H.; Biggerstaff, J.; Gardner, R.A.; Phanstiel, O. (2003). Defining the molecular requirements for the selective delivery of polyamine conjugates into cells containing active polyamine transporters. *Journal of Medicinal Chemistry*, Vol.46, 5129-5138.

Wang, X.; Levic, S.; Gratton, M.A.; Doyle, K.D.; Yamoah, E.N.; Pegg, A.E. (2009). Spermine synthase deficiency leads to deafness and a profound sensitivity to α-difluoromethylornithine. *The Journal of Biological Chemistry*, Vol.284, 930-937.

Zhang, M.; Caragine, T.; Wang, H.; Cohen, P.S.; Botchkina, G.; Soda, K.; Bianchi, M.; Ulrich, P.; Cerami, A.; Sherry, B.; Tracey, K.J. (1997). Spermine inhibits proinflammatory cytokine synthesis in human mononuclear cells: a counter regulatory mechanism that restrains the immune response. *Journal of Experimental Medicine*, Vol.185, 1759-1768.

Zou, T.; Liu, L.; Rao, J.; Marasa, B.S.; Chen, J.; Xiao, L.; Zhou, H.; Gorospe, M.; Wang, J.-Y. (2008). Polyamines modulate the subcellular localization of RNA-binding protein HuR through AMP-activated protein kinase-regulated phosphorylation and acetylation of importing α1. *Biochemical Journal*, Vol.409, 389-398.

13

Screening of some Traditionally Used Plants for Their Hepatoprotective Effect

Saleh I. Alqasoumi[1,2] and Maged S. Abdel-Kader[1]
[1]Department of Pharmacognosy, College of Pharmacy, Salman Bin Abdulaziz University,
[2]Department of Pharmacognosy, College of Pharmacy, King Saud University,
Kingdom of Saudi Arabia

1. Introduction

Liver is one of the largest organs in human body and the chief site for intense metabolism and excretion (Ram, 2001). It has a surprising role in the maintenance, performance and regulating homeostasis of the body. It is involved with almost all the biochemical pathways responsible for growth, fight against disease, nutrient supply, energy provision and reproduction (Ward & Daly, 1999). The major functions of the liver are carbohydrate, protein and fat metabolism, detoxification, blood coagulation, immunomodulation, secretion of bile and storage of vitamin.

Two major types of reactions occur in the liver in the presence of exogenous substances. The first involve chemical modification of function groups by oxidation, reduction, hydroxylation, sulfonation and dealkylation. Various enzymes including mixed oxidases, cytochromes P-450, and the glutathione S-acyltransferases are involved in such biochemical transformations that usually lead to inactivation of drugs. This step is usually followed by conversion of the resulted metabolites into more water-soluble derivatives that are excreted in the bile or urine via coupling with glucuronate, sulfate, acetate, taurine or glycine moieties (Ram, 2001).

Liver damage inflicted by hepatotoxic agents is of grave consequences (Subramoniam & Pushpangadan, 1999). Liver ailments represent a major global health problem (Baranisrinivasan et al., 2009). Liver cirrhosis is the ninth leading cause of death in the USA (Kim et al., 2002). Toxic chemicals, xenobiotics, alcohol consumption, malnutrition, anaemia, medications, autoimmune disorders (Marina, 2006), viral infections (hepatitis A, B, C, D, etc.) and microbial infections (Sharma & Ahuja, 1997) are harmful and cause damage to the hepatocytes. Hepatotoxic chemicals cause damage to the liver cells mainly by inducing lipid peroxidation and other oxidative events (Dianzani et al., 1991).

In spite of the tremendous advances in modern medicine, no effective drugs are available, which stimulate liver functions and/or offers protection to the liver from damage or help to regenerate hepatic cells (Chatterjee, 2000). In the absence of reliable liver protective drugs in modern medicine, there exists a challenge for pharmaceutical scientists to explore the potential of hepatoprotective activity of plants based on traditional use (Witte et al., 1983). A large number of medicinal preparations are recommended for the treatment of liver disorders (Chatterjee, 2000) and quite often claimed to offer significant relief. Study of many traditional plants used for liver problems led to the discovery of active compounds yet developed to successful drugs. Silymarin (Morazzoni & Bombardelli, 1995), schisandrin B (Cyong et al., 2000), phyllanthin, hypophyllanthin, picroside I and kutkoside (Ram, 2001) are examples of natural antihepatotoxic compounds derived from traditional herbs. About 600 commercial preparations with claimed liver protecting activity are available all over the world. About 100 Indian medicinal plants belonging to 40 families are components of liver herbal formulation (Handa et al., 1986). The effectiveness of most of these plant products must be scientifically verified to identify new medicaments for the management of liver disorders.

2. Silymarin, the standard antihepatotoxic drug

Silymarin, the collective name for an extract from milk thistle, *Silybum marianum* (L.) Gaertneri, is a naturally occurring flavonolignan. Silymarin is a mixture of stereoisomers mainly silybin (also called silybinin, silibin or silibinin) representing 80%, w/w of silymarin. Other minor stereoisomers include isosilybin, dihydrosilybin, silydianin and silychristin (Wagner et al., 1968). Silymarin protects experimental animals against the hepatotoxin α-amanitin (Hahn et al., 1968) and has a strong antioxidant property (Comoglio et al., 1990). Other reported biological properties of silymarin include inhibition of LOX (Fiebrich & Koch, 1979a) and PG synthetase (Fiebrich & Koch, 1979b). For decades, silymarin has been used clinically in Europe for the treatment of alcoholic liver disease and as antihepatotoxic agent (Salmi & Sarna, 1982). Silymarin is well tolerated and largely free of adverse effects (Comoglio et al., 1990). Silymarin act as an antioxidant by scavenging preoxidant free radicals and by increasing the intracellular concentration of glutathione (GSH). It also exhibits a regulatory action of cellular membrane permeability and increase its stability against xenobiotics injury, increasing the synthesis of ribosomal RNA by stimulating DNA polymerase-I, exerting a steroid like regulatory action on DNA transcription and stimulation of protein synthesis and regeneration of liver cells (Dehmlow et al., 1996; Saller et al., 2007). Silymarin efficacy is not limited to the treatment of toxic and metabolic liver damage; it is also effective in acute, chronic hepatitis and in inhibiting fibrotic activity (Saller et al., 2007). It acts as inhibitor of the transformation of stellate hepatocytes into myofibroblasts, this process is responsible for the deposition of collagen fibres leading to cirrhosis (Fraschini et al., 2002).

3. Induction of liver toxicity in experimental animals

In order to study the hepatoprotective effect of plant extracts or pure isolates it is necessary to induce liver toxicity in experimental animal models. The reported protocols for induction of liver toxicity varying greatly in terms of the used liver toxin, doses, duration and route of administration. Below is a collection of the most common experimental procedures use by different groups.

3.1 Carbon tetrachloride-induced liver toxicity

Liver damage induced by carbon tetrachloride is the most commonly used model for the screening of hepatoprotective drugs (Slater, 1965). The rise in serum levels of Glutamic

Pyruvate Transaminase (SGPT), Glutamic Oxaloacetic Transaminase (SGOT) and cholesterol following carbon tetrachloride has been attributed to the damaged structural integrity of the liver cells. These components are cytoplasmic in location and released into circulation after cellular damages (Sallie et al., 1991). Carbon tetrachloride also plays a significant role in inducing triacylgliceral accumulation, depletion of GSH, depression of protein synthesis and loss of enzymes activity (Recknagel et al., 1989). Carbon tetrachloride induces hepatotoxicity in rats following its metabolic activation in the hepatocytes. Therefore, it selectively causes toxicity in the liver cells while maintaining semi-normal metabolic function. Carbon tetrachloride is metabolically activated by the cytochrome P-450 dependent mixed oxidease in the endoplasmic reticulum to form trichloromethyl free radical ($\cdot CCl_3$) and $\cdot Cl_3COO$ which combined with critical cellular macromolecules, cellular lipids and proteins in the presence of oxygen to induce lipid peroxidation (Snyder & Andrews, 1996). Some of the lipid peroxidation products are reactive aldehydes, e.g., 4-hydroxynonenal, which can form adducts with proteins (Weber et al., 2003). These consequences lead to changes in the structures of the endoplasmic reticulum and other membranes hence to increase in plasma membrane permeability to Ca^{2+} resulting in a severe disturbances of calcium homeostasis and consequently necrotic cell death (Weber et al., 2003). The loss of metabolic enzyme activation, reduction of protein synthesis and loss of glucose-6-phosphatase activation, all lead to liver injury (Recknagel & Glende, 1973; Azri et al.,1992). In addition to the intracellular events, Kupffer cell activation can contribute to liver injury (elSisi et al., 1993). Kupffer cells are resident macrophages of the liver which constitute approximately 80% of the fixed macrophages in the body (McCuskey, 2006). They may enhance liver injury by oxidant stress (elSisi et al., 1993) or TNF-_ generation, which may lead to apoptosis (Shi et al., 1998). In more than 70% of the reviewed published data liver toxicity were experimentally induced by Carbon tetrachloride. However, the experimental procedures were considerably different.

3.1.1 Single dose carbon tetrachloride-induced liver toxicity

Acute liver toxicity can be induced by a single dose of carbon tetrachloride. However, the route of administration and dose are different from one research group to another. Intraperitoneal injection seems to be the most commonly used method for carbon tetrachloride administration due to the ease of handling and rapid onset of action. Rats are usually a popular experimental animal model and the reported doses were 3 ml/kg (Jamshidzadeh et al., 2005), 2.5 ml/kg (Sen et al., 1993; Nishigaki et al., 1992), 2 ml/kg (Channabasavaraj et al., 2008), 1.5 ml/kg (Bhadauria et al., 2009), 1.25 ml/kg (Rafatullah et al., 2008) or 0.5 ml/kg (Rao et al., 1993). In most cases, carbon tetrachloride is diluted with oils (1:1). The large variation in doses may arise from weather the stated volumes represented the volume of pure carbon tetrachloride or the total volume of the mixture. If this is the case, the wide range of doses from 3- 0.5 ml will shrink to 1 ml (1.5- 0.5 ml). In case of using mice as the experimental animal model the reported carbon tetrachloride doses were much less (0.01, 0.016. 0.02 and 0.03 ml/kg) (Amat et al., 2010; Suzuki et al., 1990; Zhou et al., 2010; Wang et al., 2008).

Induction of liver toxicity via oral routes was also reported. The used doses were 1ml/kg (Harish & Shivanandappa, 2006) 1.25 ml/Kg (Aktay et al., 2000) and 1.5 ml/kg (Gilani, & Janbaz, 1995). Subcutaneous route for administration of carbon tetrachloride was also used and the reported doses were 0.3 ml/kg (Kumar et al., 2009), 1 ml/kg (Ahmed et al., 2001) or 1.25 ml/kg (Mohamed et al., 2005).

3.1.2 Multi doses carbon tetrachloride-induced liver toxicity

The most popular multi-dose protocol for induction of liver toxicity is the subcutaneous administration of 2 ml of carbon tetrachloride/olive oil mixture (1:1) in days 2 and 3 of a five days long experiment (Zafar & Ali, 1998). In another protocol, carbon tetrachloride/olive oil (1:1) mixture was given daily via intraperitoneal injection in a 7 days long experiment. The doses were 0.5 ml (Maheswari & Rao, 2005), 0.8 ml (Özbek et al, 2004) or 1 ml/kg (Somasundaram et al., 2010). In 14 days experiment carbon tetrachloride/liquid paraffin mixture (1:1) was administered intraperitoneal every 72 hours (Christian et al., 2006). Chronic reversible cirrhosis were induced in rats by oral administration of mixture of 20% carbon tetrachloride in corn oil at 0.5mL/ kg body weight doses twice a week (Monday and Thursday) for 6 weeks (Hernandez-Munoz et al., 2001). Subcutaneous injection of 50% carbon tetrachloride in liquid paraffin (3 mL/kg) every other day for four weeks was also used to induce chronic liver toxicity (Chun-ching & Wei-Chih, 1995).

3.2 Paracetamol-induced liver toxicity

Paracetamol (acetaminophen) is a well-known antipyretic and analgesic agent. Therapeutic doses of paracetamol are safe, however, toxic doses can produce fatal hepatic necrosis in man, rats and mice (Mitchell et al., 1973). Paracetamol is eliminated mainly as sulfate and glucoronide (Eriksson et al., 1992) when administered in the regular therapeutic doses. Only 5% of the dose is converted into N-acetyl-p-benzoquineimine (NAPQI). However, upon administration of toxic doses of paracetamol the sulfation and glucoronidation routes become saturated and hence, higher percentage of paracetamol molecules are oxidized to highly reactive NAPQI by cytochrome p-450 enzymes. Semiquinone radicals, obtained by one electron reduction of NAPQI, has an extremely short half-life and is rapidly conjugated with glutathione (GSH), a sulphydryl donor which results in the depletion of liver GSH pool (Remirez et al., 1995). Under conditions of excessive NAPQI formation or reduced of glutathione store, NAPQI covalently binds to vital proteins, the lipid bilayer of hepatocyte membranes and increases the lipid peroxidation. The result is hepatocellular death and centrilobular liver necrosis (McConnachie et al., 2007). Due to liver injury caused by paracetamol overdose, the transport function of the hepatocytes gets disturbed resulting in leakage of plasma membrane (Zimmerman & Seeff, 1970), thus causing an increase in serum enzyme levels.

When rats are used as experimental animal model a single oral dose of 2 gm/kg paracetamol was used to induce liver damage (Chattopadhyay, 2003). The dose in case of using mice was 250 mg/kg (Sabir & Rocha, 2008). Intraperitoneal route of administration was also utilized. A doses of 750 mg/kg (Bhakta et al., 2001) or 835 mg/kg (Yen et al., 2007) were administered to produce liver intoxication in rats, while lower doses of 300 mg/kg (Yuan et al., 2010) were used for induction of liver damage in mice.

3.3 D-Galactosamine-induced liver toxicity

Exogenous administration of D-galactosamine (D-GalN) has been found to induce liver damage closely resembles human viral hepatitis (Decker & Keppler, 1972). A single injection of D-GalN can decrease the uracil nucleotides in the liver and heart (Wills & Asha, 2006). D-GalN markedly depletes hepatic UDP-glucuronic acid whereas extrahepatic UDP-glucuronic is minimally affected. This suggests that D-GalN predominantly inhibits hepatic glucuronidation. It disrupts the synthesis of essential uridylate nucleotides resulting in organelle injury. Depletion of these nucleotides ultimately impairs the synthesis of protein and glycoprotein, leads to progressive damage of cellular membranes. These consequences lead to change in cellular membrane permeability which leads to enzyme leakage to the circulation (Keppler et al., 1970; Abdul-Hussain & Mehendale, 1991). In addition, increased production of reactive oxygen species (ROS) has been reported in primary culture of rat hepatocytes treated with D-GalN (Quintero et al., 2002). Oxygen-derived free radicals released from activated hepatic-macrophages are also one of the primary causes of D-GalN-induced liver damage (Shiratori et al., 1988; Hu & Chen, 1992).

Experimentally induced liver damage was achieved in rats by a single dose of D-GalN 400 mg/kg (Ferenčiková et al., 2003; Kmieć et al., 2000) or 200 mg/kg (Decker & Keppler, 1974) via intrapretoneal injection. For induction of liver toxicity in mice a single dose of 15 mg D-GalN in 0.3mL saline per 20 g by intraperitoneal injection (Wang et al., 2000) was used. The use of D-GalN as liver toxin with a very small concentration of lipopolysaccharide (LPS) (10 µg/kg) was also reported (Tiegs et al., 1989).

3.4 Other methods for induction of hepatotoxicity

These methods include the use of some drugs with known side effects target the liver upon prolonged use. Rifampicin (1 g/kg in rats) (Anusuya et al., 1010), menadione (60 mg/kg in mice) (Ip et al., 2004) and anti-tubercular drugs were applied for induction of experimental liver toxicity (Tandon et al., 2008). Ethanol induced liver damage is a major cause of morbidity and mortality worldwide (Purohit et al., 2009). Consequently, ethanol was used as a liver damaging agent in some experiments (Noh et al., 2011; Sathaye et al., 2010). Natural toxins such as aflatoxins are known to have toxic effect on liver. Aflatoxin B1, under the influence of microsomal cytochrome p-450 mediated oxidation, is biotransformed into aflatoxin 8-9-epoxide, which is a reactive intermediate and highly toxic (Iyer et al., 1994). The use of aflatoxin B1 and other aflatoxins as hepatotoxic agent in experimental animal was reported (Banu et al., 2009; Naaz et al., 2007). Chemicals such as trichloroacetic acid (Celik et al., 2009), nitrobenzene (Rathi et al, 2010), thioacetamide (Khatri et al, 2009) and heavy metals such as Cadmium (Obioha et al., 2009) were also utilized to induce experimental liver injury.

Away from the use of chemicals, the hepatoprotective effect of some plant extracts was challenged against liver fibrosis caused by bile duct ligation (Fursule & Patil, 2010).

4. Assement of hepatoprotective activity

The experimental animals are usually treated with the plant extract under investigation for specified period of time. The hepatotoxic agent is usually administered near the end of the experimental period for induction of acute toxicity or in several doses during the course of the experiment for chronic toxicity. The hepatoprotective power of the tested material is assessed by measuring certain biochemical parameters, liver tissue parameters and comparing their levels with normal animals, group receiving standard drug in addition to the hepatotoxic agent and group receiving only hepatotoxic agent. The most common measured parameters are summarized below.

4.1 Serum biochemical parameters

4.1.1 Transaminases

Alanine transaminase (ALT), also called Serum Glutamic Pyruvate Transaminase (SGPT) or Alanine aminotransferase (ALAT) is an enzyme present in hepatocytes. Upon cell damaged, the enzyme leaks into the blood. SGPT level rises dramatically in acute liver damage, such as viral hepatitis or paracetamol overdose (Zimmerman & Seeff, 1970). Elevations are often measured in multiples of the upper limit of normal values. Aspartate transaminase (AST) also called Serum Glutamic Oxaloacetic Transaminase (SGOT) or aspartate aminotransferase (ASAT) is another enzyme associated with liver parenchymal cells. The level of SGOT is raised in acute liver damage, however, it is not specific as it is also present in red blood cells, heart, kidney and skeletal muscle. The ratio of SGOT to SGPT is sometimes useful in differentiating between liver damage and other conditions that elevate the levels of transaminases (Nyblom et al., 2004; Feild et al., 2008). Effective hepatoprotective agents must decrease the elevated levels of transaminases and bring them closer to the normal values as a signe for liver healing.

4.1.2 Alkaline phosphatase

Alkaline phosphatase (ALP) catalysis the hydrolysis of phosphate esters, and is found in biliary epithelium and the bile canalicular region of hepatocytes. Its function is not well established, but is thought to involve in metabolite transport across cell membranes. Elevation of the level of ALP can suggest intrahepatic, extrahepatic biliary obstruction, or infiltrative diseases of the liver (Feild et al., 2008). Agents that can lower ALP levels will be considered as useful hepatoprotective agents.

4.1.3 Bilirubin

Bilirubin (Bil) is the breakdown product of normal haem -a part of haemoglobin in red blood cells- catabolism of aged erythrocytes. Bilirubin, loosely bound to albumin in plasma to form a soluble species taken up from the Disse spaces of liver sinusoids into hepatocytes, where it is esterified at its propionyl sites with glucuronic acid under the catalytic activity of uridinediphosphoglucuronate 1A1 transferase enzymes. Esterified bilirubin is excreted into bile as water-soluble bilirubin diglucuronide. Serum concentration of bilirubin is a marker of the liver's ability to take up bilirubin from the plasma into the hepatocyte, conjugate it with glucuronic acid, and excrete bilirubin glucuronides into bile. Elevated level of serum conjugated bilirubin implies regurgitation of bilirubin glucuronides from hepatocytes back into plasma, usually because of intrahepatic or extrahepatic obstruction to bile outflow and cholestasis. The liver has substantial reserve capacity, and normal serum bilirubin levels can be maintained until there is enough injury to reduce the liver's capacity to clear bilirubin from plasma. Serum concentration of bilirubin is very specific for potentially serious liver damage, and is an important indicator of the loss of liver function (Feild et al., 2008). Reduction in the level of serum bilirubin is a strong indication of restoring normal liver function.

4.1.4 Gamma glutamyl transpeptidase (GGT)

Serum Gamma glutamyl transpeptidase (GGT) (also Gamma-glutamyl transferase) is specific to liver injury and more sensitive marker for cholestatic damage than ALP. GGT may be elevated with even minor, sub-clinical levels of liver dysfunction. GGT is raised in alcohol toxicity following several days of moderate ingestion. Rifampin, phenytoin, or barbiturates all resulted in elevation of GGT level. An isolated GGT elevation in these situations does not indicate hepatocellular injury. The GGT level will return to normal after discontinuation of the offending agent. Hepatic dysfunction should be considered if the GGT elevation is associated with other abnormalities in liver biochemistry (Owvens& Evans, 1975). Hepatoprotective agents will reduce the elevated level of GGT.

4.1.5 Total protein & albumin (Alb)

One of the most important liver functions is protein synthesis. Albumin is a major part of the total protein (TP) made specifically by the liver. Liver damage causes disruption and disassociation of polyribosomes on endoplasmic reticulum and thereby reducing the biosynthesis of protein. The TP levels including Alb levels will be depressed in hepatotoxic conditions due to defective protein biosynthesis in liver. Restoring the normal levels of TP including Alb is an important parameter for liver recovery (Navarro & Senior, 2006).

4.2 Liver tissue parameters

4.2.1 Glutathione and antioxidant enzymes

Glutathione (GSH) and its related enzymes are playing a vital role as intracellular antioxidants. GSH prevents damage to important cellular components caused by reactive oxygen species such as free radicals and peroxides (Pompella et al., 2003). Glutathione exists in both reduced (GSH) and oxidized (GSSG) states as well. In the reduced state, the thiol group of cysteine is able to donate a reducing equivalent ($H^+ + e^-$) to other unstable molecules, such as ROS. In donating an electron, GSH itself becomes reactive, but readily reacts with another reactive GSH to form glutathione disulfide (GSSG). Such a reaction is possible due to the relatively high concentration of glutathione in cells (up to 5 mM in the liver). GSH can be regenerated from GSSG by the enzyme glutathione reductase (GSR or GR) (Boyer, 1989; Tandogan & Ulusu, 2006). In healthy cells and tissues, more than 90% of the total glutathione pool is in the reduced form (GSH) and less than 10% exists in the disulfide form (GSSG). An increased GSSG-to-GSH ratio is considered indicative of oxidative stress (Pastore et al., 2003). Another protection from oxidative damage is assured by Glutathione peroxidase (GPx), an enzyme family with peroxidase activity. GPx reduce lipid hydroperoxides to their corresponding alcohols and breakdown hydrogen peroxide into water and oxygen (Castro & Freeman, 2001).

The glutathione S-transferase (GSTs) family are composed of many cytosolic, mitochondrial, and microsomal proteins. GSTs catalyze a variety of reactions and accept endogenous and xenobiotic substrates as well (Udomsinprasert et al., 2005). GSTs catalyse the conjugation of reduced glutathione - via a sulfhydryl group - to electrophilic centres on a wide variety of substrates (Douglas, 1987). This activity detoxifies endogenous compounds such as peroxidised lipids, and enable the breakdown of xenobiotics. GSTs may also bind toxins and serve as transport proteins (Leaver & George, 1998).

Plant	Dose	SGOT Test	SGOT St	SGPT Test	SGPT St	ALP Test	ALP St	T.Bil Test	T.Bil St	Ref.
Abutilon indicum	200	64.6	81.5	69.2	90.5	46.9	62.7	54.6	73.8	Porchezhian & Ansari, 2005
Abutilon indicum [a]	200	32.7	68.5	78.8	83.8	52.3	72.4	60.7	70.8	Porchezhian & Ansari, 2005
Adhatoda vasica	100	53.3	62.8	56.0	59.4	-	-	-	-	Bhattacharyya et al., 2005
Anisochilus carnosus	400	52.8	54.9	29.9	30.1	28.2	28.7	13.2	10.5	Venkatesh et al., 2011
Arachniodes exilis	750	71.9	75.8	41.7	49.3	-	-	-	-	Zhou et al., 2010
Artemisia absinthium	200	64.7	70.9	60.1	61.4	-	-	-	-	Amat et al., 2010
Azadirachta indica [a]	500	30.6	36.4	26.9	59.0	28.0	45.5	40.4	53.6	Gomase et al., 2011
Balanites aegyptiaca	500	28.7	56.9	29.9	64.5	21.5	42.8	38.4	52.0	Abdel-Kader & Alqasoumi, 2008
Bixa orellana	500	57.37	-	52.08	-	-	-	21.15	-	Ahsan et al., 2009
Butea monosperma	800	52.1	53.2	78.1	87.1	-	-	-	-	Sharma & Shukla, 2010
Byrsocarpus coccineus*	400	44.3	42.9	68.4	55.9	49.0	38.5	46.6	51.0	Akindele et al., 2010
Cajanus cajan	500	56.53	-	50.22	-	-	-	25.0	-	Akindele et al., 2010
Calotropis procera [a]	400	62.2	66.5	69.1	73.5	58.4	61.9	68.7	69.6	Setty et al., 2007
Cassia fistula [a], **	400	54.0	64.3	46.4	63.1	53.9	58.2	54.1	66.5	Bhakta et al., 2001
Castanea crenata [c]	150	54.1	-	70.6	-	-	-	-	-	Noh et al., 2011
Carduus nutans	500	44.16	-	64.68	-	-	-	-	-	Aktay et al., 2000
Chamomile capitula [a]	400	-	-	-	-	82.6	-	74.2	-	Gupta & Misra, 2006
Cichorium intybus	500	81.9	78.1	56.1	84.3	40.8	47.3	-	-	Ahmed et al., 2003
Cistanche tubulosa	1000	91.6	-	89.7	-	-	-	-	-	Morikawa et al., 2010
Clerodendrum inerme	200	31.6	40.1	83.0	85.6	88.4	89.0	-	-	Gopal & Sengottuvelu, 2008
Commiphora berryi	200	45.6	44.4	65.8	62.4	61.1	65.7	56.3	73.6	Shankar et al., 2008
C. opobalsamum	500	66.2	-	75.6	-	33.0	-	37.3	-	Al-Howiriny et al., 2004
Coptidis rhizoma	600	93.9	-	82.5	-	-	-	-	-	Ye et al., 2009
Cordia macleodii	200	84.8	86.5	77.5	82.2	63.3	60.6	40.6	42.2	Qureshi et al., 2009
Cuscuta chinensis [a]	250	86.8	-	81.6	-	31.0	-	-	-	Yen et al., 2007
Enicostemma axillare [b]	200	91.1	92.2	45.3	20.4	49.2	40.3	33.3	18.6	Jaishree & Badami, 2010
Ephedra foliata	500	42.6	55.1	39.5	66.1	21.2	39.6	46.2	63.5	Alqasoumi et al., 2008b
Euphorbia fusiformis	500	43.1	43.7	30.2	31.7	34.7	37.1	99.9	65.9	Anusuya et al., 2010
Ficus glomerata	500	44.0	30.4	72.8	57.2	68.5	74.6	-	-	Channabasavaraj et al., 2008
Filipendula ulmaria	100	58.7	-	81.9	-	-	-	-	-	Shilova et al., 2008
Fumaria indica [b]	400	72.6	-	79.0	-	68.2	-	79.7	-	Rathi et al., 2008
F. vailantii	500	60.75	-	66.93	-	-	-	-	-	Aktay et al., 2000
Ganoderma lucidum [b]	180	76.6	-	83.6	-	-	-	-	-	Shi et al., 2008
Gentiana olivieri	500	69.57	-	86.39	-	-	-	-	-	Aktay et al., 2000
Hibiscus sabdariffa	500	44.5	66.5	37.1	65.02	21.0	50.6	35.0	69.6	Alqasoumi et al., 2008b
Halenia elliptica	200	57.2	48.8	58.0	47.6	39.0	49.4	46.6	48.6	Huang et al., 2010b
Hedyotis corymbosa [a]	200	59.6	60.8	75.8	66.9	81.0	79.2	37.8	72.4	Sadasivan et al., 2006
Helminthostachys zeylanica	300	64.3	65.0	77.7	78.2	44.3	45.1	66.4	74.0	Suja et al., 2004
Hygrophila auriculata	150	40.8	43.2	24.9	23.5	28.1	26.2	53.0	60.2	Shanmugasundara & Venkataraman, 2006
Kyllinga nemoralis	200	45.6	42.5	68.3	65.5	61.3	66.0	46.6	51.1	Somasundaram et al., 2010
Laggera pterodonta	100	39.6	7.3	31.3	12.5	-	-	-	-	Wu et al., 2007
Laggera pterodonta [b, ***]	100	41.9	9.3	35.0	7.5	-	-	-	-	Wu et al., 2007
Mollugo pentaphylla	200	37.2	43.6	53.0	63.9	55.1	55.6	32.6	36.0	Valarmathi et al., 2010
Momordica balsamina	500	37.5	57.6	39.1	57.1	23.2	37.5	52.7	62.0	Alqasoumi et al., 2009b
M. dioica	200	44.7	64.0	54.3	54.6	51.9	59.7	31.1	58.5	Jain et al., 2008
Nelumbo nucifera	500	82.8	82.0	76.5	74.3	39.7	42.0	46.5	50.5	Huang et al., 2010a
Phyllanthus amarus [d]	75	16.6	21.9	28.1	31.8	-	-	-	-	Pramyothin, et al., 2007
Pittosporum neelgherrense	200	70.6	71.9	54.1	55.5	-	-	-	-	Shyamal et al., 2006
Pittosporum neelgherrense [b]	200	65.5	65.4	58.4	59.1	-	-	-	-	Shyamal et al., 2006
Propolis	500	29.4	53.4	37.3	60.2	25.5	43.5	30.1	57.0	Alqasoumi et al., 2008a
Premna corymbosa	400	-	-	-	-	61.6	52.4	-	-	Karthikeyan & Deepa, 2010
Rubus aleaefolius	35	12.7	-	-	-	-	-	-	-	Hong et al., 2010
Sida acuta [a]	100	61.9	60.7	67.7	66.9	79.6	79.2	67.3	72.4	Sreedevi et al., 2009
Smilax regelii	500	13.5	-	47.0	-	-	-	56.4	-	Rafatullah et al., 1991

[a] Paracetamol, [b] D-galactosamine, [c] ethanol, [d] aflatoxin, [e] nitrobenzene, [f] thioacetamide- induced liver toxicity, otherwise CCl₄ was used

* Livolin, ** Liver tonic, *** Silibinin were used as hepatoprotective standard, otherwise silymarin was use

Table 1. Effect of selected plants on serum biochemical parameters

Treatment of animals with hepatotoxic agents lead to depletion of GSH, reduction in the non-protein sulfhydryl moiety (NP-SH), GPx, GSR activities and ultration of GSTs activity (Naaz et al., 2007; Mitchell et al., 1973; Abdel-Kader et al., 2010; Alqasoumi et al., 2009).

Another part of the antioxidant systems in the bodies is the enzymes Superoxide dismutases (SOD) and Catalase (CAT) (Scott et al., 1991). They are an important antioxidant defence containing heavy metals in nearly all cells exposed to oxygen. SOD catalyzes the dismutation of superoxide into oxygen and hydrogen peroxide. SOD is the most efficient catalytic enzyme; its activity is only limited by the frequency of collision between itself and superoxide (Fredovich, 1997).

CAT catalyzes the decomposition of hydrogen peroxide to water and oxygen (Chelikani et al., 2004). CAT has one of the highest turnover numbers of all enzymes; one CAT enzyme can convert 40 million molecules of hydrogen peroxide to water and oxygen per second (RCSB Protein Data Bank, 2007).

Effective hepatoprotactive agents will be able to restore the normal levels of these systems in liver tissue.

4.2.2 Harmful peroxidation products

Malonaldehyde (MDA) is the main end-product of polyunsaturated fatty acid peroxidation (PUFA) following Reactive oxygen species (ROS) insult (Esterbauer et al., 1991). PUFA are essential part of biological membranes (Vaca et al., 1988). MDA is a reactive aldehyde and is one of many reactive electrophile species that cause toxic stress in cells and form covalent protein adducts (Farmer & Davoine, 2007). The production of this aldehyde is used as a biomarker to measure the level of oxidative stress in an organism (Del Rio et al., 2005). The increase in liver MDA levels induced by hepatotoxic agents suggests enhanced lipid peroxidation, leading to hepatic tissue damage and failure of endogenous antioxidant defence mechanisms to prevent formation of excessive free radicals (Souza et al., 1997).

ThioBarbituric Acid Reactive Substances (TBARS) are another harmful substances formed by lipid peroxidation. TBARS are one of the end products formed during the decomposition of lipids by ROS (Olinescu et al., 1994). The tissue concentration of TBARS increase with induced liver toxicity (Sabir & Rocha, 2008).

Physiological amounts of nitric oxide (NO) in the liver has protective effect against damage induced by tumour necrosis factor-a or Fas-dependent apoptosis (Fiorucci et al., 2001). The production of high levels of NO within the liver, via inducible NO synthase (iNOS) promote damage via interference with mitochondrial respiration (Moncada & Erusalimsky, 2002). Hepatocytes of experimental animals produce NO during chronic hepatic inflammation (Billiar et al., 1990 a, b). Human hepatocytes were also stimulated to produce NO by the same combination of endotoxin and cytokines as rat hepatocytes (Palmer et al., 1988; Nussler et al., 1992).

ROS are known to convert amino groups of protein to carbonyl moieties (Perry et al. 2000). Oxidative modification of protein leads to increased recognition and degradation by proteases and loss of enzymatic activity (Rivett & Levine, 1990). Accumulation of carbonyl derivatives of proteins (protein carbonyl) is taken as a biomarker of oxidative protein damage in aging and in various diseases (Dalle-Donne et al., 2003).

Plant	Dose	SOD	CAT	GSH	GPx	MDA	TBARS	Ref.
Abutilon indicum	200	-	-	81.4 / 82.8	-	-	-	Porchezhian & Ansari, 2005
Abutilon indicum[a]	200	-	-	75.9 / 77.3	-	-	-	Porchezhian & Ansari, 2005
Adhatoda vasica	100	-	-	-	-	-	55.4 / 55.7	Bhattacharyya et al., 2005
Arachniodes exilis	750	88.4 / 91.4	-	-	-	50.0 / 55.4	-	Zhou et al., 2010
Artemisia absinthium	200	88.0 / 90.1	-	-	71.7 / 89.0	54.9 / 58.6	-	Amat et al., 2010
Butea monosperma	800	-	-	92.3 / 92.3	-	-	-	Sharma & Shukla, 2010
Byrsocarpus coccineus *	400	92.8 / 73.6	93.7 / 73.6	104.5 / 75.5	92.2 / 96.0	82.7 / 87.3	-	Akindele et al., 2010
Calotropis procera[a]	400	-	-	58.4 / 60.5	-	-	-	Setty et al., 2007
Castanea crenata[c]	150	104.8	89.0	-	38.6	-	21.8	Noh et al., 2011
Carduus nutans	500	-	-	-	-	34.8	-	Aktay et al., 2000
Chamomile capitula[a]	400	-	-	91.0	-	-	50.2	Gupta & Misra, 2006
Clerodendrum inerme	200	-	-	92.9 / 88.2	-	-	-	Gopal & Sengottuvelu, 2008
C. opobalsamum	500	-	-	92.6	-	-	-	Al-Howiriny et al., 2004
Coptidis rhizoma	600	97.5	-	-	-	-	-	Ye et al., 2009
Cuscuta chinensis[a]	250	87.4	86.6	-	95.6	55.4	-	Yen et al., 2007
Ficus glomerata	500	62.5 / 106.3	105.0 / 101.7	-	-	-	44.1 / 45.7	Channabasavaraj et al., 2008
Filipendula ulmaria	100	66.0 / 56.1	92.9 / 73.2	-	-	-	48.4 / 35.2	Shilova et al., 2008
Fumaria indica[b]	400	-	-	-	89.8 / 93.2	48.6 / 55.1	-	Rathi et al., 2008
F. vailantii	500	-	-	-	-	33.7	-	Aktay et al., 2000
Ganoderma lucidum[b]	180	98.5	-	96.1	-	51.6	-	Shi et al., 2008
Gentiana olivieri	500	89.8	-	-	-	32.3	-	Aktay et al., 2000
Kyllinga nemoralis	200	66.1 / 51.4	81.3 / 87.3	59.0 / 57.2	-	51.1 / 52.6	-	Somasundaram et al., 2010
Memordica dioica	200	76.8 / 84.5	83.0 / 91.5	85.3 / 88.0	-	36.0 / 48.8	-	Jain et al., 2008
Nelumbo nucifera	500	85.4 / 76.5	87.9 / 55.7	126.0 / 78.7	-	-	31.0 / 31.7	Huang et al., 2010a
Phyllanthus amarus[d]	75	85.4	100.1	202.3	108.0	-	48.3	Pramyothin, et al., 2007
Rubus alaefolius	35	89.8	-	-	-	20.1	-	Hong et al., 2010
Tecomella undulata[c]	1000	-	-	134.9 / 150.9	-	50.7 / 69.4	-	Khatri et al., 2009
Tephrosia purpurea[c]	500	-	-	139.0 / 150.9	-	65.0 / 69.4	-	Khatri et al., 2009
Trichosanthes cucumerina	500	-	-	93.8 / 94.9	-	51.2 / 54.4	-	Kumar et al., 2009
Spermacoce hispida	200	85.1	82.9	-	89.9	51.7	-	Rathi et al., 2010
Uvaria chamae[a]	60	-	-	-	-	-	-	Madubunyi, 2010
Zanthoxylum armatum	400	93.7 / 99.7	90.9 / 97.9	89.0 / 94.2	-	67.3 / 70.0	-	Ranawat et al., 2010

[a] Paracetamol, [b] D-galactosamine, [c] ethanol, [d] aflatoxin, [e] thioacetamide- induced liver toxicity, otherwise CCl_4 was used

* Livolin was used as hepatoprotective standard, otherwise silymarin was use

Table 2. Effect of selected plants on liver tissue parameters

4.3 Barbiturates sleep time

Short acting barbiturates such as hexobarbiton are metabolized almost exclusively in the liver. Duration of barbiturates induced sleep in intact animals is considered as a reliable index for the activity of hepatic metabolism (Vogel, 1977). Pre-existing liver damage will result in prolongation of the sleeping time after a given dose of barbiturates due to decrease in the amount of the hypnotic broken down per unit time as a result of decreased availability of CYP2E1 contents (Singh et al., 2001). Extracts that can shorten this prolongation of barbiturates sleep time exert protective effect on CYP2E1 system.

4.4 Histopathological study of liver tissue

The histological appearance of the hepatocytes reflects their damage conditions (Prophet, et al., 1994). Exposure of hepatocytes to toxic agents such as carbon tetrachloride leads to histopathological changes from the normal histological appearance (Fig. 1). The hepatocytes of rat treated with carbon tetrachloride, showed centrilobular necrosis and extensive fatty changes observed on the midzonal or entire lobe 24 h after treatment (Fig. 1B). Liver tissues of rats treated with carbon tetrachloride and the standard drugs like silymarin showed no necrosis or fatty deposition but had only minimal portal inflammation (Fig.1C). The protective effect of tested extracts or pure materials will be expressed in histopathology as the ability to improve the histological appearance of hepatocytes and bring it closer to the normal hepatocytes of healthy liver (Fig.1A).

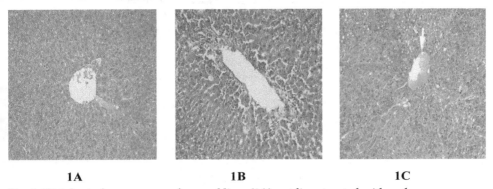

1A   **1B**   **1C**

Fig. 1. Histological appearance of normal liver (1A), rat liver treated with carbon tetrachloride (1B), rat liver treated with silymarin+ carbon tetrachloride (1C)(H & E, ×200).

5. Literature results for some promising hepatoprotective plants

Many plant extracts were tested for their hepatoprotective activity against various liver toxins. All the above mentioned parameters were used to evaluate the protective power of such plants against liver cells damage. In the following Tables some of the most promising results are presented. For handy comparative evaluation of the results percentage of protection is presented even if it was not calculate in the original article. For values where normal levels are increase due to destruction of hepatocytes integrity (SGOT, SGEPT) or over production of harmful oxidation products (MDA, TBARS) calculations were preformed based on control groups receiving the hepatotoxic agents. Percentage of reduction in the elevated values was compared to protection achieved by silymarin or any other hepatoprotective agents used in the original articles. On the other hand when experimental liver toxicity resulted in decrease in the normal levels of the measured parameters like the case of normal protective antioxidant enzymes (SOD, CAT), the protection efficacy is presented as percent recovery relative to the negative control values.

6. Summary, conclusions and future directions

Liver diseases represent a major global health problem that still has no cure in modern medicine. Some of the traditionally used plants for liver disorders provided useful therapeutic agents. A large number of such plants lack the scientific evidences supporting their effectiveness. Many groups of researchers worldwide were involved in studying the protective effects of plant extracts against experimentally induced liver toxicity. Rats and mice are the animals of choice in such experiments. Carbon tetrachloride followed by paracetamol and D-galactosamine (D-GalN) were used to induce liver toxicity in addition to ethanol and some other drugs affecting the liver on prolonged use. In most cases, positive control groups received silymarin as standard drug for liver protection. Both serum biochemical parameters, liver tissue parameters, barbiturates sleeping time and histopathological examination were used to access liver protection. The most promising data were presented in tables 1 and 2. These biological studies are extremely important to discriminate between useful and useless plants claimed to have liver healing properties. Scientific examination of all traditionally used plants for liver problems is a great goal still to be achieved. This collection of data can be a helpful guide for Phytochemists to explore the constituents of the most promising plants in order to discover new useful natural drugs for the management of liver disorders.

7. Reference

Abdel-Kader, M. S. & Alqasoumi, S. I. (2008). Evaluation of the hepatoprotective effect of the ethanol extracts of *Solanum nigrum, Cassia fistula, Balanites aegyptiaca* and *Carthamus tinctorius* against experimentally induced liver Injury in Rats. *Alexandria Journal of Pharmaceutical Sciences*, Vol 22, No.1, pp. 47- 50, ISSN 1110-1792

Abdel-Kader, M. S.; Alqasoumi, S. I.; Hefnawy, M. M. & AlSheikh, A. M. (2010). Hepatoprotective effect and safety studies of *Cleome droserifolia. Alexandria Journal of Pharmaceutical Sciences*, Vol 24, No.1, pp. 13- 21, ISSN 1110-1792

Abdul-Hussain, S. K. & Mehendale, H. M. (1991). Studies on the age dependant effect of galactosamine in primary rat hepatocyte cultures. *Toxicology and Applied Pharmacology*, Vol 107, pp. 504–513, ISSN 0041-008X

Al-Howiriny, T. A.; Al-Sohaibani, M. O.; Al-Said, M. S.; Al-Yahya, M. A.; El-Tahir, K. H. & Rafatullah, S. (2004). Hepatoprotective properties of *Commiphora opobalsamum* (Balessan, A traditional medicinal plant of Saudi Arabia. *Drugs Under Experimental & Clinical Research*, Vol XXX, No.5/6, pp. 213- 220, ISSN 0378-6501

Ahmed, B.; Alam, T. & Khan, S. A.(2001). Hepatoprotective activity of *Luffa echinata* fruits. *Journal of Ethnopharmacology*, Vol 76, No.2 ,pp. 187–189, ISSN 0378-8741

Ahmed, B.; Al-Howiriny, T. A. & Siddiqui, A. B. (2003). Antihepatotoxic activity of seeds of *Cichorium intybus. Journal of Ethnopharmacology*, Vol 87, No. 2-3, pp. 237-240, ISSN 0378-8741

Ahsan, R., Islam, K. M.; Musaddik, A. & Haque, E. (2009). Hepatoprotective activity of methanol extract of some medicinal plants against carbon tetrachloride induced hepatotoxicity in albino rats. *Global Journal of Pharmacology*, Vol 3, No.3, pp. 116-122, ISSN 1992-0075

Akindele; A. J.; Ezenwanebe, K. O.; Anunobi, C. C. & Adeyemi, O. O. (2010). Hepatoprotective and in *vivo* antioxidant effects of *Byrsocarpus coccineus* Schum. and Thonn. (Connaraceae). *Journal of Ethnopharmacology*, Vol 129, No.1, pp. 46-52, ISSN 0378-8741

Aktay, G., Deliorman, D.; Ergun, E.; Ergun, F.; Yeşilada, E. & Cevik, C. (2000). Hepatoprotective effects of Turkish folk remedies on experimental liver injury. *Journal of Ethnopharmacology*, Vol 73, pp. 121–129, ISSN 0378-8741

Alqasoumi, S. I.; El Tahir, K. E. H.; AlSheikh, A. M. & Abdel-Kader, M. S. (2009a). Hepatoprotective Effect and Safety Studies of *Juniperus phoenicea*. *Alexandria Journal of Pharmaceutical Sciences*, Vol 23, No.2, pp. 81- 88, ISSN 1110-1792

Alqasoumi, S. I.; Al-Howiriny, T. A. & Abdel-Kader, M. S. (2008a). Evaluation of the hepatoprotective effect of *Aloe Vera, Clematis hirsute, Cucumis prophetarum* and Bee Propolis against experimentally induced liver injury in rats. *International Journal of Pharmacology*, Vol 4, No.3, pp. 213- 217, ISSN 1811-7775

Alqasoumi, S. I.; Al-Dosari, M. S.; AlSheikh, A. M. & Abdel-Kader, M. S. (2009b). Evaluation of the hepatoprotective effect of *Fumaria parviflora* and *Momordica balsamina* from Saudi Folk medicine against experimentally induced liver injury in rats. *Research Journal of Medicinal Plant*, Vol 3, No.1, pp. 9- 15, ISSN 1996-0875

Alqasoumi, S. I.; Al-Rehaily, A. J.; Abdulmalik M. AlSheikh & Abdel-Kader, M. S. (2008b). Evaluation of the hepatoprotective effect of *Ephedra foliate, Alhagi maurorum, Capsella bursa-pastoris* and *Hibiscus sabdariffa* against experimentally induced liver injury in rats. *Natural Product Sciences*, Vol 14, No.2, pp. 95-99, ISSN 1226-3907

Amat, N.; Upur, H. & Blažeković, B. (2010). In *vivo* hepatoprotective activity of the aqueous extract of *Artemisia absinthium* L. against chemically and immunologically induced liver injuries in mice. *Journal of Ethnopharmacology*, Vol 131, No.2, pp. 478–484, ISSN 0378-8741

Anusuya, N.; Raju, K. & Manian, S. (2010). Hepatoprotective and toxicological assessment of an ethnomedicinal plant *Euphorbia fusiformis* Buch.-Ham.ex D.Don. *Journal of Ethnopharmacology*, Vol 127, No.2, pp. 463–467, ISSN 0378-8741

Azri, S.; Mat, H. P.; Reid, L. L.; Gandlofi, A. J. & Brendel, K. (1992). Further examination of the selective toxicity of CCl4 rat liver silices. *Toxicology and Aplied Pharmacology*, Vol 112, No.1, pp. 81- 86, ISSN 0041-008X

Banu, G. S.; Kumar, G. & Murugesan, A. G. (2009). Effect of ethanolic leaf extract of *Trianthema portulacastrum* L. on aflatoxin induced hepatic damage in rats. *Indian Journal of Clinical Biochemistry*, Vol 24, No.4, pp. 414-418, ISSN 0970-1915

Baranisrinivasan, P.; Elumalai, E. K.; Sivakumar, C.; Therasa, S. V. & David, E. (2009). Hepatoprotective effect of *Enicostemma littorale* blume and *Eclipta alba* during ethanol induced oxidative stress in albino rats. *International Journal of Pharmacology*, Vol 5, No.4, pp. 268–272, ISSN 1811-7775

Bhadauria, M.; Nirala, S. K.; Shrivastava, S.; Sharma, A.; Johri, S.; Chandan, B. K.; Singh, B.; Saxena, A. K. & Shukla, S. (2009). Emodin reverses CCl4 induced hepaticcytochrome P450 (CYP) enzymatic and ultra structural changes: the *in vivo* evidence. *Hepatology Research*, Vol 39, No.3, 290-300, ISSN 1386-6346

Bhakta, T.; Banerjee, S.; Mandal, S. C.; Maity, T. K.; Saha, B. P. & Pal, M. (2001). Hepatoprotective activity of *Cassia fistula* leaf extract. *Phytomedicine*, Vol. 8, No.3, pp. 220-224, ISSN 0944-7113

Bhattacharyya, D.; Pandit, S.; Jana, U.; Sen, S. & Sur, T. S. (2005). Hepatoprotective activity of *Adhatoda vasica* aqueous leaf extract on d-galactosamine-induced liver damage in rats. *Fitoterapia*, Vol 76, No.2, 223- 225, ISSN 0367-326X

Billiar, T.R.; Curran, R. D.; Harbrecht, B. G.; Stuehr, D. J.; Demetris, A. J. & Simmons R. L. (1990a). Modulation of nitrogen oxide synthesis *in vivo*: NG-monomethyl-L-arginine inhibits endotoxin-induced nitrate/nitrite biosynthesis while promoting hepatic damage. *Journal of Leukocyte Biology*, Vol 48, No.6, pp. 568-569, ISSN 0741-5400

Billiar, T. R.; Curran, R. D.; Stuer, D. J.; Stadler, J.; Simmons, R. L. & Murray S. A. (1990b). Inducible cytosolic enzyme activity for the production of nitrogen oxide from L-arginine in hepatocytes. *Biochemical and Biophysical Research Communications*, Vol 168, No.3, pp. 1034-1040, ISSN 0006-291X

Boyer, T. D. (1989). The glutathione S-transferases: an update. *Hepatology*, Vol 9, No.3, pp. 486-496, ISSN 0270-9139

Castro, L. & Freeman, B. A. (2001). Reactive oxygen species in human health and disease. *Nutrition*, Vol 17, No.2, pp. 161-165, ISSN: 0899-9007

Celik, I.; Temur A. & Isik, I. (2009). Hepatoprotective role and antioxidant capacity of pomegranate (*Punica granatum*) flowers infusion against trichloroacetic acid-exposed in rats. *Food and Chemical Toxicology*, Vol 47, No.1, pp. 145-149, ISSN 0278-6915

Channabasavaraj, K. P.; Badami, S. & Bhojraj, S. (2008). Hepatoprotective and antioxidant activity of methanol extract of *Ficus glomerata*. *Journal of Natural Medicines*, Vol 62, No.3, pp. 379-383, ISSN 1340-3443

Chatterjee, T. K. (2000). *Medicinal Plants with Hepatoprotective Properties in Herbal Opinions*, Vol III. 135, Books and Allied (P) Ltd., Calcutta.

Chattopadhyay, R. R. (2003). Possible mechanism of hepatoprotective activity of *Azadirachta indica* leaf extract. Part II. *Journal of Ethnopharmacology*, Vol 89, No.2-3, pp. 217-219, ISSN 0378-8741

Chelikani, P.; Fita, I. & Loewen, P. C. (2004). Diversity of structures and properties among catalases. *Cellular and Molecular Life Sciences*, Vol 61, No.2, pp. 192-208, ISSN 1420-682X

Christian, A. J.; Saraswathy, G. R.; Robert, S. J.; Kothai, R.; Chidambaranathan, N.; Nalini, G. & Therasal R. L. (2006). Inhibition of CCl4 induced liver fibrosis by *Piper longum* Linn. *Phytomedicin*, Vol 13, pp. 196- 198, ISSN 0944-7113

Chun-Ching, L. & Wei-Chih, L. (1995). Anti-inflammatory and hepatoprotective effects of *Ventilago leiocarpa*. *Phytotherapy Research*, Vol 9, No.1, pp. 11-15. ISSN 0951-418X

Comoglio, A.; Leonarduzzi, G.; Carini, R.; Busolin, D.; Basaga, H.; Albano, E.; Tomasi, A.; Poli G.; Morazzoni, P. & Magistretti M. J. (1990). Studies on the antioxidant and free radical scavenging properties of IdB 1016: a new flavanolignan complex. *Free*

Radical Research Communications, Vol 11, No.1-3, pp. 109–115, Sons. ISSN 0951-418X

Cyong, J. C.; Ki, S. M.; Iijima, K.; Kobayashi, T. & Furuya, M. (2000). Clinical and pharmacological studies on liver diseases treated with kampo herbal medicine. *The American Journal of Chinese Medicine*, Vol 28, No.3-4, pp. 351–360, ISSN 0192-415X

Dalle-Donne, I.; Rossi, R.; Giustarini, D.; Aldo Milzani, A. & Colombo, R. (2003). Protein carbonyl groups as biomarkers of oxidative stress. *Clinica Chimica Acta*, Vol 329, No.1-2, pp. 23-38, ISSN 0009-8981

Decker, K. & Keppler, D. (1972). Galactosamine induced liver injury, In: *Progress in Liver Disease*, H. Popper; F., Schaffner (Eds.) 183–199, Grune and Stratton, New York.

Decker, K. & Keppler, D. (1974). Galactosamine hepatitis: key role of the nucleotide deficiency period in the pathogenesis of cell injury and cell death. *Reviews of Physiology, Biochemistry and Pharmacology*, Vol 71, pp. 77- 106, ISSN 0303-4240

Dehmlow, C.; Erhard, J. & de Groot, H. (1996). Inhibition of Kupffer cell functions as an explanation for the hepatoprotective properties of silibinin. *Hepatology*, Vol 23, No. 4, pp. 749–754, ISSN 0270-9139

Del Rio, D.; Stewart, A. J. & Pellegrini, N. (2005). A review of recent studies on malonaldehyde as toxic molecule and biological marker of oxidative stress. *Nutrition, Metabolism & Cardiovascular Diseases*, Vol 15, No.4, pp. 316 28, ISSN 0939-4753

Dianzani, M. U.; Muzia, G.; Biocca, M. E. & Canuto, R. A. (1991). Lipid peroxidation in fatty liver induced by caffeine in rats. *International Journal of Tissue Reaction*, Vol 13, No.1, pp. 79–85, ISSN 0250-0868

Douglas, K. T. (1987). Mechanism of action of glutathione-dependent enzymes. *Advances in Enzymology & Related Areas of Molecular Biology*, Vol 59, pp. 103–167, ISSN 0065258X

elSisi, A. E.; Earnest, D. L. & Sipes, I. G. (1993). Vitamin A potentiation of carbon tetrachloride hepatotoxicity: role of liver macrophages and active oxygen species. *Toxicology and Applied Pharmacology*, Vol 119, No.2, pp. 295–301, ISSN 0041-008X

Eriksson, L.; Broome, U., Kahn, M. & Lindholm, M. (1992). Hepatotoxicity due to repeated intake of low doses of paracetamol. *Journal of Internal Medicine*, Vol 231, No.5, pp. 567-570, ISSN 0041-008X

Esterbauer, H.; Schaur, R. J. & Zollner, H. (1991). Chemistry and biochemistry of 4-hydroxynonenal, malonaldehyde and related aldehydes. *Free Radical Biology and Medicine*, Vol 11, No.1, pp. 81–128, ISSN 0891-5849

Farmer, E. E. & Davoine, C. (2007). *Reactive electrophile species.* Current Opinion in Plant Biology, Vol 10, No.4, pp. 380- 386, *ISSN* 1369-5266

Ferenčiková, R.; Červinková, Z. & Drahota, Z. (2003). Hepatotoxic effect of D-galactosamine and protective role of lipid emulsion. *Physiological research*, Vol 52, No.1, pp. 73- 78, ISSN 0862-8408

Fiebrich, F. & Koch, H. (1979a). Silymarin, an inhibitor of lipoxygenase. *Experientia*, Vol 35, No.12, pp. 1548–1550, ISSN: 0014-4754

Fiebrich, F. & Koch, H. (1979b). Silymarin, an inhibitor of prostaglandin synthetase. *Experientia*, Vol 35, No.12, pp. 1550–1552, ISSN: 0014-4754

Field, K. M.; Dow, C. & Michael, M. (2008). Liver function in oncology: biochemistry and beyond. *The Lancet Oncolog*, Vol 9, No.11, pp. 1092–1101, ISSN 0140-6736

Fiorucci, S.; Mencarelli, A.; Palazzeti, B.; Del Soldato, P.; Morelli, A. & Ignarro, L.J. (2001). An NO-derivative of ursodeoxycholic acid protects against Fas-mediated liver injury by inhibiting caspase activity. *Proceedings of the National Academy of Sciences of the United States of America,* Vol 98, No.5, pp. 2652- 2657, ISSN 0027-8424

Fraschini, F.; Demartini, G. & Esposti, D. (2002). Pharmacology of silymarin. *Clinical Drug Investigation,* Vol 22, No.1, pp. 51–65, ISSN 1173-2563

Fredovich, I. (1997). Superoxide anion radical (O2-.), superoxide dismutases, and related matters. *The Journal of Biological Chemistry,* Vol 272, No.30, pp. 18515- 18517, ISSN 0021-9258

Fursule, R. A. & Patil, S. D. (2010). Hepatoprotective and antioxidant activity of Phaseolus trilobus, Ait on bile duct ligation induced liver fibrosis in rats. *Journal of Ethnopharmacology,* Vol 129, No.3 , pp. 416–419, ISSN 0378-8741

Gilani, A. H. & Janbaz, K. H. (1995). Preventive and curative effects of *Artemisia absinthium* on acetaminophen and CCl4-induced hepatotoxicity. *General Pharmacology,*Vol 26, No.2, pp. 309–315, ISSN 0306-3623

Gomase, P. V.; Rangari V. D. & Verma P. R. (2011). Phytochemical evaluation and hepatoprotective activity of fresh juice of young stem (tender) bark of *Azadirachta indica* A. JUSS. *International Journal of Pharmacy and Pharmaceutical Sciences,* Vol 3, Suppl 2, pp. 55- 59, ISSN 0975-1491

Gopal, N. & Sengottuvelu, S. (2008). Hepatoprotective activity of Clerodendrum inerme against CCL4 induced hepatic injury in rats. *Fitoterapia,* Vol 79, No.1, pp. 24– 26, ISSN 0367-326X

Gupta, A. K. & Misra, N. (2006). Hepatoprotective Activity of Aqueous Ethanolic Extract of *Chamomile capitula* in Paracetamol Intoxicated Albino Rats. *American Journal of Pharmacology and Toxicology,* Vol 1, No.1, pp. 17-20, ISSN 1557-4962

Hahn, G.; Lehmann, H. D.; Kurten, M.; Ubel, H. & Vogel, G. (1968). Zur Pharmakologie und Toxikologie von Silymarin, des antihepatotoxischen Wirkprinzipes aus *Silybum marianum* (L.) Gaertn. *Arzneimittelforschung,* Vol 18, pp. 698– 704, ISSN 0004-4172

Handa, S. S.; Sharma, A. & Chakarborti, K. K. (1986). Natural products and plants as liver protecting drugs. *Fitoterapia,* Vol 57, No.5, pp. 307–351, ISSN 0367-326X

Harish, R. & Shivanandappa T. (2006). Antioxidant activity and hepatoprotective potential of *Phyllanthus niruri. Food Chemistry,* Vol 95, No.2 ,pp. 180– 185, ISSN 0308-8146

Hernandez-Munoz, R.; Diaz-Munoz, M.; Suarez-Cuenca, J. A.; Trejo-Solis, C.; Lopez, V.; Sanchez-Sevilla, L.; Yanez, L. & De Sanches, V. C. (2001). Adenosine reverses a preestablished CCl4-induced micronodular cirrhosis through enhancing collagenolytic activity and stimulating hepatocyte cell proliferation in rats. *Hepatology,* Vol 34, No.4, pp. 677– 687, ISSN 0270-9139

Hong, Z.; Chen, W.; Zhao, J.; Wu, Z.; Zhou, J. H.; Li, T. & Hu J. (2010). Hepatoprotective effects of *Rubus aleaefolius* Poir. And identification of its active constituents. *Journal of Ethnopharmacology,* Vol 129, No.2, pp. 267– 272, ISSN 0378-8741

Hu, H. L. & Chen, R. D. (1992). Changes in free radicals, trace elements, by d-galactosamine. *Biological Trace Element Research,* Vol 34, No.1 ,pp. 19– 25, ISSN 0163-4984

Huang, B.; Ban, X.; He, J.; Tong, H.; Zhang, J.; Tian, J. & Wang, Y. (2010a). Hepatoprotective and antioxidant activity of ethanolicextracts of edible lotus (*Nelumbo nucifera* Gaertn.) leaves. *Food Chemistry,* Vol 120, No.3, pp. 873–878, ISSN 0308-8146

Huang, B.; Ban, X.; He, J.; Zeng, H.; Zhang, P. & Wang, Y. (2010b). Hepatoprotective and antioxidant effects of the methanolic extract from *Halenia elliptica*. *Journal of Ethnopharmacology*, Vol 131, No.2, pp. 276– 281, ISSN 0378-8741

Ip, S.-P.; Woo, K.-Y.; Lau, O.-W. & Che1, C.-T. (2004). Hepatoprotective Effect of *Sabina przewalskii* against Menadione-induced Toxicity. *Phytotherapy Research*, Vol 18, No.4, pp. 329–331, ISSN 0951-418X

Iyer, R.S.; Voehler, M.W. & Harris, T.M. (1994). Adenine adduct of Aflatoxin B1 epoxide. *J. Am. Chem. Soc.*, Vol 116, No.20, pp. 8863–8869, ISSN 0002-7863

Jain, A.; Soni, M.; Deb, L.; Jain, A.; Rout, S. P.; Gupta, V. B. & Krishna, K. L. (2008). Antioxidant and hepatoprotective activity of ethanolic and aqueous extracts of *Momordica dioica* Roxb. Leaves. *Journal of Ethnopharmacology*, Vol 115, No.1, pp. 61–66, ISSN 0378-8741

Jaishree, V. & Badami, S. (2010). Antioxidant and hepatoprotective effect of swertiamarin from Enicostemma axillare against d-galactosamine induced acute liver damage in rats. *Journal of Ethnopharmacology*, Vol 130, No.1, pp. 103– 106, ISSN 0378-8741

Jamshidzadeh, A.; Fereidooni, F.; Salehi, Z. & Niknahad, H. (2005). Hepatoprotective activity of *Gundelia tourenfortii*. *Journal of Ethnopharmacology*, Vol 101, No.1-3, pp. 233-237, ISSN 0378-8741

Karthikeyan, M. & Deepa, K. (2010). Hepatoprotective effect of *Premna corymbosa* (Burn. F.) Rottl. & Willd. Leaves extract on CCl_4 induced hepatic damage in Wistar albino rats. *Asian Pacific Journal of Tropical Medicine*, Vol 3, No.1, pp. 17– 20, ISSN 16879686

Keppler, D. O.; Rudigier, J. F.; Bischoff, E. & Decker, K. (1970). The trapping of uridine phosphates by d-galactosamine, d-glucosamine, and 2-deoxy-d-galactose.Astudy on the mechanism of galactosamine hepatitis. *European Journal of Biochemistry*, Vol 17, No.2, pp. 246– 253, ISSN 0014-2956

Kim, W. R.; Brown, R. S.; Terrault, N. A. & El-Serag, H. (2002). Burden of liver disease in the United States: Summary of work-Shop. *Hepatology*, Vol 36, No.1, pp. 227-242, ISSN 0270-9139

Khatri, A.; Garg, A. & Agrawal, S. A. (2009). Evaluation of hepatoprotective activity of aerial parts of *Tephrosia purpurea* L. and stem bark of *Tecomella undulate*. *Journal of Ethnopharmacology*, Vol 122, No.1, pp. 1–5, ISSN 0378-8741

Kmieć, Z.; Ryszard Smoleński, R. T.; Zysh, M. & Myśliwski, A. (2000). The effects of galactosamine on UTP levels in the livers of young, adult and old rats. *Acta Biochimica Polonica*, Vol 47, No.2, pp. 349- 353, ISSN 0001-527X

Kumar, S. S.; Kumar, B. R. & Mohan G. K. (2009). Hepatoprotective effect of *Trichosanthes cucumerina* Var *cucumerina* L. on carbon tetrachloride induced liver damage in rats. *Journal of Ethnopharmacology*, Vol 123, No.2, pp. 347–350, ISSN 0378-8741

Leaver, M. J. & George, S. G. (1998). A piscine glutathione S-transferase which efficiently conjugates the end-products of lipid peroxidation. *Marine Environmental Research*, Vol 46, No.1-5, pp. 71–74, ISSN 0141-1136

Madubunyi, I. I. (2010). Hepatoprotective activity of *Uvaria chamae* root bark methanol extract against acetaminophen-induced liver lesions in rats. *Comparative Clinical Pathology*, In Press, ISSN 1618-5641

Maheswari, M. U. & Rao, P. G. M. (2005). Anti hepatotoxic effect of grape seed oil. *Indian Journal of Pharmacology*, Vol 37, No.3, pp. 179- 182, ISSN 0253-7613

Marina, N. (2006). Hepatotoxicity of antiretrovirals: incidence, mechanisms and management. *Journal of Hepatology*, Vol 44, No.1, pp. S132–S139, ISSN 0168-8278

McConnachie, L. A.; Mohar, I.; Hudson, F. N.; Ware, C. B.; Ladiges, W. C.; Fernandez, C.; Chatterton-Kirchmeier, S.; White, C. C.; Pierce, R. H. & Kavanagh, T. J. (2007). Glutamate cysteine ligase modifier subunit deficiency and gender as determinants of acetaminophen-induced hepatotoxicity in mice. *Toxicological Scinces*, Vol 99, No.2, pp. 628–636, ISSN 1096-6080

McCuskey, R. S. (2006). Anatomy of the liver. In: *Zakim and Boyer's Hepatology*, T. D. Boyer; T. L. Wright; M. Manns, (Eds.), 37, 5th ed., Saunders–Elsevier, Philadephia.

Mitchell, J. R.; Jollow, D. J.; Potter, W. Z.; Gillete, J. R. & Brrodle, B.N. (1973). Acetaminophen induced hepatic necrosis. I. Role of drug metabolism. *Journal of Pharmacology and Experimental Therapeutics*, Vol 187, No.1, pp. 185–194, ISSN 0022-3565

Mohamed, M. A.; Marzouk, M. S. A.; Moharram, F. A.; El-Sayed, M. M. & Baiuomy A. R. (2005). Phytochemical constituents and hepatoprotective activity of *Viburnum tinus*. *Phytochemistry*, Vol 66, No.23, pp. 2780–2786, ISSN 1819-3471

Moncada, S. & Erusalimsky, J. D. (2002). Does nitric oxide modulate mitochrondrial energy generation and apoptosis? *Nature Reviews Molecular Cell Biology*, Vol 3, pp. 214–220, ISSN 1471-0072

Morazzoni, P. & Bombardelli, E. (1995). *Silybum marianum. Fitoterapia*, Vol 66, No.1, pp. 3–42, ISSN 0367-326X

Morikawa, T.; Pan, Y.; Ninomiya, K.; Imura, K.; Matsuda, H.; Yoshikawa, M.; Yuan, D. & Muraoka, O. (2010). Acylated phenylethanoid oligoglycosides with hepatoprotective activity from the desert plant *Cistanche tubulosa. Bioorganic & Medicinal Chemistry*, Vol 18, No.5, pp. 1882–1890, ISSN 0960-894X

Naaz, F.; Javed, S. & Abdin, M. Z. (2007). Hepatoprotective effect of ethanolic extract of *Phyllanthus amarus* Schum. et Thonn. on aflatoxin B1-induced liver damage in mice. *Journal of Ethnopharmacology*, Vol 113, No.3, pp. 503–509, ISSN 0378-8741

Navarro, V. J. & Senior, J. R. (2006). Drug-related hepatotoxicity. *New England Journal of Medicine*, Vol 35, No.4, pp. 731–739, ISSN 0028-4793

Nishigaki, I.; Kuttan, R.; Oku, H.; Ashoori, F.; Abe, H. & Yagi, K. (1992). Suppressive effect of curcumin on lipid peroxidation induced in rats by CCl_4 or ^{60}Co irradiation. *Journal of Clinical Biochemistry and Nutrition*, Vol 13, pp. 23- 30, ISSN 0912-0009

Noh J.-R.; Kim, Y.-H.; Gang, G.-T.; Hwang, J. H.; Lee, H.-S.; Ly, S,-Y.; Oh, W.-K.; Song, K.-S.& Lee, C.-H. (2011). Hepatoprotective effects of chestnut (*Castanea crenata*) inner shell extract against chronic ethanol-induced oxidative stress in C57BL/6 mice. *Food and Chemical Toxicology*, In Press, ISSN 0278-6915

Nussler, A.; DiSilvio, M.; Billiar, T. R.; Hoffman, R. A.; Geller, D. A.; Selby, R.; Madariaga, J. & Simmons R. L. (1992). Stimulation of the nitric oxide synthase pathway in human hepatocytes by cytokines and endotoxin. *Journal of Experimental Medicine*, Vol 176, pp. 261-264, ISSN 0022-1007

Nyblom, H.; Berggren, U.; Balldin, J. & Olsson, R. (2004). High AST/ALT ratio may indicate advanced alcoholic liver disease rather than heavy drinking. *Alcohol & Alcoholism*, Vol 39, No.4, pp. 336- 339, ISSN 0735-0414

Obioha, U. E.; Suru, S. M.; Ola-Mudathir, K. F. & Faremi, T. Y. (2009). Hepatoprotective potentials of Onion and Garlic extracts on Cadmium-Induced oxidative damage in rats. *Biological Trace Element Research*, Vol 129, No.1-3, pp. 143–156, ISSN 0163-4984

Olinescu, R.; Alexandrescu, R.; Hulea, S. A. & Kummerow, F. A. (1994). Tissue lipid peroxidation may be triggered by increased formation of bilirubin *in vivo*. *Research Communications in Chemical Pathology & Pharmacology*, Vol 84, No.1, pp. 27-34, ISSN 0034-5164

Owvens, D. & Evans, J. (1975). Population studies on Gilbert's syndrome. *Journal of Chemical Genetics*, Vol 12, pp. 152- 156, ISSN 0104-6632

Özbek, H.; Çitoğlu, G. S.; Dülger, H.; Uğraş, S. & Sever, B. (2004). Hepatoprotective and anti-inflammatory activities of *Ballota glandulosissima*. *Journal of Ethnopharmacology*, Vol 95, No.2-3, pp. 143–149, ISSN 0378-8741

Palmer, R. M. J.; Ashton, D. S.; & Moncada, S. (1988). Vascular endothelial cells synthesis nitric oxide from L-arginine. *Nature*, Vol 333, No.6174, pp. 664-666, ISSN 0028-0836

Pastore, A.; Piemonte, F.; Locatelli, M.; Russo, A. L.; Gaeta, L. M.; Tozzi, G.& Federici, G. (2003). Determination of blood total, reduced, and oxidized glutathione in pediatric subjects. *Clinical Chemistry*, Vol 47, No.8, pp. 1467–1469, ISSN 0009-9147

Perry, G.; Raina, A. K.; Nunomura, A.; Wataya T.; Sayre, L. M. & Smith M. A. (2000). How important is oxidative damage? Lessons from Alzheimer's disease. *Free Radical Biology and Medicine*, Vol 28, No.5, pp. 831-834, ISSN 0891-5849

Pompella, A.; Visvikis, A.; Paolicchi, A.; de Tata, V. & Casini, A. F. (2003). The changing faces of glutathione, a cellular protagonist. *Biochemical Pharmacology*, Vol 66, No.8, pp. 1499–503, ISSN 0006-2952

Porchezhian, E. & Ansari, S. H. (2005). Hepatoprotective activity of *Abutilon indicum* on experimental liver damage in rats. *Phytomedicine*, Vol 12, No.1-2, pp. 62–64, ISSN 0944-7113

Pramyothin, P.; Ngamtin, C.; Poungshompoo, S. & Chaichantipyuth, C. (2007). Hepatoprotective activity of *Phyllanthus amarus* Schum. et. Thonn. extract in ethanol treated rats: *In vitro* and *in vivo* studies. *Journal of Ethnopharmacology*, Vol 114, No.2, pp. 169–173, ISSN 0378-8741

Prophet, E. P.; Mills, B.; Arrington, J. B. & Sobin, L. H. (1994). *Laboratory Methods in Histology*. 1st Ed, American Registry of Pathology, Washington, D.C.

Purohit, V.; Gao, B. & Song, B.-J. (2009). Molecular Mechanisms of Alcoholic Fatty Liver. *Alcohol.: Clin. Exp. Res.*, Vol 33, No.2, pp. 191–205, ISSN 1530-0277

Quintero, A.; Pedraza, C. A.; Siendones, E.; Kamal, E. A. M.; Colell, A.; García -Ruiz, C.; Montero, J. L.; Dela, M. M.; Fernández-Checa, J. C.; Miño, G.; Muntane´ , J.; Kamal, E. A. M. & Colell, A. (2002). PGE1 protection against apoptosis induced by D-galactosamine is not related to the modulation of intracellular free radical production in primary culture of rat hepatocytes. *Free Radical Research*, Vol 36, No.3, pp. 345–355, ISSN 1071-5762

Qureshi, N. N.; Kuchekar, B. S.; Logade, N. A. & Haleem, M. A. (2009). Antioxidant and hepatoprotective activity of *Cordia macleodii* leaves. *Saudi Pharmaceutical Journal*, Vol 17, No.4, pp. 299- 302, ISSN 1319-0164

Rafatullah, S.; Al-Sheikh, A.; Alqasoumi, S.; Al-Yahya, M.; El-Tahir, K. & Galal, A. (2008). Protective effect of fresh radish juice (*Raphanus sativus* L.) against carbon tetrachloride-induced hepatotoxicity. *International Journal of Pharmacology*, Vol 4, No.2, pp. 130- 134. ISSN 1811-7775.

Rafatullah, S.; Mossa, J. S.; Ageel, A. M.; Al-Yahya, M. A. & Tariq, M. (1991). Hepatoprotective and safety evaluation studies on Sarsaparilla. *International Journal of Pharmacognosy (Now Pharmaceutical Biology)*, Vol 29, No.4, pp. 296- 301, ISSN 1388-0209

Ram, V. J. (2001). Herbal preparations as a source of hepatoprotective agents. *Drug News and Perspective*, Vol 14, No.6, pp. 353-363. ISSN 0214-0934

Ranawat, L.; Bhatt, J. & Patel J. (2010). Hepatoprotective activity of ethanolic extracts of bark of *Zanthoxylum armatum* DC in CCl4 induced hepatic damage in rats. *Journal of Ethnopharmacology*, Vol 127, No.3, pp. 777–780, ISSN 0378-8741

Rao, P. G. M.; Rao, S. G. & Kumar, V. (1993). Effects of hepatogard against carbon tetrachloride induced liver damage in rats. *Fitoterapia*, Vol 64, No.2, pp. 108-113, ISSN 0367-326X

Rathi, M. A.; Thirumoorthi, L.; Sunitha, M.; Meenakshi, P.; Gurukumar, D. & Gopalakrishnan, V. K. (2010). Hepatoprotective activity of *Spermacoce hispida* Linn. extract against nitrobenzene induced hepatotoxicity in rats. (2010). *Journal of Herbal Medicine and Toxicology*, Vol 4, No.2, pp. 201-205, ISSN 0973-4643.

Rathi, A., Srivastava, A. K.; Shirwaikar, A.; Rawat, A. K. S. & Mehrotra S. (2008). Hepatoprotective potential of *Fumaria indica* Pugsley whole plant extracts, fractions and an isolated alkaloid protopine. *Phytomedicine*, Vol 15, pp. 470– 477, ISSN 0944-7113

RCSB Protein Data Bank. Catalase. *Molecule of the Month*. (2004-09-01). Retrieved on 2007-02-11, http://www.pdb.org/pdb/101/motm.do?momID=57

Recknagel, R. O. & Glende, E. A. Jr. (1973). Carbon tetrachloride hepatotoxicity: an example of lethal cleavage. CRC (*Critical Reviews in Toxicology*). Vol. 2, No.3, pp. 263-297, ISSN 1040-8444

Recknagel, R. O.; Glonde, E. A.; Dolak, J. A. & Walter, R. L. (1989). Mechanism of carbon tetrachloride toxicity. *Pharmacology and Therapeutics*, Vol 43, No.1, pp. 139–154, ISSN 0163-7258

Remirez, D.; Commandeur, J. N. M.; Ed Groot, E. & Vermeulen, N. P. E. (1995). Mechanism of protection of *Lobenzarti* against paracetamol-induced toxicity in rat hepatocytes. *European Journal of Pharmacology: Environmental Toxicology and Pharmacology*, Vol 293, No.4, pp. 301- 308, ISSN 0926-6917

Rivett, A. J. & Levine, R. L. (1990): Metal-catalyzed oxidation of Escherichia coli glutamine synthetase: correlation of structural and functional changes. *Archives of Biochemistry and Biophysics*. Vol 278, No.1, pp. 26- 34, ISSN 0003-9861

Sabir, S. M.& Rocha, J. B. T. (2008). Antioxidant and hepatoprotective activity of aqueous extract of *Solanum fastigiatum* (false "Jurubeba") against paracetamol-induced liver damage in mice. *Journal of Ethnopharmacology*, Vol 120, No.2, pp. 226– 232, ISSN 0378-8741

Sadasivan, S.; Latha, P. G.; Sasikumar, J. M.; Rajashekaran, S.; Shyamal, S. & Shine, V. J. (2006). Hepatoprotective studies on *Hedyotis corymbosa* (L.) Lam. *Journal of Ethnopharmacology*, Vol 106, No.2, pp. 245– 249, ISSN 0378-8741

Saller, R.; Melzer, J.; Reichling, J.; Brignoli, R. & Meier, R. (2007). An updated systematic review of the pharmacology of silymarin. *Forschende Komplementmedizin (Research in Complementary Medicine)*, Vol 14, No.2, pp. 70- 80, ISSN 1661-4119

Sallie, R.; Tredger, J. M. & William, R. (1991). *Drugs and the liver. Part I. Testing liver function. Biopharmaceutics & Drug Disposition*, Vol 12, No.4, pp. 251- 259, ISSN 0142-2782

Salmi, H. A. & Sarna S. (1982). Effect of silymarin on chemical, functional, and morphological alterations of the liver. A double-blind controlled study. *Scandinavian Journal of Gastroenterology*, Vol17, No.4, pp. 517- 521, ISSN 0036-5521

Sathaye, S., Bagul, Y.; Gupta, S.; Kaur, H. & Roopali Redkar, R. (2010). Hepatoprotective effects of aqueous leaf extract and crude isolates of *Murraya koenigii* against *in vitro* ethanol-induced hepatotoxicity model. *Experimental and Toxicologic Pathology*, In Press, ISSN 0940-2993

Scott, M. D.; Lubin, B. H.; Zuo, L. & Kuypers, F. A. (1991). Erythro-cyte defense against hydrogen peroxide: preeminent importance of catalase. *Journal of Laboratory and Clinical Medicine*, Vol 118, No.1, 7- 16, ISSN 0022-2143

Sen, T.; Basu, A.; Ray, R. N. & Nag Shaudhuri, A. K. (1993). Hepatoprotective effects of *Pluchea indica* (Lees) extract in experimental acute liver damage in rodents. *Phytotherapy Research*, Vol 7, No.5, pp. 352-355, ISSN 0951-418X

Setty, S. R.; Quereshi, A. A.; Swamy, A. H. M. V.; Patil, T.; Prakash, T.; Prabhu, K. & Gouda, A. V. (2007). Hepatoprotective activity of *Calotropis procera* flowers against paracetamol-induced hepatic injury in rats. *Fitoterapia*, Vol 78, pp. 451- 454, ISSN 0367-326X

Shankar, N. L. G.; Manavalan, R.; Venkappayya, D. & Raj, C. D. (2008). Hepatoprotective and antioxidant effects of *Commiphora berryi* (Arn) Engl bark extract against CCl4-induced oxidative damage in rats. *Food and Chemical Toxicology*, Vol 46, No.9, pp. 3182- 3185, ISSN 0278-6915

Shanmugasundaram, P. & Venkataraman, S. (2006). Hepatoprotective and anti oxidant effects of *Hygrophila Auriculta* (K. Schum) Heine Acanthaceae root extract. *Journal of Ethnopharmacology*, Vol 104, No.1-2, pp. 124- 128, ISSN 0378-8741

Sharma, N. & Shukla, S. (2010). Hepatoprotective potential of aqueous extract of *Butea monosperma* against CCl4 induced damageinrats. *Experimental and Toxicologic Pathology*, In Press, ISSN 0940-2993

Shi, J.; Aisaki, K.; Ikawa, Y. & Wake, K., (1998). Evidence of hepatocyte apoptosis in rat liver after administration of carbon tetrachloride. *American Journal of Pathology*, Vol 153, No.2, 515- 525, ISSN 0002-9440

Shi, Y.; Sun J.; He, H.; Guo, H. & Zhang, S. (2008). Hepatoprotective effects of *Ganoderma lucidum* peptides against d-galactosamine-induced liver injury in mice. *Journal of Ethnopharmacology*, Vol 117, No.3, pp. 415- 419, ISSN 0378-8741

Shilova, I. V.; Zhavoronok, T. V.; Souslov, N. I.; Novozheeva, T. P.; Mustafin, R. N. & Losseva, A. M. (2008). Hepatoprotective Properties of Fractions from Meadowsweet Extract during Experimental Toxic Hepatitis. *Bulletin of Experimental Biology and Medicine, Pharmacology and Toxicology*, Vol. 146, No.1, pp. 49- 51, ISSN 1535-3702

Shiratori, Y.; Kawase, T.; Shiina, S.; Okano, K.; Sugimoto, T.; Teraoka, H.; Matano, S.; Matsumoto, K. & Kamii, K. (1988). Modulation of hepatotoxicity by macrophages in the liver. *Hepatology*, Vol 8, No.4, pp. 815- 821, ISSN 0270-9139

Shyamal, S.; Latha, P. G.; Shine, V. J.; Suja, S. R.; Rajasekharan S. & Devi, T. G. (2006). Hepatoprotective effects of *Pittosporum neelgherrense* Wight&Arn., a popular Indian ethnomedicine. *Journal of Ethnopharmacology*, Vol 107, No.1, pp. 151– 155, ISSN 0378-8741

Singh, B; Saxena, A. K.; Chandan, B. K.; Agrawal, S. G. & Anand, K. K. (2001). In vivo hepatoprotective activity of active fraction from ethanolic extract of *Eclipta alba* leaves. *Indian Journal of Physiology and Pharmacology*, Vol 45, No.4, pp. 435– 441, ISSN 0019-5499

Slater, T. F. (1965). *Biochemical mechanism of liver injury*. London: Academic Press.

Snyder, R. & Andrews, L. S. (1996). Toxic effects of solvents and vapors. In: *Toxicology: the Basic Science of Poisons*, C. D. Klassen, (Ed.), 737–772, McGraw-Hill, New York.

Somasundaram, A.; Karthikeyan, R.; Velmurugan, V.; Dhandapani, B. & Raja, M. (2010). Evaluation of hepatoprotective activity of *Kyllinga nemoralis* (Hutch & Dalz) rhizomes. *Journal of Ethnopharmacology*, Vol 127, No.2, pp. 555– 557, ISSN 0378-8741

Souza, M. F.; Rao, V. S. N. & Silveira, E. R. (1997). Inhibition of lipid peroxidation by ternatin, a tetramethoxyflavone from *Egletes viscosa* L. *Phytomedicine*, Vol 4, pp. 25– 9, ISSN 0944-7113

Sreedevi, C. D.; Latha, P. G.; Ancy, P.; Suja, S. R.; Shyamal, S.; Shine, V. J.; Sini, S.; Anuja, G. I. & Rajasekharan, S. (2009). Hepatoprotective studies on *Sida acuta* Burm. f. *Journal of Ethnopharmacology*, Vol 124, No.2, pp. 171– 175, ISSN 0378-8741

Subramoniam, A. & Pushpangadan, P. (1999). Development of phytomedicine for liver diseases. *Indian Journal of Pharmacology*, Vol 31, No.3, pp. 166–175, ISSN 0253-7613

Suja, S. R.; Latha, P. G.; Pushpangadan, P. & Rajasekharan, S. (2004). Evaluation of hepatoprotective effects of *Helminthostachys zeylanica* (L.) Hook against carbon tetrachloride-induced liver damage in Wistar rats. *Journal of Ethnopharmacology*, Vol 92, No.1, pp. 61– 66, ISSN 0378-8741

Suzuki, I.; Tanaka, H.; Yajima, H.; Fukuda, H.; Sezaki, H.; Koga, K.; Hirobe, M. & Nakajima, T. (1990). *Pharmaceutical Research and Development*, Vol 19, 227, Hirokawa Publishing, Tokyo.

Tandogan, B. & Ulusu, N. N. (2006). Kinetic Mechanism and Molecular Properties of Glutathione Reductas, *FABAD Journal of Pharmaceutical Sciences*, Vol 31, pp. 230-237. ISSN 1300-4182.

Tandon, V. R.; Khajuria, V.; Kapoor, B.; Kour, D. & Gupta, S. (2008). Hepatoprotective activity of *Vitex negundo* leaf extract against anti-tubercular drugs induced hepatotoxicity. *Fitoterapia*, Vol 79, pp. 533– 538, ISSN 0367-326X

Tiegs, G., Wolter, M. & Wendel, A. (1989). Tumor necrosis factor is a terminal mediator in galactosamine/endotoxin-induced hepatitis in mice. *Biochemical Pharmacology*, Vol 38, No.4, pp. 627– 631, ISSN 0006-2952

Udomsinprasert, R.; Pongjaroenkit, S.; Wongsantichon, J.; Oakley, A. J.; Prapanthadara, L. A.; Wilce, M. C. & Ketterman, A. J. (2005). Identification, characterization and structure of a new Delta class glutathione transferase isoenzyme. *Biochemical Journal*, Vol 388, No.3, pp. 763 – 771, ISSN 0264-6021

Vaca, C. E.; Wilhelm, J. & Harms-Rihsdahl, M. (1988). Interaction of lipid peroxidation product with DNA. A review. *Mutation Research-Reviews in Genetic Toxicology*, Vol 195, No.2, pp. 137– 149, ISSN 0165-1110

Valarmathi, R.; Rajendran, A.; Gopal, V.; Senthamarai, R.; Akilandeswari, S. & Srileka, B. (2010). Protective Effcet of the whole plant of *Mollugo pentaphylla* Linn. against Carbon Tetrachloride induced Hepatotoxicity in Rats. *International Journal of PharmTech Research*, Vol 2, No.3, pp. 1658-1661, ISSN 0974-4304

Venkatesh, P.; Dinakar, A. & Senthilkumar, N. (2011). Hepatoptotective activity of an ethanolic extract of stems of *Anisochilus carnosus* against carbon tetrachloride induced hepatotoxicity in rats. *International Journal of Pharmacy and Pharmaceutical Sciences*, Vol 3, No.1, pp. 243- 245, ISSN- 0975-1491

Vogel, G. (1977). Natural substances with effects on the liver, In: *New natural products and plant drugs with pharmacological, biological or therapeutic activity*. H. Wagner & P. Wolff (eds), pp 249–265, Springer-Verlag, Berlag, Heidelberg, New York.

Wagner, H.; Seligmann, O.; Horhammer, L. & Munster, R. (1968). The chemistry of silymarin (silybin), the active principle of the fruits of *Silybum marianum* (L.) Gaertn. [*Carduus marianus* (L.)]. *Arzneimittelforschung*, Vol 18, No.6, pp. 688– 696, ISSN 0004-4172

Wang, M. Y.; Liu, Q.; Che, Q. M. & Lin, Z. B. (2000). Effects of triterpenoids from *Ganoderma lucidum* (Leyss. Ex fr.) karst on three different experimental liver injury models in mice. *Acta Pharmaceutica Sinica*, Vol 35, No.5, pp. 326– 329, ISSN 0513-4870

Wang, N.; Li, P.; Wang, Y.; Peng, W.; Wu, Z.; Tan, S.; Liang, S.; Shen, X. & Su, W. (2008). Hepatoprotective effect of *Hypericum japonicum* extract and its fractions. *Journal of Ethnopharmacology*, Vol 116, No.1, pp. 1– 6, ISSN 0378-8741

Ward, F. M. & Daly, M. J. (1999). Hepatic Disease. In: *Clinical Pharmacy and Therapeutics*, R. Walker & C.Edwards (Eds.), 195- 212, Churchill Livingstone, New York.

Weber, L.W.; Boll, M. & Stampfl, A. (2003). Hepatotoxicity and mechanism of action of haloalkanes: carbon tetrachloride as a toxicological model. *Critical Reviews in Toxicology*, Vol 33, No.2, pp. 105– 136, ISSN 1040-8444

Wills, P. J. & Asha, V. V. (2006). Protective effect of *Lygodium.exuosum* (L.) Sw. (Lygodiaceae) against d-galactosamine induced liver injury in rats. *Journal of Ethnopharmacology*, Vol 108, No.1, pp. 116–123, ISSN 0378-8741

Witte, I.; Berlin, J.; Wray, V.; Schubert, W.; Kohl, W.; Hofle, G. & Hammer, J. (1983). Mono and diterpins from cell culture or *Thuja Occidenalis*. *Planta Medica*, Vol 49, pp. 216-221, ISSN 00320943

Wu, Y.; Yang, L.; Wang, F.; Wu, X.; Zhou, C.; Shi, S.; Mo, J. & Zhao, Y. (2007). Hepatoprotective and antioxidative effects of total phenolics from *Laggera pterodonta* on chemical-induced injury in primary cultured neonatal rat hepatocytes. *Food and Chemical Toxicology*, Vol 45, No.8, pp. 1349– 1355, ISSN 0278-6915

Ye, X.; Feng, Y.; Tong, Y.; Ng, K.-M.; Tsao, S.; Lau, G. K. K.; Sze, C.; Zhang, Y.; Tang, J.; Shen, J. & Kobayashi, S. (2009). Hepatoprotective effects of *Coptidis rhizoma* aqueous extract on carbon tetrachloride-induced acute liver hepatotoxicity in rats. *Journal of Ethnopharmacology*, Vol 124, No.1, pp. 130– 136, ISSN 0378-8741

Yen, F.-L.; Wu, T.-H.; Lin, L.-T. & Lin, C.-C. (2007). Hepatoprotective and antioxidant effects of *Cuscuta chinensis* against acetaminophen-induced hepatotoxicity in rats. *Journal of Ethnopharmacology*, Vol 111, No.1, pp. 123–128, ISSN 0378-8741

Yuan, H.-D., Jin, G.-Z. & Piao, G.-C. (2010). Hepatoprotective effects of an active part from *Artemisia sacrorum* Ledeb. against acetaminophen-induced toxicity in mice. *Journal of Ethnopharmacology*, Vol 127, No.2, pp. 528– 533, ISSN 0378-8741

Zafar, R. & Ali, S. M. (1998). Anti-hepatotoxic effects of root and root callus extracts of *Cichorium intybus* L. *Journal of Ethnopharmacology*, Vol 63, No.3, pp. 227–231, ISSN 0378-8741

Zhou, D.; Ruan, J.; Cai, Y.; Xiong, Z.; Fu, W. & Wei, A. (2010). Antioxidant and hepatoprotective activity of ethanol extract of *Arachniodes exilis* (Hance) Ching. *Journal of Ethnopharmacology*, Vol 129, No.2, pp. 232– 237, ISSN 0378-8741

Zimmerman, H. J. & Seeff, L. B. (1970). Enzymes in hepatic disease. In: *Diagnostic Enzymology*. E. I. Goodly (Ed.), 1, Lea and Febiger, Philadelphia, USA.

14

The Dichapetalins
– Unique Cytotoxic Constituents
of the Dichapetalaceae

Dorcas Osei-Safo[1], Mary A. Chama[1],
Ivan Addae-Mensah[1] and Reiner Waibel[2]
[1]Chemistry Department, University of Ghana, Legon,
[2]Institute of Pharmacy and Food Chemistry,
Department of Pharmaceutical Chemistry, University of Erlangen,
[1]Ghana,
[2]Germany

1. Introduction

The Dichapetalaceae (syn. Chailletiaceae) is a small family of plants comprising 3 genera and about 165 species. *Dichapetalum* Thouars is the most prominent genus, with 124 species, and is mostly found in the world's tropical and subtropical regions. Irvine lists eight species as occurring in West Africa and Ghana. *D. madagascariensis* (syn. *D. guineense*) and *D. toxicarium* are the commonest and most widely distributed (Irvine, 1961). Hall and Swaine also describe eight species as occurring in Ghana and other parts of West Africa, four of which - *D. barteri*, *D. crassifolium*, *D. filicaule* and *D. heudelotii* - were not mentioned by Irvine. The first two are likely to be new species identified after Irvine. According to Hall and Swaine, *D. heudelotii* includes *D. johnstonii* and *D. kumansiense* which appear on Irvine's list while *D. filicaule* also includes *D. cymulosum* described by Irvine (Hall and Swaine, 1981). Irvine's *D. oblongum* is not mentioned by Hall and Swaine. Several species of the *Dichapetalum* are poisonous to livestock due to the presence of fluorinated compounds, mainly fluorocarboxylic acids (Hall, 1972; O'Hagan *et al.*, 1993). These include *D. toxicarium*, *D. cymosum*, *D. tomentosum* and to a lesser extent *D. barteri*.

D. madagascariensis is one of the less toxic species of the genus. It can grow up to 25m high and about 1.5m in girth. The bark is dry and stringy and peels off in scales. Drooping oval-shaped smooth leaves are arranged alternately in branchlets and grow to about 8 - 16cm long and are 3 - 7cm broad. The numerous tiny flowers occurring in dense heads are yellowish-white in colour and are also fragrant. The orange-yellow ripe fruits are spherical in shape (Irvine, 1961). In the various tropical African communities where it occurs, *D. madagascariensis* finds use in traditional and folk medicine for the treatment of viral hepatitis, jaundice (Lewis and Elvin-Lewis, 1977), sores and urethritis (Burkill, 1985). The fruit pulp and seeds are edible while the plant wood, due to its hardness, is used for domestic purposes (Irvine, 1961).

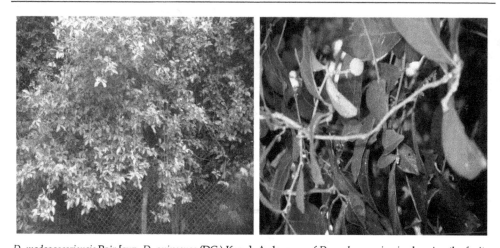

D. madagascariensis Poir [syn. *D. guineense* (DC.) Keay]   A close-up of *D. madagascariensis*, showing the fruit

D. gelonioides (Roxb.) **Engler** [syn. *Moacurra gelonioides* Roxb.] represents another of the less toxic species and it occurs in wet evergreen forests of South East Asia. In the Philippines, it is reported as treatment for amenorrhea (Fang *et al.* 2006).

Recent separate investigations of *D. madagascariensis* and *D. gelonioides* have led to the isolation and characterization of a novel and unique class of triterpenoids in which a 2-phenylpyrano moiety is annellated to ring A of a dammarane-triterpene skeleton. Biogenetically, their basic structure is characterized by the addition of a C_6-C_2 unit, which might probably be derived from the shikimic acid pathway, to a 13, 30-cyclodammarane-type skeleton (Figure 1). Thirteen dichapetalins, named dichapetalins A – M, have so far been isolated from these two species of the Dichapetalaceae (Achenbach *et al.*, 1995; Addae-Mensah *et al.*, 1996; Fang *et al.* 2006; Osei-Safo *et al.* 2008).

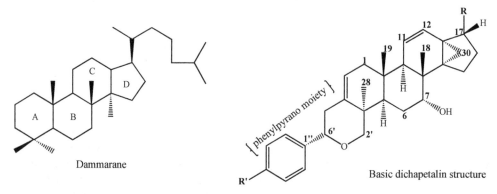

Fig. 1. Structures of dammarane and the dichapetalin skeleton

2. Isolation and characterization

Chromatographic separation of the acetone extract of the whole roots of *D. madagascariensis* collected in Ghana afforded dichapetalin A as the major constituent, together with the minor components dichapetalins B – H (Achenbach *et al.*, 1995; Addae-Mensah *et al.*, 1996). A separate collection from the same locality gave dichapetalin A and yet another member of the series, dichapetalin M. The absolute configuration of dichapetalin A (Figure 2), the first in the series to be isolated, was determined by single-crystal X-ray diffraction analysis, and has been established to be 4*R*,5*R*,7*R*,8*R*,9*R*,10*S*,13*R*,14*S*,17*S*,20*S*,23*R*,6′*S*. Its systematic name is therefore [(4α,6′α,7α,17α,20*S*,23*R*,24*E*)-2′,3′,5′,6′-tetrahydro-7,23,26-trihydroxy-6′-phenyl-13,30-cyclo-29-nordammara-2,11,24-tri-eno[4,3-c] pyran-21-oic acid γ-lactone]. Dichapetalin A is the dextrorotatory isomer, $[\alpha]_D^{21} = +35°$, (Weckert *et al.*,1996).

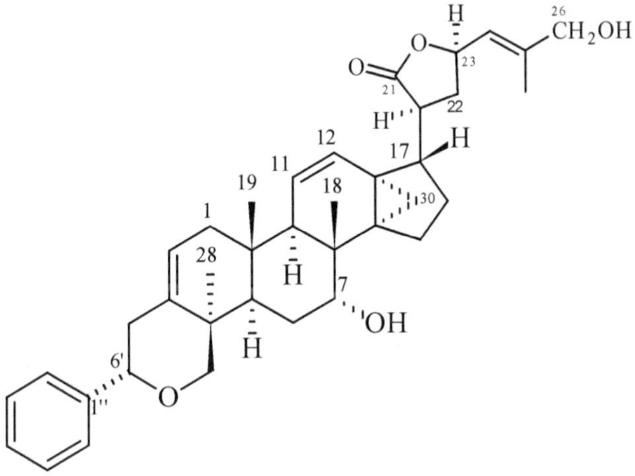

Fig. 2. Dichapetalin A

Meanwhile, between the two investigations of *D. madagascariensis*, Fang and co-workers, on fractionation of the ethyl acetate-soluble extract of the stem bark of *D. gelonioides* (Philippines), isolated dichapetalins A, I and J in one collection and in a re-collection, dichapetalins K and L (Fang *et al.* 2006). The structures of all the compounds were determined on the basis of spectroscopic data interpretation.

So far, only two species of the genus *Dichapetalum* - *D. madagascariensis* (roots) and *D. gelonioides* (stem bark), have produced dichapetalins. The stem bark of *D. madagascariensis* only indicated the presence of dichapetalin A on TLC as part of a complex mixture. The isolated compounds were friedo-oleananes and zeylanol (Darbah, 1994). Zeylanol has been isolated from *D. gelonioides* (Fang *et al.* 2006). Chemical investigation of both the stem and the roots of *D. barteri* did not show any dichapetalins – the isolated compounds were friedelins, including 2β-hydroxy-3-oxo-D:A-friedooleanan-29-oic-acid, a new triterpene belonging to the friedo-oleanane group, ferulic acid derivatives and the known anticancer lupane triterpenes, betulinic acid and betulonic acid (Addae-Mensah, 2007). *D. gelonioides* also produced betulinic acid (Fang *et al.* 2006).

Basically, the dichapetalins can be distinguished by the nature of the side chain at C-17 which may be grouped into two – the lactone side chain (Figure 3) and the methyl ester side chain (Figure 5). Dichapetalins A, B, I, J, K, L and M possess a lactone side chain while a

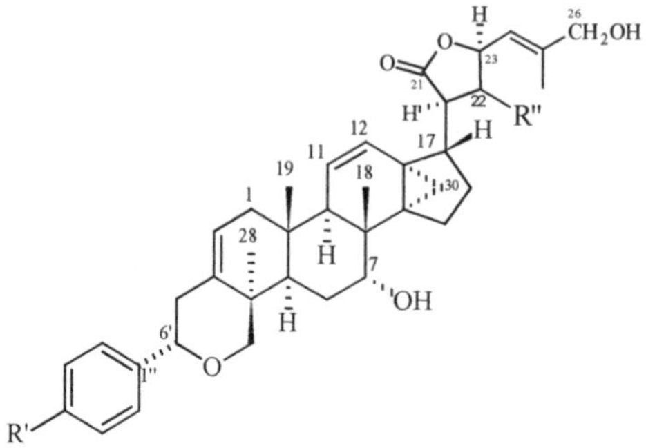

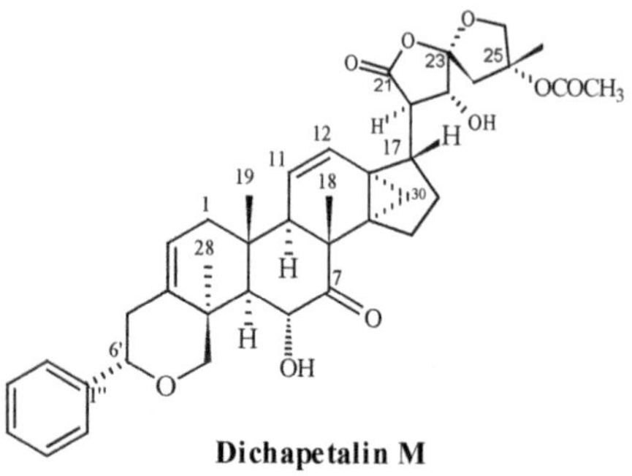

Dichapetalin M

Fig. 3. Dichapetalins with a lactone side chain

Dichapetalin	R'	R''	Other
A	H	H	-
B	H	22α-OH	-
I	H	H	11,12-dihydro 12-β-OH
J	OMe	H	11,12-dihydro 12-β-OH
K	OMe	H	-
L	H	H	11,12-dihydro

methyl ester side chain can be found in dichapetalins C, D, E, F, G and H. Five members of the lactone group, dichapetalins A, I, J, K and L, have an identical side chain comprising a 5-membered lactone with an allyl alcohol substituent. Their structural differences arise from the presence or otherwise of the 11,12-double bond, a 12β-OH group and a methoxy on the benzene ring of the phenylpyrano moiety. Dichapetalins J and K are methoxylated variants of dichapetalins I and A respectively. According to Fang and co-workers, they are likely to be extraction artifacts due to the initial use of methanol as a solvent. Dichapetalin B on the other hand, is a hydroxylated variant of dichapetalin A.

The uniqueness of the side chain in dichapetalin M is evident in the spiroketal moiety and the C-25 acetoxy group. The oxygenation of C-6 in the basic skeleton is also peculiar to dichapetalin M. A close examination of the side chains of dichapetalins B and M reveals a possible biosynthetic conversion of the former to the latter. Initial hydroxylation and phosphorylation followed by cyclisation could convert the allyl alcohol into a dihydrofuran. Subsequent hydration to the hydroxyl furan followed by acetylation of the hydroxyl by acetyl-CoA could then give the side chain of dichapetalin M (Figure 4).

The methyl ester group consists on one hand, of an open chain terminating in a primary alcohol (dichapetalins C and F) or its stearic acid esterified analogue (dichapetalin D). On the other hand, the primary alcohol cyclizes with the oxo substituent at C-23, to give either a 3-methylfuranyl moiety (dichapetalin E) or a cyclic methyl ketal (dichapetalins G and H). Dichapetalins G and H are isomeric methyl ketals with the 11,12-dihydro basic skeleton (Figure 5).

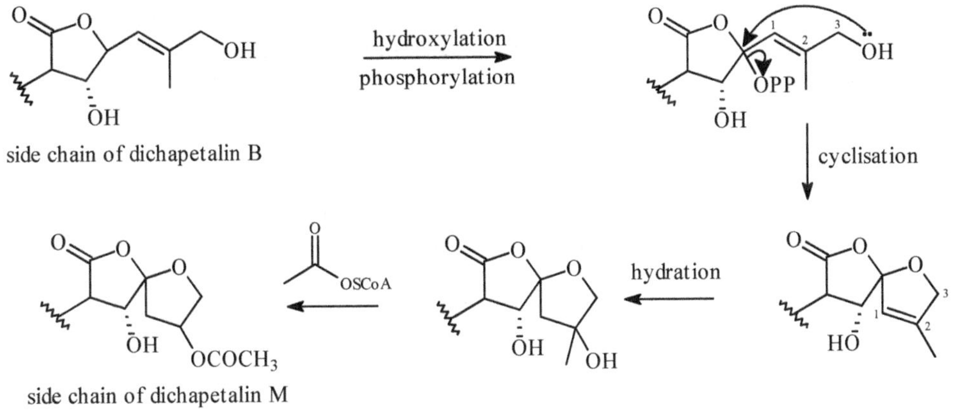

side chain of dichapetalin B

hydroxylation
phosphorylation

cyclisation

side chain of dichapetalin M

hydration

Fig. 4. Proposed biosynthetic pathway for the side chain of dichapetalin M

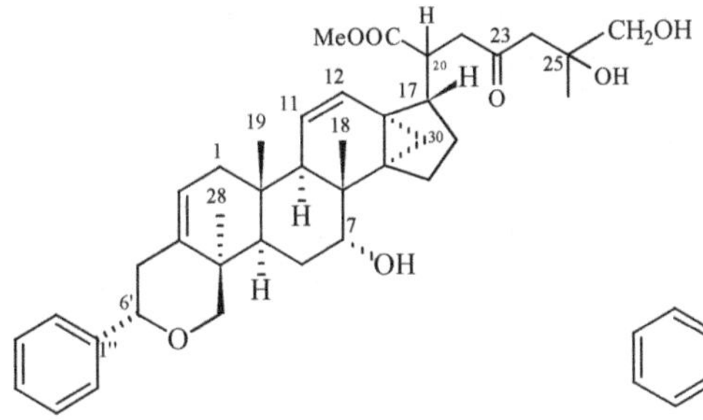

Dichapetalin C
Dichapetalin F – 11,12-dihydro

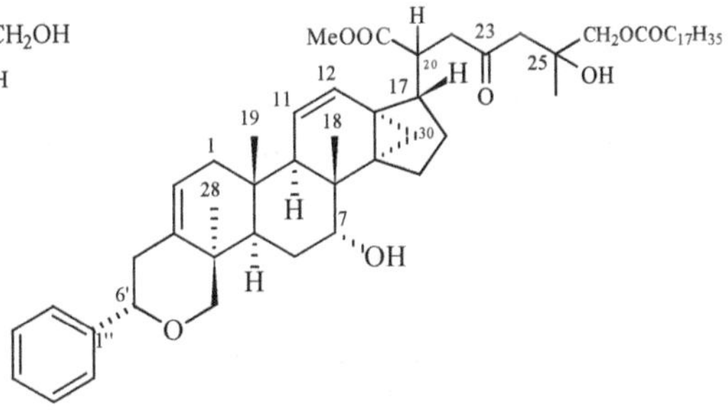

Dichapetalin D

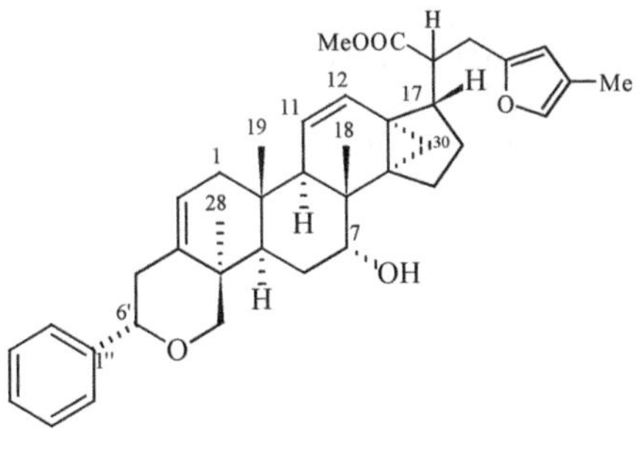

Dichapetalin E

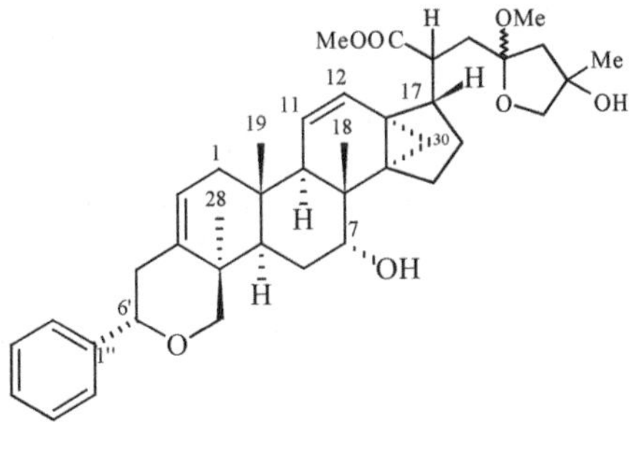

Dichapetalins G & H – 11,12-dihydro

Fig. 5. Dichapetalins with a methyl ester side chain

3. Biological activity

Biological assays including brine shrimp and anticancer studies have so far shown significant activity only with dichapetalins possessing a lactone side chain. None of the methyl ester side chain dichapetalins exhibited significant cytotoxicity.

3.1 Brine shrimp test

The dichapetalins were assayed in the Brine Shrimp Lethality Test according to established protocols (Meyer et al., 1982; Anderson et al., 1991). Dichapetalin A exhibited pronounced cytotoxicity (LC_{50} = 0.31µg/ml), exceeding that of podophyllotoxin by 7-fold while dichapetalin M was 28-fold (LC_{50} = 0.011 µg/ml) more potent than dichapetalin A. Dichapetalin C was active to a lesser extent while dichapetalins D & F were almost inactive.

3.2 Antitumour studies

Dichapetalin A showed significant inhibition to cell growth in various cancer cell systems *in vitro*. The sensitivity of the respective systems was however, highly different. L1210 murine leukaemia cells were extremely sensitive (EC_{90} <0.0001µg/ml) while human KB carcinoma and murine bone marrow stimulated with GM-CSF were affected by concentrations four orders of magnitude higher. *In vivo* tests were also not encouraging (Achenbach et al., 1995; Addae-Mensah et al., 1996). Fang and co-workers further demonstrated selective and significant cytotoxicity in dichapetalins A, I and J (IC_{50} = 0.2 - 0.5 µg/mL) against the SW626 human ovarian cancer cell line. Dichapetalins K and L showed broader cytotoxicity against the same cell line. Their study confirmed the loss of activity of dichapetalin A when evaluated in the *in vivo* hollow fiber model (Fang et al. 2006). Loss of activity of dichapetalin A *in vivo* is likely to be due to enzymatic hydrolysis of the lactone to an open chain carboxylic acid (methyl ester side chain). Dichapetalin M is yet to be evaluated for its anti tumour potential which, based on its extremely high toxicity towards the brine shrimp, is expected to be more potent than that of dichapetalin A. Moreover, it is envisaged that the unique spiroketal bicyclic side chain of dichapetalin M will confer stability on the lactone, reducing the possibility of ring opening and hence, likely to result in retention of activity *in vivo*.

3.3 Anti-HIV assay

The Tetrazolium-based colorimetric selective assay was employed in the anti-HIV activity test of dichapetalins A and M against HIV-1/IIIB in MT-4 cells as previously published (Ayisi et al., 1991). They both elicited activity at concentrations that were toxic to the cells and therefore did not exhibit any appreciable selectivity in its anti-HIV activity. The aqueous extract of the plant, however, gave an antiviral index of 4.7, an indication of the presence of some level of anti-HIV principle. This may be an indication that the plant contains other compounds that may either be anti-HIV on their own, or in combination with the dichapetalins.

4. Dichapetalins from other sources

The isolation of five new dichapetalin-type triterpenoids, acutissimatriterpenes A – E, from the aerial parts of *Phyllanthus acutissima* (Euphorbiacea) by Tuchinda and co-workers

(Tuchinda P. *et al*, 2008) has been reported (Figure 6). This finding of the dichapetalins from a different plant family is of significant taxonomic importance.

Like the dichapetalins, the C-17 side chain is a distinguishing structural feature among the acutissimatriterpenes. Another structural difference is the presence or otherwise of a methylenedioxy unit in the phenylpyrano moiety. This structural unit is peculiar to the acutissimatriterpenes – it has so far not occurred in the dichapetalins. Acutissimatriterpenes A and C are methylenedioxy analogues of acutissimatriterpenes B and D respectively.

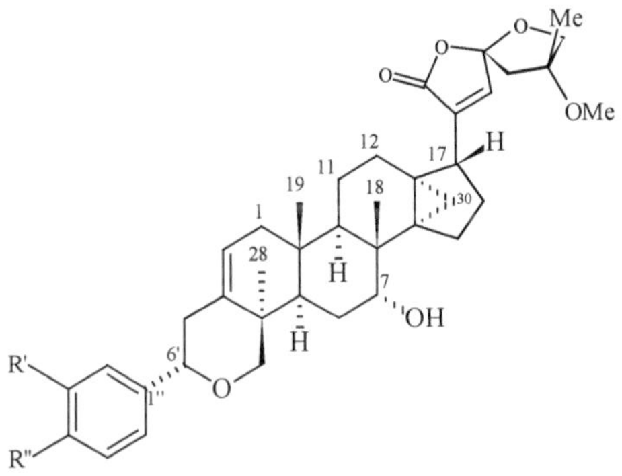

Acutissimatriterpene A: R', R'' = O-CH$_2$-O
Acutissimatriterpene B: R', R'' = H

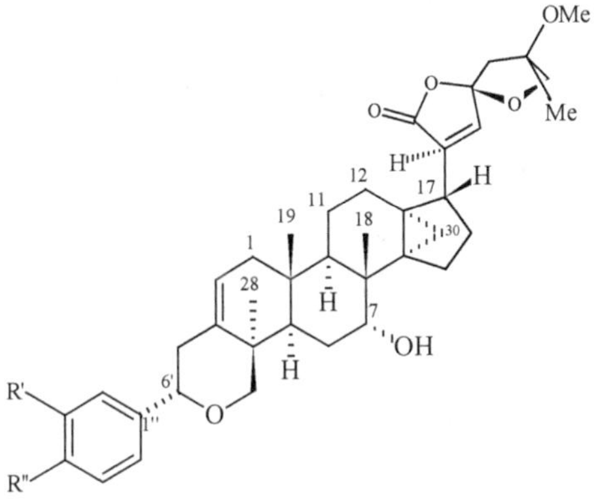

Acutissimatriterpene C: R', R'' = O-CH$_2$-O
Acutissimatriterpene D: R', R'' = H

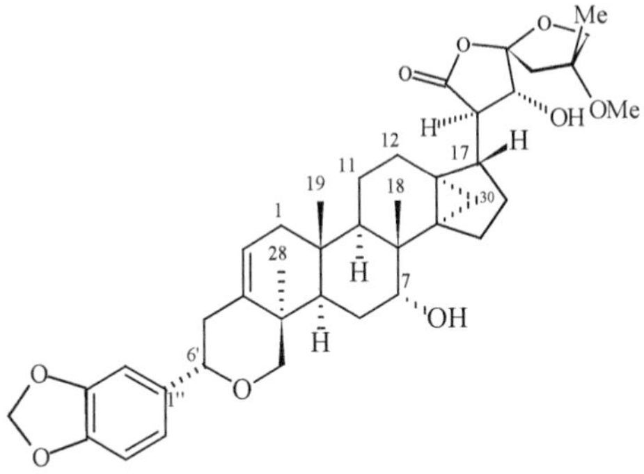

Acutissimatriterpene E

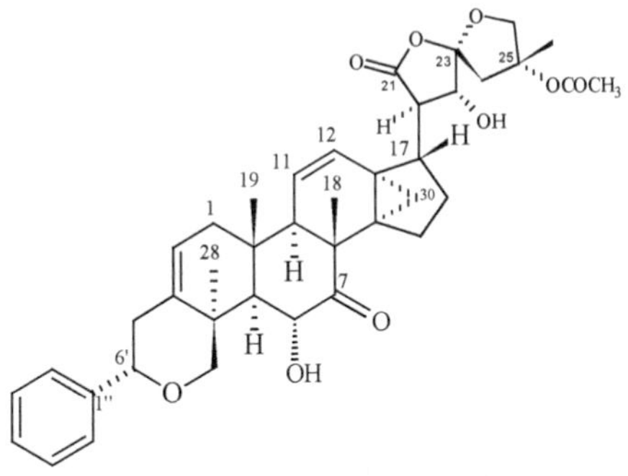

Dichapetalin M

Fig. 6. Acutissimatriterpenes A - E

Based on the side chain alone, acutissimatriterpenes A and B are isomeric ketals of acutissimatriterpenes C and D. In terms of the tetrahydrofuran configuration, acutissimatriterpenes A, B and E bear similar side chains – the difference is the hydroxylated alkene in the latter. It is interesting to note the resemblance of their spiroketal side chain to that of dichapetalin M where the acetoxy group at C-25 in the latter has been replaced with a methoxy substituent. Thus, the acutissimatriterpenes can be categorized into the lactone side chain group of the dichapetalins.

As mentioned earlier, structure-activity relationship (SAR) studies revealed significant cytotoxic activity with dichapetalins in the lactone side chain group. Results of biological testing of the acutissimatriterpenes for cytotoxic effects against a panel of six cancer cell lines (P-388 murine lymphocytic leukaemia, human KB nasopharyngeal carcinoma, MCF-7 human breast cancer, Lu-1 human lung cancer, Col-2 human colon cancer and ASK rat glioma) is reported (Tuchinda P. *et al*, 2008). Acutissimatriterpene E exhibited significant activities against P-388 murine lymphocytic leukaemia (EC_{50} = 0.005μg/ml), MCF-7 human breast cancer (EC_{50} = 1.1μg/ml) and Lu-1 human lung cancer (EC_{50} = 3.1μg/ml). Acutissimatriterpenes A and B gave EC_{50} = 0.4 and 0.5μg/ml respectively against P-388 murine lymphocytic leukaemia. The remaining cell lines did not show activity. Insignificant activities (EC_{50} > 5μg/ml) were reported for acussimatriterpenes C and D against all the cell lines tested. A comparison of these results with those obtained from cytotoxicity test of the dichapetalins indicate that dichapetalin A was ten-fold more sensitive (EC_{90} <0.0001μg/ml) than acutissimatriterpene E against a different strain of murine leukaemia cells. Human KB nasopharyngeal carcinoma exhibited low sensitivity against all the acutissimatriterpenes (EC_{50} > 5μg/ml) whereas in a different study, human KB squamous carcinoma was affected by dichapetalin A at EC_{90} = 1.8μg/ml.

SAR consideration of the acutisimmatriperpenes suggests that the methylenedioxy moiety may not be required for activity but rather, the tetrahydrofuran configuration in the side chain of acutissimatriterpenes A, B and E.   All three compounds gave encouraging cytotoxicity against some of the cell lines tested. Both acutissimatriterpenes C and D possess identical side chains, with a tetrahydrofuran configuration opposite that of acutissimatriterpenes A, B and E. Acutissimatriterpene C is the methylenedioxy variant of acutissimatriterpene D, and both did not exhibit appreciable cytotoxic activity against any of the cancer cells. Possibly, the presence of the hydroxylated alkene found in acutissimatriterpene E alone, also enhances cytotoxicity. These deductions confirm the earlier predicted activity of dichapetalin M. It seems to possess all the appropriate structural features for activity – the hydroxylated alkene, the required orientation of the spiro-lactone and the absence of the methylenedioxy unit. The effect of the acetoxy substituent on activity, however, remains to be tested.

Anti-HIV-1 activity employing cell-based assays against MC99 virus and 1A2 cell line system showed various levels of activity with acutissimatriterpenes A – E (Selectivity index = >1.5 - >8.1). In an HIV-1 RT assay, acutissimatriterpenes A and B were moderately sensitive (> 50 to 70% inhibition at 200μg/ml) followed by acutissimatriterpenes D and C at 37% and 11% inhibition respectively. Acutissimatriterpene E was the least active (-0.5% inhibition). Both dichapetalins A and M also failed to exhibit any appreciable selectivity in anti-HIV activity against HIV-1/IIIB in MT-4 cells.

5. References

Achenbach, H., Asunka, S. A., Waibel, R., Addae-Mensah, I., Oppong, I. V. (1995). Dichapetalin A, A novel plant constituent from *Dichapetalum madagascariense*. *Nat. Prod. Lett.*, 7, 93-100.

Addae-Mensah, I., Adu-Kumi, S., Waibel, R., Asunka, S. A., Oppong, I. V. (2007). A novel D:A-friedooleanane triterpenoid and other constituents of the stem bark of *Dichapetalum barteri* Engl. *ARKIVOK (Archives of Organic Chemistry)* IX, 71-79. Web version: www.arkat-usa.org or www.arkivoc.com

Addae-Mensah, I., Waibel, R., Asunka, S. A., Oppong, I. V., Achenbach, H. (1996). The Dichapetalins – A new class of triterpenoids. *Phytochemistry*, 43(3), 649-656.

Anderson, J. E., Goetz, C. M., McLauglin, J. L., Suffness, M. (1991). A blind comparison of simple bench-top bioassays and human tumour cell cytotoxicities as antitumour prescreens. *Phytochemical analysis*, 2, 107-111.

Ayisi, N. (1991). Modified tetrazolium-based colorimetric method for determining the activities of anti-HIV compounds. *J. Virol Methods*, 33, 335-344

Burkill, H. M. (1985). The useful plants of West Tropical Africa, vol. 1. Royal Botanic Gardens, Kew, pp 647-648.

Darbah, V. F., (1994). Chemical investigation of the stem bark of *Dichapetalum madagascariense*. M. Phil (Chemistry) Thesis. Unpublished.

Fang, F., Ito, A., Chai, H., Mi, Q., Jones, W. P., Madulid, D. R., Oliveros, M. B., Gao, Q., Orjala, J., Farnsworth, N. R., Soejarto, D. D., Cordell, G. A., Swanson, S. M., Pezzuto, J. M., Kinghorn, A. D. (2006). Cytotoxic constituents from the stem bark of *Dichapetalum gelonoides* collected in the Philippines. *J. Nat. Prod.* 69, 332-337.

Hall, J. B. and Swaine, M. D., (1981). Distribution and Ecology of Vascular Plants in a tropical rain forest. Forest Vegetation in Ghana. Dr. W. Junk Publishers. The Hague, Biston, London, pp 175 -177.

Hall, R. J. (1972). *D. barteri* as a potential rodenticide. *New Phytologist*, 71, 855-871.

Irvine F.R. (1961). Woody Plants of Ghana. Oxford University Press, pp 266-269.

Lewis, W. H., Elvin-Lewis, M. P. F. (1977). Medical Botany, Plants affecting man's health. *Wiley Interscience* City, pp 234.

Meyer, B. N., Ferrigni, N. R., Putnam, J. E., Jacobsen, L. B., Nichols, D. E., McLauglin, J. L. (1982). Brine Shrimp: A convenient general bioassay for active plant constituents. *Planta Med.*, 45, 31-34.

O'Hagan, D., Perry, R., Lock, J. M., Meyer, J. J. M., Dasaradhi, L., Hamilton, J. T. G., Harper, D. B. (1993). High levels of monofluoroacetate in *Dichapetalum braunii*. *Phytochemistry*, 33, 1043-1045.

Osei-Safo, D., Chama, M. A., Addae-Mensah, I., Waibel, R., Asomaning, W. A., Oppong, I. V. (2008). Dichapetalin M from *Dichapetalum madagascariense*. *Phytochemistry Letters* 1, 147-150.

Tuchinda P, Kornsakulkarn J, Pohmakotr M, Kongsaeree P, Prabpai S, Yoosook C, Kasisit J, Napaswad C, Sophasan S, Reutrakul V. (2008). Dichapetalin-type triterpenoids and lignans from the aerial parts of *Phyllanthus acutissima*. *J. Nat. Prod.*, 71(4):655-663.

Weckert, E., Hümmer, K., Addae-Mensah, I., Waibel, R., Achenbach, H. (1996). The absolute configuration of Dichapetalin A. *Phytochemistry*, 43, 657–660.

Permissions

The contributors of this book come from diverse backgrounds, making this book a truly international effort. This book will bring forth new frontiers with its revolutionizing research information and detailed analysis of the nascent developments around the world.

We would like to thank Dr. A. V. Rao, for lending his expertise to make the book truly unique. He has played a crucial role in the development of this book. Without his invaluable contribution this book wouldn't have been possible. He has made vital efforts to compile up to date information on the varied aspects of this subject to make this book a valuable addition to the collection of many professionals and students.

This book was conceptualized with the vision of imparting up-to-date information and advanced data in this field. To ensure the same, a matchless editorial board was set up. Every individual on the board went through rigorous rounds of assessment to prove their worth. After which they invested a large part of their time researching and compiling the most relevant data for our readers. Conferences and sessions were held from time to time between the editorial board and the contributing authors to present the data in the most comprehensible form. The editorial team has worked tirelessly to provide valuable and valid information to help people across the globe.

Every chapter published in this book has been scrutinized by our experts. Their significance has been extensively debated. The topics covered herein carry significant findings which will fuel the growth of the discipline. They may even be implemented as practical applications or may be referred to as a beginning point for another development. Chapters in this book were first published by InTech; hereby published with permission under the Creative Commons Attribution License or equivalent.

The editorial board has been involved in producing this book since its inception. They have spent rigorous hours researching and exploring the diverse topics which have resulted in the successful publishing of this book. They have passed on their knowledge of decades through this book. To expedite this challenging task, the publisher supported the team at every step. A small team of assistant editors was also appointed to further simplify the editing procedure and attain best results for the readers.

Our editorial team has been hand-picked from every corner of the world. Their multi-ethnicity adds dynamic inputs to the discussions which result in innovative outcomes. These outcomes are then further discussed with the researchers and contributors who give their valuable feedback and opinion regarding the same. The feedback is then collaborated with the researches and they are edited in a comprehensive manner to aid the understanding of the subject.

Apart from the editorial board, the designing team has also invested a significant amount of their time in understanding the subject and creating the most relevant covers. They scrutinized every image to scout for the most suitable representation of the subject and create an appropriate cover for the book.

The publishing team has been involved in this book since its early stages. They were actively engaged in every process, be it collecting the data, connecting with the contributors or procuring relevant information. The team has been an ardent support to the editorial, designing and production team. Their endless efforts to recruit the best for this project, has resulted in the accomplishment of this book. They are a veteran in the field of academics and their pool of knowledge is as vast as their experience in printing. Their expertise and guidance has proved useful at every step. Their uncompromising quality standards have made this book an exceptional effort. Their encouragement from time to time has been an inspiration for everyone.

The publisher and the editorial board hope that this book will prove to be a valuable piece of knowledge for researchers, students, practitioners and scholars across the globe.

List of Contributors

Xirley Pereira Nunes, Fabrício Souza Silva, Jackson Roberto Guedes da S. Almeida, Julianeli Tolentino de Lima and Luciano Augusto de Araújo Ribeiro
Universidade Federal do Vale do São Francisco, Brazil

Lucindo José Quintans Júnior
Universidade Federal de Sergipe, Brazil

José Maria Barbosa Filho
Universidade Federal da Paraíba, Brazil

Orlando A. Abreu
Faculty of Chemistry, University of Camagüey, Cuba

Guillermo Barreto
Faculty of Veterinary Sciences, University of Camagüey, Cuba

Lukeman Adelaja Joseph Shittu
Department of Anatomy, Benue State University College of Medicine
Medical Microbiology Unit, Jireh International Foundation Laboratories, Abuja, Gwagwalada, Nigeria

Remilekun Keji Mary Shittu
Medical Microbiology Unit, Jireh International Foundation Laboratories, Abuja, Gwagwalada, Nigeria

Elita Scio, Renata F. Mendes, Erick V.S. Motta, Paula M.Q. Bellozi, Danielle M.O. Aragão, Josiane Mello, Rodrigo L. Fabri, Jussara R. Moreira, Isabel V.L. de Assis and Maria Lúcia M. Bouzada
Federal University of Juiz de Fora, Laboratory of Bioactive Natural Products, Brazil

G.O. Adeshina, J.A. Onaolapo and J.O. Ehinmidu
Department of Pharmaceutics and Pharmaceutical Microbiology, Ahmadu Bello University, Zaria, Nigeria

O.F. Kunle
Department of Medicinal Plant Research, National Institute for Pharmaceutical Research and Development, Idu – Abuja, Nigeria

L.E. Odama
Department of Biological Sciences, Kogi State University, Anyingba, Nigeria

Simona Ioana Vicas
University of Oradea, Faculty of Environmental Protection, Oradea, Romania

Dumitrita Rugina and Carmen Socaciu
University of Agricultural Sciences and Veterinary Medicine, Department of Chemistry and Biochemistry, Cluj-Napoca, Romania

Se-Jae Kim, Joon-Ho Hwang, Hye-Sun Shin, Mi-Gyeong Jang, Hee-Chul Ko and Seong-Il Kang
Department of Biology and Sasa Industry Development Agency, Jeju National University, Jeju, Republic of Korea

Leseilane J. Mampuru, Pirwana K. Chokoe, Maphuti C. Madiga and Matlou P. Mokgotho
Department of Biochemistry, Microbiology and Biotechnology, Faculty of Science and Agriculture, University of Limpopo, Sovenga

Annette Theron and Ronald Anderson
Medical Research Council Unit for Inflammation and Immunity, Department of Immunology, Faculty of Health Sciences, University of Pretoria and Tshwane Academic Division of the NHLS, Pretoria, South Africa

Sanda Vladimir-Knežević, Biljana Blažeković, Maja Bival Štefan and Marija Babac
University of Zagreb, Faculty of Pharmacy and Biochemistry, Croatia

Nour-Eddine Es-Safi
Mohammed V-Agdal University, Ecole Normale Supérieure, Rabat, Morocco

A. Al-Weshahy and V.A. Rao
Department of Nutritional Sciences, Faculty of Medicine, University of Toronto, Toronto, Ontario, Canada

Denise C. Hunter and David J. Burritt
Food & Wellness Group, The New Zealand Institute for Plant & Food Research Limited, Auckland
The Department of Botany, The University of Otago, Dunedin, New Zealand

Saleh I. Alqasoumi
Department of Pharmacognosy, College of Pharmacy, Salman Bin Abdulaziz University, Kingdom of Saudi Arabia
Department of Pharmacognosy, College of Pharmacy, King Saud University, Kingdom of Saudi Arabia

Maged S. Abdel-Kader
Department of Pharmacognosy, College of Pharmacy, Salman Bin Abdulaziz University, Kingdom of Saudi Arabia

Dorcas Osei-Safo, Mary A. Chama and Ivan Addae-Mensah
Chemistry Department, University of Ghana, Legon, Ghana

Reiner Waibel
Institute of Pharmacy and Food Chemistry, Department of Pharmaceutical Chemistry, University of Erlangen, Germany

Printed in the USA
CPSIA information can be obtained
at www.ICGtesting.com
JSHW011456221024
72173JS00005B/1098

9 781632 392855